ATS-109   ADMISSION TEST SERIES

*This is your*
*PASSBOOK for...*

# Certified Personal Trainer (CPT)

*Test Preparation Study Guide*
*Questions & Answers*

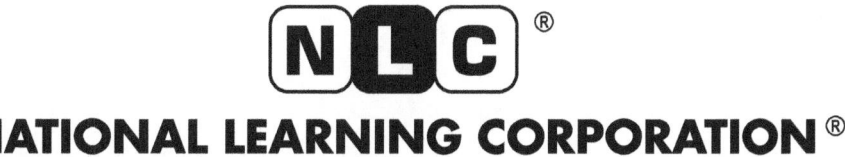

# COPYRIGHT NOTICE

This book is SOLELY intended for, is sold ONLY to, and its use is RESTRICTED to individual, bona fide applicants or candidates who qualify by virtue of having seriously filed applications for appropriate license, certificate, professional and/or promotional advancement, higher school matriculation, scholarship, or other legitimate requirements of education and/or governmental authorities.

This book is NOT intended for use, class instruction, tutoring, training, duplication, copying, reprinting, excerption, or adaptation, etc., by:

1) Other publishers
2) Proprietors and/or Instructors of "Coaching" and/or Preparatory Courses
3) Personnel and/or Training Divisions of commercial, industrial, and governmental organizations
4) Schools, colleges, or universities and/or their departments and staffs, including teachers and other personnel
5) Testing Agencies or Bureaus
6) Study groups which seek by the purchase of a single volume to copy and/or duplicate and/or adapt this material for use by the group as a whole without having purchased individual volumes for each of the members of the group
7) Et al.

Such persons would be in violation of appropriate Federal and State statutes.

PROVISION OF LICENSING AGREEMENTS – Recognized educational, commercial, industrial, and governmental institutions and organizations, and others legitimately engaged in educational pursuits, including training, testing, and measurement activities, may address request for a licensing agreement to the copyright owners, who will determine whether, and under what conditions, including fees and charges, the materials in this book may be used them. In other words, a licensing facility exists for the legitimate use of the material in this book on other than an individual basis. However, it is asseverated and affirmed here that the material in this book CANNOT be used without the receipt of the express permission of such a licensing agreement from the Publishers. Inquiries re licensing should be addressed to the company, attention rights and permissions department.

All rights reserved, including the right of reproduction in whole or in part, in any form or by any means, electronic or mechanical, including photocopying, recording, or by any information storage and retrieval system, without permission in writing from the Publisher.

Copyright © 2025 by
# National Learning Corporation

212 Michael Drive, Syosset, NY 11791
(516) 921-8888 • www.passbooks.com
E-mail: info@passbooks.com

# PASSBOOK® SERIES

THE *PASSBOOK® SERIES* has been created to prepare applicants and candidates for the ultimate academic battlefield – the examination room.

At some time in our lives, each and every one of us may be required to take an examination – for validation, matriculation, admission, qualification, registration, certification, or licensure.

Based on the assumption that every applicant or candidate has met the basic formal educational standards, has taken the required number of courses, and read the necessary texts, the *PASSBOOK® SERIES* furnishes the one special preparation which may assure passing with confidence, instead of failing with insecurity. Examination questions – together with answers – are furnished as the basic vehicle for study so that the mysteries of the examination and its compounding difficulties may be eliminated or diminished by a sure method.

This book is meant to help you pass your examination provided that you qualify and are serious in your objective.

The entire field is reviewed through the huge store of content information which is succinctly presented through a provocative and challenging approach – the question-and-answer method.

A climate of success is established by furnishing the correct answers at the end of each test.

You soon learn to recognize types of questions, forms of questions, and patterns of questioning. You may even begin to anticipate expected outcomes.

You perceive that many questions are repeated or adapted so that you can gain acute insights, which may enable you to score many sure points.

You learn how to confront new questions, or types of questions, and to attack them confidently and work out the correct answers.

You note objectives and emphases, and recognize pitfalls and dangers, so that you may make positive educational adjustments.

Moreover, you are kept fully informed in relation to new concepts, methods, practices, and directions in the field.

You discover that you are actually taking the examination all the time: you are preparing for the examination by "taking" an examination, not by reading extraneous and/or supererogatory textbooks.

In short, this PASSBOOK®, used directedly, should be an important factor in helping you to pass your test.

# CERTIFIED PERSONAL TRAINER

**EXAM CONTENT OUTLINE**

**Domain I: Client Interviews and Assessments - 31%**

1. Obtain health, medical, and exercise history and lifestyle information (e.g., personal, physical, environmental, nutritional, and occupational factors) using questionnaires, interviews, and available documents to determine risk stratification, identify the need for medical clearance and referrals, and facilitate program design.
2. Assess clients' current attitudes, preferences, goals, and readiness for behavior change using questionnaires and interviews to identify potential barriers, motivators, and expectations necessary to set appropriate program goals.
3. Identify and evaluate the quality of client movement (e.g., balance, stability, and mobility) through observations and assessments, to develop appropriate exercise programming designed to improve movement efficiency and enhance activities of daily living, overall physical performance, and injury prevention and recovery.
4. Select and conduct physiological assessments (e.g., cardiorespiratory fitness, muscular strength and endurance, flexibility, body composition, heart rate, blood pressure) based on client interviews, questionnaires, and standardized protocols to facilitate safe and effective program design and to monitor changes over time.

**Domain II: Program Design and Implementation - 33%**

1. Interpret the results of the client interview and assessment data (e.g., client goals, attitudes, motivations), define program goals, and design safe and effective exercise and lifestyle programs.
2. Apply appropriate exercise parameters (e.g., frequency, intensity, duration, type) and principles (e.g., overload, specificity, and progression) for cardiorespiratory fitness, muscular strength and endurance, and flexibility using current guidelines to develop safe and effective exercise programs.
3. Incorporate skill-related exercises (e.g., stability, mobility, coordination, balance, power, speed, agility) and appropriate equipment into client programs, in accordance with scientific research, to improve movement efficiency and enhance activities of daily living, overall physical performance, and injury prevention and recovery.
4. Instruct clients on safe and effective exercise techniques (e.g., intensity, breathing, tempo, movement patterns, and postural alignment) and equipment use, using a variety of cues (e.g., verbal, visual, kinesthetic) to achieve program goals.

**Domain III: Progression and Modifications - 19%**

1. Promote program adherence through reinforcement of client motivators, education regarding the benefits of exercise and leading a healthy lifestyle, and modification of program parameters to achieve program goals.
2. Recognize and respond to lapses in program adherence by identifying client barriers and helping to establish and implement support systems and/or solutions.
3. Routinely evaluate client exercise programs by using assessment data, observations, and client feedback to progress and modify programs as needed.

## Domain IV: Professional Conduct, Safety, and Risk Management -17%

1. Apply risk-management strategies in accordance with recognized standards, guidelines, laws, and regulations to protect the client, personal trainer, and other relevant parties in order to reduce the risk of injury and liability.
2. Document client-related data, communications, and progress using a secure record-keeping system in accordance with legal and regulatory requirements to maintain confidentiality and continuity of care, and to minimize liability.
3. Use credible resources to maintain and enhance competency by staying current with scientifically based research, theories, and practices in order to provide safe and effective services.
4. Conduct assessments of the exercise space, equipment, and environment in order identify potential hazards and undertake necessary modifications to provide a safe environment for clients and the personal trainer.

# HOW TO TAKE A TEST

You have studied long, hard and conscientiously.

With your official admission card in hand, and your heart pounding, you have been admitted to the examination room.

You note that there are several hundred other applicants in the examination room waiting to take the same test.

They all appear to be equally well prepared.

You know that nothing but your best effort will suffice. The "moment of truth" is at hand: you now have to demonstrate objectively, in writing, your knowledge of content and your understanding of subject matter.

You are fighting the most important battle of your life—to pass and/or score high on an examination which will determine your career and provide the economic basis for your livelihood.

What extra, special things should you know and should you do in taking the examination?

I. YOU MUST PASS AN EXAMINATION

A. WHAT EVERY CANDIDATE SHOULD KNOW
Examination applicants often ask us for help in preparing for the written test. What can I study in advance? What kinds of questions will be asked? How will the test be given? How will the papers be graded?

B. HOW ARE EXAMS DEVELOPED?
Examinations are carefully written by trained technicians who are specialists in the field known as "psychological measurement," in consultation with recognized authorities in the field of work that the test will cover. These experts recommend the subject matter areas or skills to be tested; only those knowledges or skills important to your success on the job are included. The most reliable books and source materials available are used as references. Together, the experts and technicians judge the difficulty level of the questions.
Test technicians know how to phrase questions so that the problem is clearly stated. Their ethics do not permit "trick" or "catch" questions. Questions may have been tried out on sample groups, or subjected to statistical analysis, to determine their usefulness.
Written tests are often used in combination with performance tests, ratings of training and experience, and oral interviews. All of these measures combine to form the best-known means of finding the right person for the right job.

## II. HOW TO PASS THE WRITTEN TEST

### A. BASIC STEPS

1) Study the announcement

How, then, can you know what subjects to study? Our best answer is: "Learn as much as possible about the class of positions for which you've applied." The exam will test the knowledge, skills and abilities needed to do the work.

Your most valuable source of information about the position you want is the official exam announcement. This announcement lists the training and experience qualifications. Check these standards and apply only if you come reasonably close to meeting them. Many jurisdictions preview the written test in the exam announcement by including a section called "Knowledge and Abilities Required," "Scope of the Examination," or some similar heading. Here you will find out specifically what fields will be tested.

2) Choose appropriate study materials

If the position for which you are applying is technical or advanced, you will read more advanced, specialized material. If you are already familiar with the basic principles of your field, elementary textbooks would waste your time. Concentrate on advanced textbooks and technical periodicals. Think through the concepts and review difficult problems in your field.

These are all general sources. You can get more ideas on your own initiative, following these leads. For example, training manuals and publications of the government agency which employs workers in your field can be useful, particularly for technical and professional positions. A letter or visit to the government department involved may result in more specific study suggestions, and certainly will provide you with a more definite idea of the exact nature of the position you are seeking.

3) Study this book!

## III. KINDS OF TESTS

Tests are used for purposes other than measuring knowledge and ability to perform specified duties. For some positions, it is equally important to test ability to make adjustments to new situations or to profit from training. In others, basic mental abilities not dependent on information are essential. Questions which test these things may not appear as pertinent to the duties of the position as those which test for knowledge and information. Yet they are often highly important parts of a fair examination. For very general questions, it is almost impossible to help you direct your study efforts. What we can do is to point out some of the more common of these general abilities needed in public service positions and describe some typical questions.

1) General information

Broad, general information has been found useful for predicting job success in some kinds of work. This is tested in a variety of ways, from vocabulary lists to questions about current events. Basic background in some field of work, such as sociology or economics, may be sampled in a group of questions. Often these are principles which have become familiar to most persons through exposure rather than through formal training. It is difficult to advise you how to study for these questions; being alert to the world around you is our best suggestion.

2) Verbal ability

An example of an ability needed in many positions is verbal or language ability. Verbal ability is, in brief, the ability to use and understand words. Vocabulary and grammar tests are typical measures of this ability. Reading comprehension or paragraph interpretation questions are common in many kinds of civil service tests. You are given a paragraph of written material and asked to find its central meaning.

## IV. KINDS OF QUESTIONS

1. Multiple-choice Questions

Most popular of the short-answer questions is the "multiple choice" or "best answer" question. It can be used, for example, to test for factual knowledge, ability to solve problems or judgment in meeting situations found at work.

A multiple-choice question is normally one of three types:
- It can begin with an incomplete statement followed by several possible endings. You are to find the one ending which best completes the statement, although some of the others may not be entirely wrong.
- It can also be a complete statement in the form of a question which is answered by choosing one of the statements listed.
- It can be in the form of a problem – again you select the best answer.

Here is an example of a multiple-choice question with a discussion which should give you some clues as to the method for choosing the right answer:

When an employee has a complaint about his assignment, the action which will best help him overcome his difficulty is to
- A. discuss his difficulty with his coworkers
- B. take the problem to the head of the organization
- C. take the problem to the person who gave him the assignment
- D. say nothing to anyone about his complaint

In answering this question, you should study each of the choices to find which is best. Consider choice "A" – Certainly an employee may discuss his complaint with fellow employees, but no change or improvement can result, and the complaint remains unresolved. Choice "B" is a poor choice since the head of the organization probably does not know what assignment you have been given, and taking your problem to him is known as "going over the head" of the supervisor. The supervisor, or person who made the assignment, is the person who can clarify it or correct any injustice. Choice "C" is, therefore, correct. To say nothing, as in choice "D," is unwise. Supervisors have and interest in knowing the problems employees are facing, and the employee is seeking a solution to his problem.

2. True/False

3. Matching Questions

Matching an answer from a column of choices within another column.

## V. RECORDING YOUR ANSWERS

Computer terminals are used more and more today for many different kinds of exams.

For an examination with very few applicants, you may be told to record your answers in the test booklet itself. Separate answer sheets are much more common. If this separate answer sheet is to be scored by machine – and this is often the case – it is highly important that you mark your answers correctly in order to get credit.

## VI. BEFORE THE TEST

### YOUR PHYSICAL CONDITION IS IMPORTANT

If you are not well, you can't do your best work on tests. If you are half asleep, you can't do your best either. Here are some tips:

1) Get about the same amount of sleep you usually get. Don't stay up all night before the test, either partying or worrying—DON'T DO IT!
2) If you wear glasses, be sure to wear them when you go to take the test. This goes for hearing aids, too.
3) If you have any physical problems that may keep you from doing your best, be sure to tell the person giving the test. If you are sick or in poor health, you relay cannot do your best on any test. You can always come back and take the test some other time.

Common sense will help you find procedures to follow to get ready for an examination. Too many of us, however, overlook these sensible measures. Indeed, nervousness and fatigue have been found to be the most serious reasons why applicants fail to do their best on civil service tests. Here is a list of reminders:

- Begin your preparation early – Don't wait until the last minute to go scurrying around for books and materials or to find out what the position is all about.
- Prepare continuously – An hour a night for a week is better than an all-night cram session. This has been definitely established. What is more, a night a week for a month will return better dividends than crowding your study into a shorter period of time.
- Locate the place of the exam – You have been sent a notice telling you when and where to report for the examination. If the location is in a different town or otherwise unfamiliar to you, it would be well to inquire the best route and learn something about the building.
- Relax the night before the test – Allow your mind to rest. Do not study at all that night. Plan some mild recreation or diversion; then go to bed early and get a good night's sleep.
- Get up early enough to make a leisurely trip to the place for the test – This way unforeseen events, traffic snarls, unfamiliar buildings, etc. will not upset you.
- Dress comfortably – A written test is not a fashion show. You will be known by number and not by name, so wear something comfortable.
- Leave excess paraphernalia at home – Shopping bags and odd bundles will get in your way. You need bring only the items mentioned in the official notice you received; usually everything you need is provided. Do not bring reference books to the exam. They will only confuse those last minutes and be taken away from you when in the test room.

- Arrive somewhat ahead of time – If because of transportation schedules you must get there very early, bring a newspaper or magazine to take your mind off yourself while waiting.
- Locate the examination room – When you have found the proper room, you will be directed to the seat or part of the room where you will sit. Sometimes you are given a sheet of instructions to read while you are waiting. Do not fill out any forms until you are told to do so; just read them and be prepared.
- Relax and prepare to listen to the instructions
- If you have any physical problem that may keep you from doing your best, be sure to tell the test administrator. If you are sick or in poor health, you really cannot do your best on the exam. You can come back and take the test some other time.

## VII. AT THE TEST

The day of the test is here and you have the test booklet in your hand. The temptation to get going is very strong. Caution! There is more to success than knowing the right answers. You must know how to identify your papers and understand variations in the type of short-answer question used in this particular examination. Follow these suggestions for maximum results from your efforts:

1) Cooperate with the monitor

The test administrator has a duty to create a situation in which you can be as much at ease as possible. He will give instructions, tell you when to begin, check to see that you are marking your answer sheet correctly, and so on. He is not there to guard you, although he will see that your competitors do not take unfair advantage. He wants to help you do your best.

2) Listen to all instructions

Don't jump the gun! Wait until you understand all directions. In most civil service tests you get more time than you need to answer the questions. So don't be in a hurry. Read each word of instructions until you clearly understand the meaning. Study the examples, listen to all announcements and follow directions. Ask questions if you do not understand what to do.

3) Identify your papers

Civil service exams are usually identified by number only. You will be assigned a number; you must not put your name on your test papers. Be sure to copy your number correctly. Since more than one exam may be given, copy your exact examination title.

4) Plan your time

Unless you are told that a test is a "speed" or "rate of work" test, speed itself is usually not important. Time enough to answer all the questions will be provided, but this does not mean that you have all day. An overall time limit has been set. Divide the total time (in minutes) by the number of questions to determine the approximate time you have for each question.

5) Do not linger over difficult questions

If you come across a difficult question, mark it with a paper clip (useful to have along) and come back to it when you have been through the booklet. One caution if you do this – be sure to skip a number on your answer sheet as well. Check often to be sure that you have not lost your place and that you are marking in the row numbered the same as the question you are answering.

6) Read the questions

Be sure you know what the question asks! Many capable people are unsuccessful because they failed to read the questions correctly.

7) Answer all questions

Unless you have been instructed that a penalty will be deducted for incorrect answers, it is better to guess than to omit a question.

8) Speed tests

It is often better NOT to guess on speed tests. It has been found that on timed tests people are tempted to spend the last few seconds before time is called in marking answers at random – without even reading them – in the hope of picking up a few extra points. To discourage this practice, the instructions may warn you that your score will be "corrected" for guessing. That is, a penalty will be applied. The incorrect answers will be deducted from the correct ones, or some other penalty formula will be used.

9) Review your answers

If you finish before time is called, go back to the questions you guessed or omitted to give them further thought. Review other answers if you have time.

10) Return your test materials

If you are ready to leave before others have finished or time is called, take ALL your materials to the monitor and leave quietly. Never take any test material with you. The monitor can discover whose papers are not complete, and taking a test booklet may be grounds for disqualification.

## VIII. EXAMINATION TECHNIQUES

1) Read the general instructions carefully. These are usually printed on the first page of the exam booklet. As a rule, these instructions refer to the timing of the examination; the fact that you should not start work until the signal and must stop work at a signal, etc. If there are any special instructions, such as a choice of questions to be answered, make sure that you note this instruction carefully.

2) When you are ready to start work on the examination, that is as soon as the signal has been given, read the instructions to each question booklet, underline any key words or phrases, such as least, best, outline, describe and the like. In this way you will tend to answer as requested rather than discover on reviewing your paper that you listed without describing, that you selected the worst choice rather than the best choice, etc.

3) If the examination is of the objective or multiple-choice type – that is, each question will also give a series of possible answers: A, B, C or D, and you are called upon to select the best answer and write the letter next to that answer on your answer paper – it is advisable to start answering each question in turn. There may be anywhere from 50 to 100 such questions in the three or four hours allotted and you can see how much time would be taken if you read through all the questions before beginning to answer any. Furthermore, if you

come across a question or group of questions which you know would be difficult to answer, it would undoubtedly affect your handling of all the other questions.

4) If the examination is of the essay type and contains but a few questions, it is a moot point as to whether you should read all the questions before starting to answer any one. Of course, if you are given a choice – say five out of seven and the like – then it is essential to read all the questions so you can eliminate the two that are most difficult. If, however, you are asked to answer all the questions, there may be danger in trying to answer the easiest one first because you may find that you will spend too much time on it. The best technique is to answer the first question, then proceed to the second, etc.

5) Time your answers. Before the exam begins, write down the time it started, then add the time allowed for the examination and write down the time it must be completed, then divide the time available somewhat as follows:
    - If 3-1/2 hours are allowed, that would be 210 minutes. If you have 80 objective-type questions, that would be an average of 2-1/2 minutes per question. Allow yourself no more than 2 minutes per question, or a total of 160 minutes, which will permit about 50 minutes to review.
    - If for the time allotment of 210 minutes there are 7 essay questions to answer, that would average about 30 minutes a question. Give yourself only 25 minutes per question so that you have about 35 minutes to review.

6) The most important instruction is to read each question and make sure you know what is wanted. The second most important instruction is to time yourself properly so that you answer every question. The third most important instruction is to answer every question. Guess if you have to but include something for each question. Remember that you will receive no credit for a blank and will probably receive some credit if you write something in answer to an essay question. If you guess a letter – say "B" for a multiple-choice question – you may have guessed right. If you leave a blank as an answer to a multiple-choice question, the examiners may respect your feelings but it will not add a point to your score. Some exams may penalize you for wrong answers, so in such cases only, you may not want to guess unless you have some basis for your answer.

7) Suggestions
    a. Objective-type questions
        1. Examine the question booklet for proper sequence of pages and questions
        2. Read all instructions carefully
        3. Skip any question which seems too difficult; return to it after all other questions have been answered
        4. Apportion your time properly; do not spend too much time on any single question or group of questions
        5. Note and underline key words – all, most, fewest, least, best, worst, same, opposite, etc.
        6. Pay particular attention to negatives
        7. Note unusual option, e.g., unduly long, short, complex, different or similar in content to the body of the question
        8. Observe the use of "hedging" words – probably, may, most likely, etc.

9. Make sure that your answer is put next to the same number as the question
10. Do not second-guess unless you have good reason to believe the second answer is definitely more correct
11. Cross out original answer if you decide another answer is more accurate; do not erase until you are ready to hand your paper in
12. Answer all questions; guess unless instructed otherwise
13. Leave time for review

  b. Essay questions
  1. Read each question carefully
  2. Determine exactly what is wanted. Underline key words or phrases.
  3. Decide on outline or paragraph answer
  4. Include many different points and elements unless asked to develop any one or two points or elements
  5. Show impartiality by giving pros and cons unless directed to select one side only
  6. Make and write down any assumptions you find necessary to answer the questions
  7. Watch your English, grammar, punctuation and choice of words
  8. Time your answers; don't crowd material

8) Answering the essay question

Most essay questions can be answered by framing the specific response around several key words or ideas. Here are a few such key words or ideas:

M's: manpower, materials, methods, money, management
P's: purpose, program, policy, plan, procedure, practice, problems, pitfalls, personnel, public relations

a. Six basic steps in handling problems:
  1. Preliminary plan and background development
  2. Collect information, data and facts
  3. Analyze and interpret information, data and facts
  4. Analyze and develop solutions as well as make recommendations
  5. Prepare report and sell recommendations
  6. Install recommendations and follow up effectiveness

b. Pitfalls to avoid
1. Taking things for granted – A statement of the situation does not necessarily imply that each of the elements is necessarily true; for example, a complaint may be invalid and biased so that all that can be taken for granted is that a complaint has been registered
2. Considering only one side of a situation – Wherever possible, indicate several alternatives and then point out the reasons you selected the best one
3. Failing to indicate follow up – Whenever your answer indicates action on your part, make certain that you will take proper follow-up action to see how successful your recommendations, procedures or actions turn out to be
4. Taking too long in answering any single question – Remember to time your answers properly

# EXAMINATION SECTION

# ANATOMY & KINESIOLOGY

# EXAMINATION SECTION
# TEST 1

DIRECTIONS: Each question or incomplete statement is followed by several suggested answers or completions. Select the one that BEST answers the question or completes the statement. *PRINT THE LETTER OF THE COERECT ANSWER IN THE SPACE AT THE RIGHT.*

1. Which of the following anatomical reference terms refers to the midline of the body toward the attached end of the limb?  1.____

    A. Medial   B. Lateral   C. Proximal   D. Distal

2. The imaginary longitudinal line that divides the body into right and left parts is called the _____ plane.  2.____

    A. sagittal   B. frontal
    C. transverse   D. dorsal

3. Microscopic blood vessels where the exchange of nutrients and metabolic waste products take place are called  3.____

    A. venuoles   B. arterioles
    C. capillaries   D. none of the above

4. If torn or stressed beyond its ability to recoil, this connective tissue remains loose and nonfunctional until repaired by a physician.  4.____

    A. Tendon   B. Ligament
    C. Cartilage   D. Synovial capsule

5. Which of the following are movements in the frontal plane?  5.____

    A. Abduction, adduction   B. Elevation, depression
    C. Lateral flexion   D. All of the above

6. Most muscles are arranged in opposing pairs. When one muscle is contracting to achieve a desired movement (agonist), its opposite muscle (antagonist) is being stretched.
The antagonist to the muscles biceps femoris, semitendinosus, and semimembranosus is  6.____

    A. rectus femoris   B. psoas
    C. gluteus maximus   D. none of the above

7. Flexion of the knee joint is caused by  7.____

    A. sartorius   B. vastus medialis
    C. gastroenemius   D. all of the above

8. Twisting bent-knee situps will effectively strengthen the  8.____

    A. rectus abdominis
    B. transverse abdominis

C. external and internal obliques
D. erector spinae

9. In addition to the deltoid, which muscle functions to extend the elbow during a military press?

   A. Triceps
   B. Supra spinatus
   C. Trapezius
   D. Biceps

10. The latissimus dorsi's PRIMARY function includes

    A. extension
    B. adduction
    C. medial rotation
    D. all of the above

11. The MOST effective position for work is when the bone-muscle angle is closest to _____ degrees.

    A. 160
    B. 180
    C. 120
    D. 90

12. Shoulder shrugs with resistance will utilize the

    A. rhomboids
    B. latissimus dorsi
    C. trapezius
    D. all of the above

13. A pivot joint responsible for supination-pronation of the forearm is the

    A. elbow
    B. wrist
    C. radioulnar
    D. none of the above

14. Rotation of the foot to the outside so the plantar surface tends to face away from the midline of the body is called

    A. inversion
    B. eversion
    C. supination
    D. pronation

15. The muscles involved in shoulder adduction are
    I. pectoralis major
    II. latissimus dorsi
    III. middle deltoid

    The CORRECT answer is:

    A. I and II
    B. II *only*
    C. I and III
    D. II and III

16. The gluteus maximus is responsible for
    I. medial rotation
    II. hip extension.
    III. hip flexion
    IV. lateral rotation

    The CORRECT answer is:

    A. I and II
    B. I, III, and IV
    C. II and III
    D. II and IV

17. According to _____, bone is capable of adjusting its strength in proportion to the amount of stress placed on it.   17.____

    A. Collagen Law
    B. osteoporosis
    C. Wolff's Law
    D. the Amenorrheic Rule

18. Maintaining the natural curves of the back without flexion, extension, rotation, or excessive anterior pelvic tilt is referred to as   18.____

    A. neutral position
    B. base of support
    C. gravitational pull
    D. antigravity position

19. In a case of *impingement syndrome,* the performance of _____ should be restricted.   19.____

    A. side lateral raises
    B. military press
    C. pull downs
    D. bleep curls

20. If adductors and internal rotators are tight or scapular adductors are weak and overstretched, or pectoralis minor is tight, _____ may be exhibited.   20.____

    A. lordosis
    B. round-shouldered posture
    C. rotator cuff injury
    D. impingement syndrome

21. Blood flow through the heart is as follows:   21.____

    A. RA-RV-LA-LV
    B. LA-LV-RV-RA
    C. RA-biscuspid valves-RV-LV tricuspid v LA
    D. superior vena cava-RA, RV-pulmonary veins, CA-LV-lunges

22. The exchange of $O_2$ and $CO_2$ between the atmosphere and the blood within the capillaries in the lungs is called _____ respiration.   22.____

    A. internal
    B. external
    C. asthmatic
    D. cellular

23. Which are rotation cuff muscles?   23.____

    A. Supraspinatus
    B. Subscapularis
    C. Teres minor
    D. All of the above

24. The internal oblique muscle fibers run   24.____

    A. anteriorly downward and toward the midline
    B. horizontally
    C. posteriorly downward
    D. vertically from pubis to rib cage

25. Nerve cells that carry impulses from the CNS to respond to perceived changes in the internal and external environment of the body are called _____ cells.   25.____

    A. motor nerve
    B. sensory nerve
    C. receptor
    D. all of the above

# KEY (CORRECT ANSWERS)

| | | | |
|---|---|---|---|
| 1. | C | 11. | D |
| 2. | A | 12. | C |
| 3. | C | 13. | C |
| 4. | B | 14. | B |
| 5. | D | 15. | A |
| 6. | A | 16. | D |
| 7. | D | 17. | C |
| 8. | C | 18. | A |
| 9. | A | 19. | B |
| 10. | D | 20. | B |

21. D
22. B
23. D
24. C
25. A

---

# TEST 2

DIRECTIONS: Each question or incomplete statement is followed by several suggested answers or completions. Select the one that BEST answers the question or completes the statement. *PRINT THE LETTER OF THE CORRECT ANSWER IN THE SPACE AT THE RIGHT.*

1. Choose the correct pair of the muscle tissue matched with the appropriate contraction:  1.____
    I. Skeletal - voluntary
    II. Cardiac - voluntary
    III. Visceral - voluntary
   The CORRECT answer is:

   A. I *only*  B. I and II
   C. II and III  D. I, II, and III

2. Which of the following is CORRECT?  2.____
   _____ cervical, _____ thoracic, _____ lumbar, _____ .

   A. 7; 5; 7; 5 coccyx
   B. 5; 12; 7; 5 coccyx
   C. 7; 12; 5; 5 sacral, 4 coccyx
   D. 12; 7; 7; 5 sacral fused

3. Within the sagittal plane flexion and extension occurrences, _____ the angle between the articulating bones.  3.____
    I. flexion decreases
    II. flexion increases
    III. extension decreases
    IV. extension increases
   The CORRECT answer is:

   A. II *only*  B. II and III *only*
   C. I and III *only*  D. I and IV *only*

4. Of the joint structures below, the one that names NO joint cavity and includes all of the joints where bones are held together by fibrous connective tissue is  4.____

   A. fibrous joints  B. synovial joints
   C. cartilaginous joints  D. all skeletal articulations

5. Which of the following muscles are bi-articulate?  5.____

   A. Vastus medius  B. Soleus
   C. Hamstring muscles  D. All of the above

Questions 6-11.

DIRECTIONS: In Questions 6 through 11, refer to the following diagram and write the label of the numbered structure in the appropriate space at the right.

5

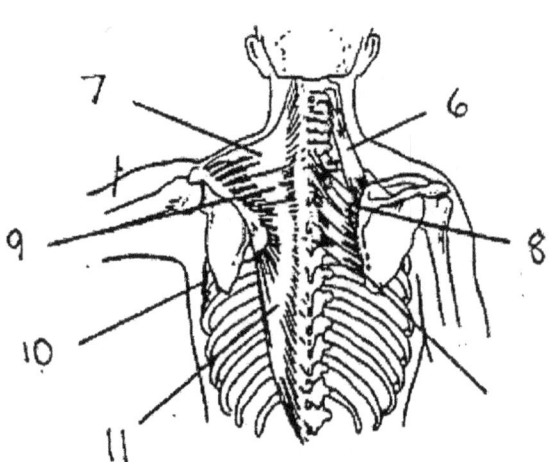

6. ___
7. ___
8. ___
9. ___
10. ___
11. ___

Questions 12-14.

DIRECTIONS: In Questions 12 through 14, refer to the following diagram and write the label of the numbered structure in the appropriate space at the right.

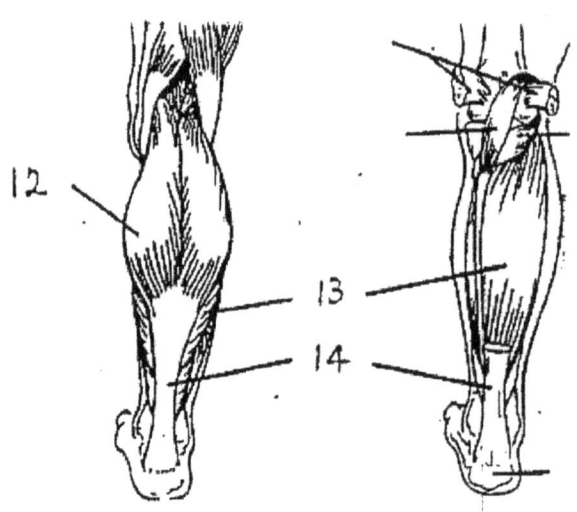

12. ___
13. ___
14. ___

Questions 15-25.

DIRECTIONS: In Questions 15 through 25, refer to the following diagram and write the label of the numbered structure in the appropriate space at the right.

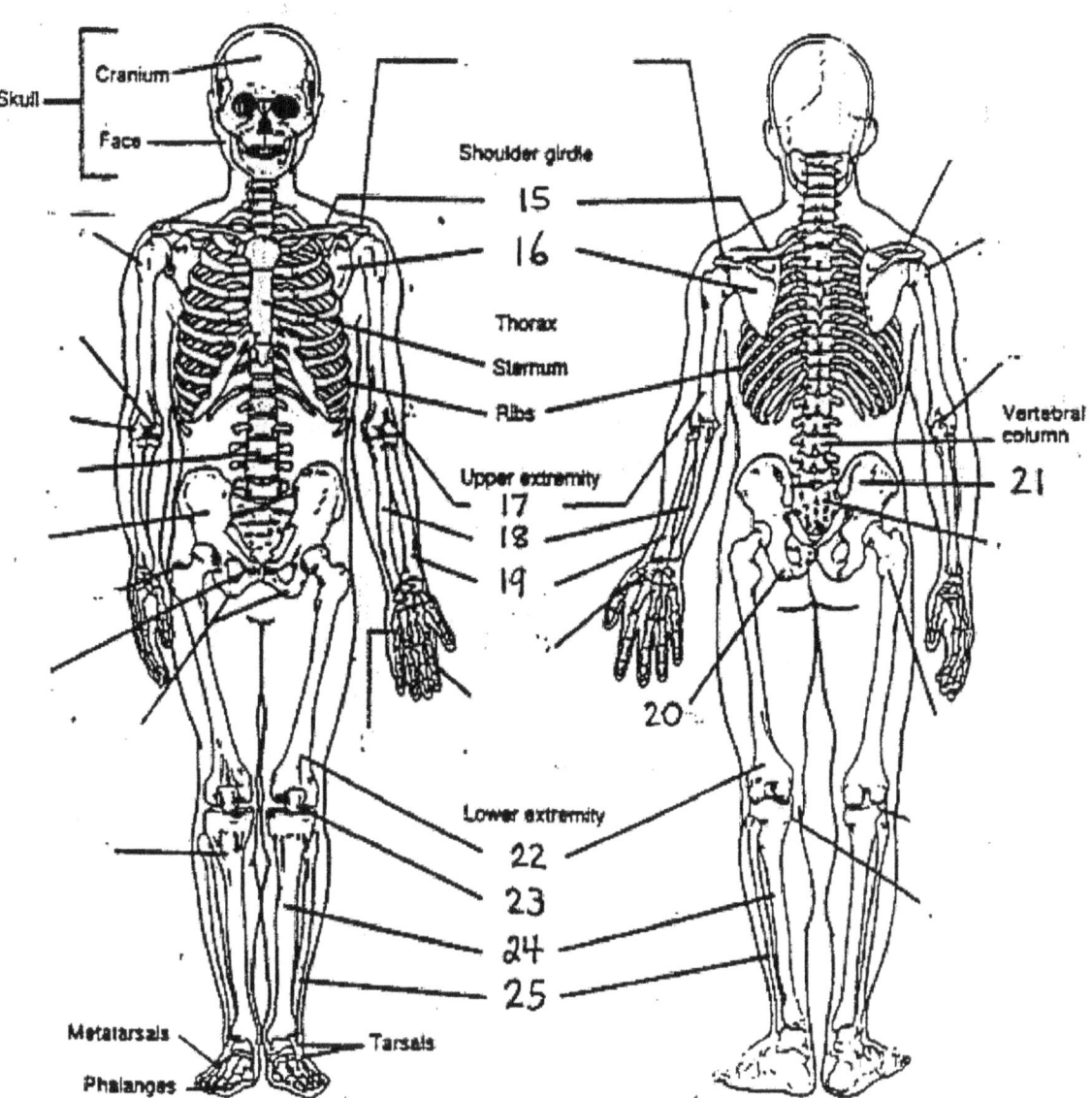

15. _____
16. _____
17. _____
18. _____
19. _____
20. _____
21. _____
22. _____
23. _____
24. _____
25. _____

# KEY (CORRECT ANSWERS)

1. B
2. C
3. D
4. A
5. C

6. levatator scapulae
7. upper trapezius
8. rhomboids
9. middle trapezius
10. serratus anterior

11. lower trapezius
12. gastroenciumis
13. soleus
14. achilles tendon
15. clavicle

16. scapula
17. humerus
18. ulna
19. radius
20. ishium

21. illium
22. femur
23. patella
24. tibia
25. fibula

# ANATOMIC SCIENCES
## EXAMINATION SECTION
## TEST 1

DIRECTIONS: Each question or incomplete statement is followed by several suggested answers or completions. Select the one that BEST answers the question or completes the statement. *PRINT THE LETTER OF THE CORRECT ANSWER IN THE SPACE AT THE RIGHT.*

1. The cell that is MOST capable of mitotic division in the adult is the    1.____

    A. fibroblast
    B. odontoblast
    C. nerve cell
    D. epithelial cell
    E. smooth muscle cell

2. Movement of the head about its vertical axis (rotation to right or left) occurs at the _____ joint.    2.____

    A. atlantoaxial
    B. atlanto-occipital
    C. spheno-occipital
    D. third to the seventh cervical vertebrae
    E. all of the above

3. The smooth muscle cell shows no striations because it has no myofilaments in its cytoplasm.    3.____

    A. Both statement and reason are correct and related.
    B. Both statement and reason are correct but not related.
    C. The statement is correct but the reason is not.
    D. The statement is not correct but the reason is an accurate statement.
    E. Neither statement nor reason is correct.

4. Abdominal organs supplied by the three unpaired branches of the aorta include all of the following EXCEPT the    4.____

    A. spleen
    B. stomach
    C. pancreas
    D. vermiform appendix
    E. suprarenal (adrenal)

5. An osteoclast is a(n)    5.____

    A. cell that forms bone
    B. cell of the endosteum
    C. multinucleated giant cell
    D. osteoblast which has become surrounded by a bony matrix
    E. cell of the periphery of bone which forms from the fibroblasts of the periosteum

6. Which of the following statements apply to DNA?    6.____
    I. It is found as a component of the nucleoli.
    II. It can be distinguished from RNA by the Feulgen reaction.
    III. In polyploidy, it is a multiple of the normal cell chromosome content.
    IV. It is not confined to the chromosomes.

    The CORRECT answer is:

    A. I, II    B. I, III    C. I, IV    D. II, III    E. II, IV

7. The fate of the epithelial rests of Malassez is that they may
    I. undergo calcification
    II. form into cementicles
    III. become fibrous
    IV. form cartilaginous nodules
   The CORRECT answer is:

   A. I, II
   B. I, II, III
   C. II, III
   D. II, III, IV
   E. III, IV

8. Spleen, thymus, and lymph nodes are SIMILAR in that they all

   A. filter blood
   B. contain lymphocytes
   C. have a medulla and a cortex
   D. serve as filters for tissue fluid
   E. have afferent and efferent lymphatic vessels

9. Epithelial cells of the small intestine show surface modification known as

   A. stereocilia
   B. the ciliary border
   C. the striated border
   D. the cuticular border
   E. none of the above

10. The layer of the skin that forms the epithelial root sheaths of the hair follicle is the stratum

    A. corneum
    B. lucidum
    C. granulosum
    D. germinativum
    E. lacrimum

11. Which of the following is characteristic of heart muscle?

    A. Nodes of Ranvier
    B. Rod-shaped nuclei
    C. Spindle-shaped fibers
    D. Centrally-placed nuclei
    E. None of the above

12. Pressure receptors in the carotid sinus are associated with which cranial nerve?

    A. Glossopharyngeal
    B. Trigeminal
    C. Accessory
    D. Facial
    E. Zygomatic

13. Cell membranes are best described as one layer of

    A. charged (polar) lipids
    B. protein on the inside and one layer of neutral lipids on the outside
    C. protein on either side of a layer of neutral lipids
    D. charged (polar) lipids on either side of a layer of neutral lipids
    E. neutral lipids

14. The structure that passes through the foramen rotundum is the      14.____

    A. maxillary nerve          B. zygomatic nerve
    C. lacrimal artery          D. maxillary artery
    E. trigeminal nerve

15. Each of the following cell types secretes the substance with which it is paired EXCEPT      15.____

    A. Sertoli's cells - testosterone
    B. corpus luteum - progesterone
    C. alpha cells of the pancreas - glucagon
    D. chromaffin cells of the adrenal - catecholamine
    E. all of the above are correct

16. In H & E stained sections, the large, deeply stained granules found in the cytoplasm of epithelial cells in keratinized oral mucosa are *most likely*      16.____

    A. glycogen                 B. desmosomes
    C. tonofibrils              D. keratohyaline
    E. basophils

17. The diploid number of chromosomes is perpetuated in somatic cells by a process of      17.____

    A. meiosis                  B. mitosis
    C. amitosis                 D. cytokinesis
    E. pinocytosis

18. The bone that is NOT formed by endochondral ossification is the      18.____

    A. nasal                    B. ethmoid
    C. sphenoid                 D. temporal
    E. jugular

19. The tentorium cerebelli contains all of the following dural venous sinuses EXCEPT the      19.____

    A. straight                 B. transverse
    C. superior petrosal        D. inferior petrosal
    E. superior nasal

20. All of the following are located in the nasopharynx EXCEPT the      20.____

    A. piriform recess          B. eustachian canal
    C. pharyngeal tonsil        D. pharyngeal recess
    E. lacrimal artery

21. An endocrine gland of ectodermal origin in the abdomen is the      21.____

    A. liver
    B. corpus luteum
    C. medulla of the adrenal
    D. cortical portion of the adrenal
    E. interstitial cells of the testis

22. The middle cardiac vein empties into the        22.___

    A. left atrium                B. right atrium
    C. coronary sinus             D. great cardiac vein
    E. anterior cardiac vein

23. Which of the following does NOT occur during contraction of the left ventricle of a normal    23.___
    heart?

    A. The aortic similunar valve opens.
    B. Blood enters the coronary arteries.
    C. The pulmonary semilunar valve opens.
    D. The left atrioventricular valve closes.
    E. The right atrioventricular valve closes.

24. The transverse diameter of the pleural cavity is *increased* during inspiration by    24.___

    A. contraction of the diaphragm
    B. relaxation of the scalene muscles
    C. elevation of the arched shaft of the ribs
    D. depression of the anterior ends of the ribs
    E. contraction of the external abdominal oblique muscle

25. The vertical dimension of the thoracic cavity is increased *chiefly* by contraction of the    25.___

    A. diaphragm
    B. quadratus lumborum muscles
    C. external intercostal muscles
    D. serratus posterior inferior muscles
    E. transversus thoracis (sternocostalis) muscle

## KEY (CORRECT ANSWERS)

1. D
2. A
3. C
4. E
5. C

6. D
7. A
8. B
9. C
10. D

11. D
12. A
13. D
14. A
15. A

16. D
17. B
18. A
19. D
20. A

21. C
22. C
23. B
24. C
25. A

# TEST 2

DIRECTIONS: Each question or incomplete statement is followed by several suggested answers or completions. Select the one that BEST answers the question or completes the statement. *PRINT THE LETTER OF THE CORRECT ANSWER IN THE SPACE AT THE RIGHT.*

1. Progesterone production in the ovary is *primarily* by                              1._____

    A. stroma
    B. corpora lutea
    C. mature follicles
    D. corpora albicans
    E. growing follicles

2. From an anatomic standpoint, an emergency airway may be established MOST readily by an opening into the trachea                              2._____

    A. at the level of the jugular notch
    B. through the thyrohyoid membrane
    C. through the median cricothyroid ligament
    D. between the thyroid cartilages
    E. none of the above

3. Systemic arteries and veins DIFFER in that                              3._____

    A. veins have more elastic tissue
    B. arteries have a relatively thinner tunica media
    C. valves are often present in veins
    D. arteries have larger endothelial pores
    E. elastic membranes are less pronounced in arteries

4. A small bronchus differs from a bronchiole by possessing                              4._____

    A. stratified squamous epithelium and rings or plates of cartilage
    B. stratified squamous epithelium and no rings or plates of cartilage
    C. stratified columnar epithelium and rings or plates of cartilage
    D. pseudostratified columnar epithelium and no rings or plates of cartilage
    E. pseudostratified columnar epithelium and rings or plates of cartilage

5. The basic framework or stroma of ALL lymphoid tissues except thymus consists of                              5._____

    A. reticular fibers primarily and a lesser amount of collagen fibers
    B. a combination of epithelioid cells and reticular fibers
    C. a combination of smooth muscle and reticular fibers
    D. some smooth muscle and trabeculae of collagen fibers
    E. collagen fibers primarily and some elastic fibers

6. In a double vertical fracture through the mental foramina, muscle action will cause the small fragment to move                              6._____

    A. inferiorly *only*
    B. superiorly *only*
    C. anteriorly and superiorly
    D. posteriorly and inferiorly
    E. posteriorly and superiorly

7. The organelle that binds and releases calcium during relaxation and contraction of skeletal muscle is a

   A. nucleus
   B. lysosome
   C. mitochondrion
   D. transverse tubule
   E. sarcoplasmic reticulum

8. The foramen ovale is an embryological opening between

   A. right and left atria
   B. right and left ventricles
   C. right atrium and right ventricle
   D. umbilical vein and inferior vena cava
   E. pulmonary artery and arch of the aorta

9. A sarcomere is the part of the myofibril enclosed between

   A. two consecutive H bands
   B. two consecutive I bands
   C. two consecutive Z bands
   D. an I band and the next A band
   E. a Z band and the next H band

10. Mucosa of all parts of the small intestine is characterized by possessing

    A. rugae
    B. villi
    C. haustra
    D. teniae coli
    E. appendices epiploicae

11. Ribonucleic acid that is involved in protein synthesis is found *primarily* in the

    A. nucleolus
    B. mitochondria
    C. Golgi complex
    D. fluid ground substance
    E. granular endoplasmic reticulum

12. The normal percentage of neutrophilic leukocytes in a differential blood count is *approximately* _____ percent.

    A. 0.5-1
    B. 2-5
    C. 8-15
    D. 20-25
    E. 60-70

13. The parasympathetic fibers to the pterygopalatine ganglion come from the _____ nerve.

    A. maxillary
    B. mandibular
    C. deep petrosal
    D. glossopharyngeal
    E. greater petrosal

14. Production of bile takes place in

    A. the hepatic duct
    B. the gallbladder
    C. von Kupffer's cell
    D. the common bile duct
    E. none of the above

15. The component of bone tissue that gives a bone tensile strength is the

    A. calcified cement substance
    B. interconnecting canaliculi
    C. collagenous fibrils of matrix
    D. periosteal connective tissue
    E. elastic fibers

16. Long bones of the skeleton *increase* in length because of

    A. mitotic division of osteocytes
    B. mitotic division of osteoblasts
    C. resorption of primary bone by osteoclasts
    D. appositional growth on the cartilaginous epiphyseal plate
    E. interstitial growth in the cartilaginous epiphyseal plate

17. In an adult, the site of origin of the thyroid gland is seen as the

    A. copula
    B. foramen cecum
    C. eustachian tube
    D. palatine tonsil
    E. tuberculum impar

18. In the adult, cerebrospinal fluid can be aspirated most safely by inserting the needle between the third and the fourth lumbar vertebrae because

    A. there is more space between the laminae of these two vertebrae
    B. the subarachnoid space does not extend below lumbar 4
    C. the spinal cord usually does not extend below lumbar 2
    D. there is less danger of entering the internal vertebral plexus at this level
    E. there are no important nerves in this part of the vertebral canal

19. The visual center of the cerebral cortex is located in the

    A. hypothalamus
    B. parietal lobe
    C. occipital lobe
    D. indusium griseum
    E. medulla oblongata

20. In normal light microscopy of striated muscle, the dark portion of the striation is caused by the presence of

    A. actin
    B. myosin
    C. Cohnheim's fields
    D. an intercalated disk
    E. fibers in the endomysium

21. Stereocilia are characteristic of the

    A. epididymis
    B. seminal vesicle
    C. ejaculatory duct
    D. proximal convoluted tubule
    E. ampulla of the ductus deferens

22. The principal fibrous elements of the periodontal ligament in adults consist *chiefly* of _____ fibers.

    A. elastic
    B. collagen
    C. reticular
    D. a mixture of elastic and collagen
    E. a mixture of elastic and reticular

23. Mucus-secreting cells are found in the
    I. parotid gland
    II. submandibular gland
    III. mucosa of the trachea
    IV. mucosa of the ureter
    V. glands of the esophagus

    The CORRECT answer is:

    A. I, III
    B. I, V
    C. II, III, IV
    D. II, III, V
    E. II, IV

24. Each of the following structures is derived from ectoderm EXCEPT

    A. hair
    B. enamel
    C. dentin
    D. sweat gland
    E. salivary gland

25. Testosterone is produced by the

    A. epididymis
    B. Sertoli cells
    C. sustenacular cells
    D. seminiferous tubules
    E. interstitial cells of Leydig

## KEY (CORRECT ANSWERS)

1. B
2. C
3. C
4. E
5. A

6. D
7. E
8. A
9. C
10. B

11. E
12. E
13. E
14. E
15. C

16. E
17. B
18. C
19. C
20. B

21. A
22. B
23. D
24. C
25. E

# EXERCISE PHYSIOLOGY

# EXAMINATION SECTION
## TEST 1

DIRECTIONS: Each question or incomplete statement is followed by several suggested answers or completions. Select the one that BEST answers the question or completes the statement. *PRINT THE LETTER OF THE CORRECT ANSWER IN THE SPACE' AT THE RIGHT.*

1. The intensity at which adequate oxygen is UNAVAILABLE is referred to as  1._____
    A. aerobic glycolysis
    B. PNF
    C. anaerobic threshold
    D. specificity

2. Excess _____ are stored as glycogen in the muscle or liver cells for energy.  2._____
    A. proteins
    B. carbohydrates
    C. fats
    D. lactic acids

3. Oxygenated blood is carried away from the heart to be delivered to the various cells and tissues of the body by the  3._____
    A. veins
    B. vena cava
    C. arteries
    D. ventricles

4. Lean body mass is made up of  4._____
    A. muscles, bones, skin, organs
    B. muscles, bones, adipose tissue, nervous tissue
    C. muscles, bones, adipose tissue, organs
    D. skin, organs, nervous tissue, adipose tissue

5. Movement patterns requiring a sudden burst of energy for relatively short periods of time would be classified as  5._____
    I. aerobic glycolysis
    II. anaerobic glycolysis
    III. fast twitch muscle fibers
    The CORRECT answer is:
    A. I only
    B. II only
    C. I and III
    D. II and III

6. The contraction phase when the heart pumps the blood to the body is called  6._____
    A. systolic
    B. diastolic
    C. cardiac output
    D. ejection fraction

7. _____ are used for growth and repair of cellular structures.  7._____
    A. Fats
    B. Carbohydrates
    C. Proteins
    D. Lipids

8. Which of the following stages of ATP production produce lactic acid as a by-product?

   A. Phosphogen system
   B. Fatty acid oxidation
   C. Aerobic glycolysis
   D. Anaerobic glycolysis

9. Benefits from regular weight-bearing aerobic exercise include increased

   A. bone density, decreased body fat, increased cardiovascular benefits
   B. cardiovascular benefits, increased lean mass, increased insulin
   C. bone density, increased cardiovascular benefits, osteoporosis
   D. bone density, cardiovascular benefits, increased body fat

10. _____ fibers have a large number of mitochondria and are primarily recruited for low intensity, longer duration activities, such as jogging, walking, and swimming.
    I. Slow twitch
    II. Fast twitch
    III. Intermediate

    The CORRECT answer is:

    A. I only
    B. III only
    C. I and III
    D. II and III

11. Contractile proteins involved in muscular contraction include
    I. myosin
    II. actin
    III. mitochondria

    The CORRECT answer is:

    A. II only
    B. II and III
    C. III only
    D. I and II

12. When the muscle visibly shortens and joint movement occurs, the contraction described is
    I. isometric
    II. isotonic
    III. isokinetic

    The CORRECT answer is:

    A. I only
    B. III only
    C. II and III
    D. I, II, and III

13. Flexibility is thought to be related to
    I. acute muscle injury
    II. delayed muscle soreness
    III. increased muscle mass

    The CORRECT answer is:

    A. I, II, and III
    B. II and III
    C. II only
    D. I and II

14. For MAXIMUM results, it is usually recommended that muscular endurance training be completed

    A. 2-3 times per week
    B. 3-5 times per week
    C. 5-7 times per week
    D. every day

15. When training outdoors in the cold, it is recommended that you wear     15.____

    A. layers, hat and gloves
    B. cottons and reflective materials
    C. nylon and dark colors
    D. loose-fitting clothing so you can move

16. When the muscle develops tension as it lengthens against resistance during contraction,     16.____
    the contraction is called
        I.   eccentric
        II.  concentric
        III. isometric
    The CORRECT answer is:

    A. I only                B. I or II
    C. II or III             D. I, II, or III

17. An increase in the size of the muscle itself is known as     17.____

    A. hypertrophy
    B. atrophy
    C. sliding filament theory
    D. contractile protein content

18. The function of the force generated by the heart during its contraction phase and the     18.____
    force generated by the vessels on the blood flowing through them is called

    A. systolic              B. diastolic
    C. stroke volume         D. blood pressure

19. Strength exercises using a fixed amount of external resistance are referred to as _____     19.____
    resistance.

    A. dynamic variable      B. dynamic constant
    C. isometric             D. isokinetic

20. The connective tissues that connect bone to bone are     20.____

    A. tendons               B. muscles
    C. ligaments             D. cartilage

21. When we exercise in the heat,     21.____

    A. blood vessels near the skin open
    B. we sweat more
    C. we increase water consumption
    D. all of the above

22. Exercise intensity should be APPROXIMATELY _____% of oxygen consumption to     22.____
    improve cardiovascular endurance.

    A. 40-75      B. 50-85      C. 60-90      D. 60-80

23. The product of stroke volume x heart rate is     23.____

    A. cardiac output        B. blood pressure
    C. hemoglobin count      D. systolic reading

24. Which of the following stretches involves holding a non-moving position so the specified joint is immobilized in a position that places the desired muscles and connective tissues passively at their greatest length?
    I. Ballistic
    II. PNF
    III. Static
    The CORRECT answer is:

    A. I only
    B. I or II
    C. III only
    D. II or III

25. _____ training involves exercise at high intensity levels for relatively brief periods with intervening rest periods to allow the heart rate to decline.

    A. Overload
    B. Continuous
    C. Circuit
    D. Interval

## KEY (CORRECT ANSWERS)

1. C
2. B
3. C
4. A
5. D
6. A
7. C
8. D
9. A
10. A
11. D
12. C
13. D
14. B
15. A
16. A
17. A
18. D
19. B
20. C
21. D
22. B
23. A
24. C
25. D

# TEST 2

DIRECTIONS: Each question or incomplete statement is followed by several suggested answers or completions. Select the one that BEST answers the question or completes the statement. *PRINT THE LETTER OF THE CORRECT ANSWER IN THE SPACE AT THE RIGHT.*

1. The *transport* system through which gases, nutrients, and by-products are exchanged between the blood and cells is referred to as  1.____

   A. capillaries  
   B. arteries  
   C. veins  
   D. ventricles

2. Oxygen is carried in the blood on protein called  2.____

   A. amino acid  
   B. glucose  
   C. hemoglobin  
   D. glycogen

3. Increased stroke volume, decreased arterial blood pressure, and increased glucose utilization are some of the results of  3.____

   A. strength training  
   B. stretching  
   C. plyometrics  
   D. cardiovascular exercise

4. Improved cardiovascular fitness consists of _____ heart rate at a given workload and _____ return of heart rate to normal after work.  4.____

   A. lower; slower  
   B. lower; quicker  
   C. higher; slower  
   D. higher; quicker

5. Slow twitch muscle fibers  5.____
   I. have a high density of mitochondria
   II. contract slower than fast twitch fibers
   III. are specifically designed for power moves
   The CORRECT answer is:

   A. I, II, and III  
   B. I *only*  
   C. II *only*  
   D. I and II

6. Three of the PRIMARY risk factors for developing C.A.D. are  6.____

   A. obesity, hypertension, smoking  
   B. hypertension, smoking, poor lipid profile  
   C. diabetes, obesity, hypertension  
   D. hypertension, poor lipid profile, obesity

7. Which of the following are MOST likely to increase in response to an aerobic exercise program?  7.____

   A. High density lipoproteins (HDL's)  
   B. Low density lipoproteins (LDL's)  
   C. Fatty acids  
   D. Triglycerides

8. Fatigue is associated with
   A. accumulation of lactic acid
   B. anaerobic energy production
   C. depletion of glycogen stores
   D. all of the above

9. Of the following, _____ is NOT one of the five components of physical fitness.
   A. strength
   B. endurance
   C. agility
   D. body composition

10. A motor unit consists of
    A. myosin and actin
    B. a motor neuron and the muscle cells it innervates
    C. sensory and motor neurons
    D. CNS and motor end plate

11. The _____ principle states that training adaptations will gradually decline if not regularly reinforced.
    A. all or none
    B. specificity
    C. reversibility
    D. F.I.T.

12. Which of the following statements about ATP is NOT true? ATP
    A. is not produced anaerobically
    B. is stored in the muscle cells
    C. fuels all biological work
    D. is produced in the mitochondria of muscle cells

13. With the commencement of exercise, a(n) _____ would normally be expected.
    I. constriction of blood vessels
    II. increase in stroke volume
    III. increase in systolic pressure
    The CORRECT answer is:
    A. I, II, and III
    B. II only
    C. I and III
    D. II and III

14. Fast twitch fibers are
    A. adapted for endurance activities
    B. characteristically smaller than slow twitch fibers
    C. higher in mitochondrial density than slow twitch fibers
    D. adapted for power activities

15. There are three basic types of connective tissues. They are
    A. cartilage, ligaments, tendons
    B. muscles, bones, tendons
    C. tendons, bones, ligaments
    D. muscles, tendons, ligaments

16. The PRIMARY physiological adaptation to progressive resistance exercise is an increase in the

    A. number of individual muscle fibers
    B. size of the individual muscle fibers
    C. tensile strength of muscle
    D. all of the above

17. Plyometrics refers to a system of training designed to enhance muscular

    A. endurance    B. strength    C. power    D. flexibility

18. At the first 3-4 weeks of training of a novice weight lifter, initial strength gains are believed to be induced PRIMARILY by

    A. an increase in the number of muscle fibers
    B. an increase in the size and strength of the ligaments
    C. muscular-neural pathway development
    D. excited participation in a new activity

19. A dynamic state of stability in which supply equals demand is called

    A. ATP production
    B. metabolic waste production
    C. homeostasis
    D. overload

20. ESSENTIAL body fat percentages for women lie between _____%, and for men, between _____%.

    A. 15-18; 6-9    B. 8-12; 3-6    C. 8-12; 6-9    D. 15-18; 3-6

21. The body will use significant amounts of fatty acids to produce energy during _____ intensity exercise for _____ duration.

    A. moderate to high; long
    B. moderate to high; short
    C. low to moderate; long
    D. low to moderate; short

22. Which of the following is NOT a factor affecting flexibility?

    A. Age    B. Gender    C. Inactivity    D. Agility

23. Of the following, the gland MOST closely related to muscular efficiency is the

    A. adrenal    B. gonads    C. pituitary    D. thyroid

24. When oxygen consumption momentarily does NOT meet the physiological demand for oxygen, it is known as

    A. oxygen debt
    B. oxygen deficit
    C. tidal volume
    D. respiratory rate

25. Heat cramps are a sign of

    A. not hydrating properly
    B. not eating well
    C. exercising in the cold
    D. altitude changes

# KEY (CORRECT ANSWERS)

| | | | |
|---|---|---|---|
| 1. | A | 11. | C |
| 2. | C | 12. | A |
| 3. | D | 13. | D |
| 4. | B | 14. | D |
| 5. | D | 15. | A |
| 6. | B | 16. | B |
| 7. | A | 17. | C |
| 8. | D | 18. | C |
| 9. | C | 19. | C |
| 10. | B | 20. | B |

21. C
22. D
23. A
24. B
25. A

# NUTRITION & WEIGHT CONTROL

## EXAMINATION SECTION
## TEST 1

DIRECTIONS: Each question or incomplete statement is followed by several suggested answers or completions. Select the one that BEST answers the question or completes the statement. *PRINT THE LETTER OF THE CORRECT ANSWER IN THE SPACE AT THE RIGHT.*

1. Minerals are responsible for

    A. regulation of muscle contraction and heart rhythm
    B. conduction of nerve impulses
    C. clotting of blood
    D. all of the above

    1._____

2. All of the following are major minerals EXCEPT

    A. iron    B. calcium    C. sodium    D. magnesium

    2._____

3. Fat soluble vitamins include A, D

    A. E and K    B. C and B    C. E and C    D. K and B

    3._____

4. Complete proteins contain all ESSENTIAL amino acids, numbering

    A. 13
    C. 20
    B. 9
    D. none of the above

    4._____

5. One gram of fat supplies _____ kilocalories.

    A. 4    B. 3    C. 9    D. 12

    5._____

6. At room temperature, _____ fat is solid.

    A. polyunsaturated
    C. saturated
    B. unsaturated
    D. monounsaturated

    6._____

7. Fats

    A. insulate and protect the body's organs
    B. are a source of linoleic acid
    C. perform absorption and transport of fat-soluble vitamins
    D. all of the above

    7._____

8. The RDA for vitamin C is _____ mg.

    A. 10    B. 60    C. 80    D. 20

    8._____

9. According to the 1977 Senate Select Committee, the TOTAL number of calories consumed in the form of complex carbohydrates should be _____%.

    A. 58    B. 48    C. 30    D. 12

    9._____

10. Which of the following meals represents ALL four basic food groups?

   A. Turkey sandwich on whole wheat with lettuce and tomato and a glass of chocolate milk
   B. Lasagna dinner with a glass of iced tea
   C. Chef's salad with whole wheat toast and a cup of coffee
   D. Steak, potatoes, broccoli, and a coke

11. Which food below has vitamins A, K, and B?
   I. Milk
   II. Liver
   III. Green leafy vegetables

   The CORRECT answer is:

   A. I and II
   B. III *only*
   C. II and III
   D. I, II, and III

12. An inadequate supply of _____ is one of the MAJOR contributing factors to osteoporosis.

   A. iron
   B. phosphorus
   C. potassium
   D. calcium

13. The RDA for calcium is _____ mg.

   A. 800
   B. 1500
   C. 1200
   D. 900

14. To increase iron intake, you can

   A. eat foods rich in vitamin C
   B. drink tea or coffee with meals
   C. use cast iron cookware
   D. all of the above

15. Which of the following remove cholesterol from the system?

   A. Cholesterol
   B. High density lipoproteins
   C. Low density lipoproteins
   D. All of the above

16. An appropriate meal before exercising is

   A. high in protein one hour prior to exercising
   B. high in fat to speed up transit time
   C. high in carbohydrates several hours before exercising
   D. heavy just before exercising to increase muscle glycogen stores

17. The BEST fluid for exercisers is

   A. Gatorade
   B. fruit juice
   C. coffee
   D. cold water

18. The protein requirement for a 160 1b. man would be _____ grams.

   A. 45.7
   B. 50.5
   C. 57.6
   D. none of the above

19. Body weight will stay the same when calorie intake equals calorie expenditure. 19.____
    This theory is called

    A. set point theory        B. obesity
    C. energy balance          D. thermo-regulation

20. To lose one pound of fat, a deficit of _____ Kcals is necessary. 20.____

    A. 3500      B. 3000      C. 1500      D. 1000

21. Self-imposed starvation to the point of emaciation is called 21.____

    A. bulimia        B. obesity
    C. cellulite      D. anorexia nervosa

22. The rate of sustained weight loss per week should NOT exceed _____ lb(s). 22.____

    A. one       B. two       C. three     D. four

23. According to the _____ theory, the body strives to main-tain a certain level of body fat. 23.____

    A. energy balance     B. set point
    C. spot reduction     D. ketosis

24. A person's water intake is governed by the thirst mechanism, which is regulated by the 24.____

    A. mitochondria      B. motor neuron
    C. hypothalamus      D. medulla

25. The ratio between HDL-C and total cholesterol is the single most important factor in 25.____
    determining risk for heart disease.
    This ratio for women is

    A. 5.0       B. 4.0       C. 5.5       D. 4.4

26. To incorporate more calcium into the diet, clients might 26.____

    A. add nonfat dry milk to soups, stews, and casseroles
    B. add grated low fat cheese to salads, tacos, and pasta dishes
    C. have yogurt as a snack
    D. all of the above

27. The DESIRABLE level of blood cholesterol is _____ mg/dl. 27.____

    A. less than 200     B. 200-239
    C. 240               D. more than 240

28. A triglyceride is made up of 28.____

    A. 3 fatty acids and one glycerol    B. 3 glycerols and one fatty acid
    C. 3 HDLs and one LDL                D. 1 HDL and three LDLs

29. The lacto-ovo vegetarian eats 29.____

    A. fish and poultry but excludes red meat
    B. only foods from plant sources
    C. milk and eggs but excludes meat, fish, and poultry
    D. beans and rice

30. Which of the following are nutrient dense foods?

    A. Soda, potato chips
    B. Cookies, cake
    C. Yogurt, beans, and peas
    D. None of the above

31. The protein requirement for a 154 1b. man would be _____ grams.

    A. 90      B. 100      C. 105      D. 95

32. Which of the following factors affect a person's BMR?

    A. Age, height, and gender
    B. Fasting and dieting
    C. Environmental temperature
    D. All of the above

33. Guidelines for fluid replacement recommend _____ ounces every 10-15 minutes during a workout.

    A. 2-4      B. 3-6      C. 5-7      D. 6-8

34. Decreasing training intensity while increasing carbohy-drate intake over a one week period prior to competition would be an example of

    A. ketosis
    B. hypoglycemia
    C. carbohydrate depletion
    D. carbohydrate loading

35. Water is important in the daily intake of the body CHIEFLY because it

    A. causes the oxidation of food in the body
    B. is a transporting medium for all body substances
    C. cools the air in the lungs
    D. gives off minerals when it is digested

## KEY (CORRECT ANSWERS)

1. D
2. A
3. A
4. B
5. C

6. C
7. D
8. B
9. B
10. A

11. C
12. D
13. C
14. D
15. B

16. C
17. D
18. D
19. C
20. A

21. D
22. B
23. B
24. C
25. D

26. D
27. A
28. A
29. C
30. C

31. C
32. D
33. B
34. D
35. B

# TEST 2

DIRECTIONS: Each question or incomplete statement is followed by several suggested answers or completions. Select the one that BEST answers the question or completes the statement. *PRINT THE LETTER OF THE CORRECT ANSWER IN THE SPACE AT THE RIGHT.*

1. Food satisfies the body's need for

   A. energy
   B. new tissue and growth repair
   C. regulating metabolic function
   D. all of the above

   1.____

2. The six classes of nutrients are

   A. triglycerides, polyunsaturated fat, monounsaturated fat, polyunsaturated fat, and cholesterol
   B. water, carbohydrates, protein, fat, vitamins, and minerals
   C. dairy, fruits, vegetables, grains, proteins, and fats
   D. meat, fish, poultry, dry beans, eggs, and nuts

   2.____

3. When the supply of calcium in the body is too low, the body

   A. excretes more urinary calcium
   B. increases iron supply
   C. withdraws calcium from the bones
   D. none of the above

   3.____

4. Good sources of calcium include
   - I. whole milk, cottage cheese, frozen yogurt, swiss cheese
   - II. pudding, ice cream, cream cheese
   - III. ice cream, feta cheese, skim milk, low-fat yogurt

   The CORRECT answer is:

   A. I and III
   B. II and III
   C. I, II, and III
   D. I *only*

   4.____

5. Hemochromatosis is a disease defined as

   A. chromium overload
   B. iron overload
   C. chromium deficiency
   D. iron deficiency

   5.____

6. The adult body cannot make _____ for itself; therefore, it needs to be included in the diet.
   - I. vitamin K
   - II. essential nutrients
   - III. linoleic acid

   The CORRECT answer is:

   A. I *only*
   B. I and II
   C. I and III
   D. II and III

   6.____

7. The quantitative analysis of the amount of nutrients versus the amount of calories in a given food is called  7.____

   A. calorie deficit
   B. nutritional analysis
   C. nutrient density
   D. quality evaluation

8. What used to be known as the four food groups is now known as the  8.____

   A. food guide pyramid
   B. food groups of America
   C. 2-2-4-4 plan
   D. none of the above

9. The laboratory test that measures storage iron is  9.____
   I. total iron binding capacity
   II. serum ferritin
   III. serum iron
   The CORRECT answer is:

   A. I only
   B. II only
   C. II and III
   D. I, II, and III

10. The dietary goals for Americans consist of  10.____
    I. 10% simple carbohydrates, 15% saturated fat, 12% protein
    II. 48% complex carbohydrates, 10% monounsaturated fat, 12% protein
    III. 58% total carbohydrates, 12% protein, 30% total fat
    The CORRECT answer is:

    A. I and II
    B. II only
    C. I and III
    D. II and III

11. Scientific evidence proves that athletes should consume  11.____

    A. chromium picolinate
    B. glucose tolerance factor
    C. amino acid
    D. none of the above

12. A fat-like, waxy substance in the blood that is an ESSENTIAL component of cell structures and hormones is  12.____

    A. triglyceride
    B. linoleic acid
    C. cholesterol
    D. fat-soluble vitamins

13. The *good* cholesterol is known as  13.____

    A. triglycerides
    B. LDL (low density lipoprotein)
    C. HDL (high density lipoprotein)
    D. MDL (medium density lipoprotein)

14. Dietary fat contains a mixture of 3 fatty acids:  14.____

    A. Saturated, polyunsaturated, and biosaturated
    B. Saturated, monounsaturated, and triglyceride
    C. Unsaturated, saturated, and semisaturated
    D. None of the above

15. Weight loss during an exercise session is PRIMARILY the result of  15.____

    A. fat metabolism
    B. dehydration
    C. protein synthesis
    D. glycogen depletion

16. Linoleic acid is needed for

    A. calcium absorption
    B. growth and skin maintenance
    C. fat transport
    D. all of the above

17. Excessive protein or amino acid intake causes
    I. excessive weight gain
    II. dehydration
    III. excessive loss of urinary calcium

    The CORRECT answer is:

    A. I and II              B. II only
    C. I and III             D. I, II, and III

18. Three ounces of chicken has _____ grams of protein.

    A. 3        B. 7        C. 21        D. 36

19. Ketosis, an abnormal increase of ketone bodies in the body, is USUALLY the result of

    A. an excessively low carbohydrate diet
    B. lowfat diet
    C. both A and B
    D. none of the above

20. Hypoglycemia (low blood sugar) may be caused by too

    A. much insulin
    B. little glucose
    C. much exercise in the insulin-dependent diabetic
    D. all of the above

21. Muscle cramps may be caused by

    A. inadequate salt intake
    B. excess water loss through sweating
    C. drinking water during exercise
    D. none of the above

22. The ingestion of caffeine before an athletic event may result in
    I. an increased heart rate
    II. decreased urine production
    III. dehydration

    The CORRECT answer is:

    A. I only               B. II only
    C. I and II             D. I and III

23. Weight loss of MORE than 1-3 pounds/week is USUALLY

    A. lean body mass       B. fat
    C. both A and B         D. none of the above

24. _____ contain high amounts of iron and hemoglobin, which are found in red blood cells.   24.\_\_\_\_

    A. Hemochromatosis  B. Brown fat cells
    C. White fat cells   D. Mitochondria

25. According to ACSM, which of the following is NOT true about steroids?   25.\_\_\_\_

    A. The prolonged use of steroids has resulted in liver disorders in some people.
    B. Steroids given to males may result in increased testicular size.
    C. Steroids given to males may result in decreased sperm production.
    D. Steroid use does not bring about any significant improvements in strength, aerobic endurance, lean body mass, or body weight.

26. The basal metabolic rate (BMR) of a 30-year-old man who weighs 200 pounds is _____ calories.   26.\_\_\_\_

    A. 2,000   B. 2,304   C. 2,352   D. 2,400

27. The energy needed by a 220-pound, 5' 9" man lifting weights (3 METS) for 1 hour equals _____ calories.   27.\_\_\_\_

    A. 105   B. 210   C. 315   D. 525

Questions 28-30.

DIRECTIONS: Questions 28 through 30 are to be answered on the basis of the following information.

Haagen Dazs Vanilla Chocolate Crunch Frozen Yogurt bar has the following food label:

> Serving Size: 1
> Calories: 210
> Total Fat: 11 grams
> Polyunsaturated Fat: 2 grams
> Saturated Fat: 6 grams
> Carbohydrate: 23 grams

28. What is the percentage of total fat in 1 yogurt bar?   28.\_\_\_\_

    A. 21%
    B. 34%
    C. 47%
    D. Cannot calculate with the information given

29. What is the percentage of saturated fat in 2 yogurt bars?   29.\_\_\_\_

    A. 18%
    B. 26%
    C. 51%
    D. Cannot calculate with the information given

30. How many calories come from simple carbohydrates?

    A. 23
    B. 92
    C. 207
    D. Cannot calculate with the information given

30._____

---

## KEY (CORRECT ANSWERS)

| | | | |
|---|---|---|---|
| 1. | D | 16. | B |
| 2. | B | 17. | A |
| 3. | C | 18. | C |
| 4. | A | 19. | A |
| 5. | B | 20. | D |
| 6. | D | 21. | B |
| 7. | C | 22. | D |
| 8. | A | 23. | A |
| 9. | B | 24. | B |
| 10. | D | 25. | B |
| 11. | D | 26. | C |
| 12. | C | 27. | C |
| 13. | C | 28. | C |
| 14. | D | 29. | B |
| 15. | B | 30. | D |

# EXAMINATION SECTION
## TEST 1

DIRECTIONS: Each question or incomplete statement is followed by several suggested answers or completions. Select the one that BEST answers the question or completes the statement. *PRINT THE LETTER OF THE CORRECT ANSWER IN THE SPACE AT THE RIGHT.*

1. Fuel value of foods is determined by use of a(n)

    A. caloric unit
    B. calorific unit
    C. calciferol
    D. calorimeter

2. Folacin is necessary for

    A. digestion of carbohydrates
    B. metabolism of sterols
    C. synthesis of chlorophyll
    D. hematopoiesis

3. Avidin is a(n)

    A. vitamin B. protein C. fiber D. fabric

4. Baking powders are a mixture of cornstarch, baking soda, and a(n)

    A. acid B. alkali C. gas D. neutralizer

5. The CORRECT method of cooking green-colored vegetables is to

    A. pressure cook
    B. add a small amount of baking soda
    C. release the steam occasionally while cooking in a covered saucepan
    D. keep the saucepan tightly covered

6. Popovers and cream puffs are PRINCIPALLY leavened by

    A. steam
    B. air
    C. carbon dioxide
    D. nitrous oxide

7. Compared with the recommended figure of 50%, the actual percentage of food calories derived from protective foods in the American diet is

    A. 20% B. 25% C. 33% D. 45%

8. A bacteriostatic method of food preservation is

    A. open kettle canning
    B. pressure canning
    C. dehydration
    D. irradiation

9. For the average American, minerals of value as food supplements for the diet are calcium,

    A. phosphorus, sodium, and choline
    B. chlorine, magnesium, and iron
    C. phosphorus, iron, and iodine
    D. chlorine, iron, and manganese

37

10. For the average American, the vitamins of value as food supplements are thiamine, pyro-   10._____
    doxine, riboflavin, calciferol, ascorbic acid, and

    A. niacin, $B_{12}$, A                B. $B_6$, $B_{12}$, folic acid
    C. $B_{12}$, K and A                  D. $B_{12}$, A and E

11. The critical temperatures for eggs in storage are                                            11._____

    A. 28° and 68°                        B. 32° and 75°
    C. 38° and 60°                        D. 25° and 75°

12. When they are to form an ingredient in cake, eggs blend with the batter better if they are  12._____

    A. new laid
    B. chilled thoroughly
    C. brought to room temperature
    D. candled

13. Of the following, the HIGHEST in caloric value is 1 cupful                                   13._____

    A. strained honey                     B. orange juice
    C. sugar                              D. homogenized milk

14. Among the following, the BEST food source of thiamine is                                     14._____

    A. refined sugars                     B. fats
    C. egg white                          D. pork

15. In the list below, the BEST source of vitamin A is                                           15._____

    A. wheat germ     B. pork             C. milk            D. spinach

16. A disadvantage resulting from the intake of mineral oil is that it                           16._____

    A. adds calories                      B. reduces weight
    C. impairs the appetite               D. dissolves vitamin A

17. The leavening power of baking powders results from chemical action which releases            17._____

    A. carbon monoxide                    B. carbon dioxide
    C. cream of tartar                    D. lactic acid

18. The diet prescribed in diverticulitis is one that is                                         18._____

    A. high in calorie value              B. high in roughage content
    C. low residue, bland                 D. high protein, bland

19. In typhoid fever, the diet should be                                                         19._____

    A. *high* in calories and residue
    B. *low* in calories, high in residue
    C. *high* in calories, low in residue
    D. *high* in fruit juice content

20. Allspice is derived from

    A. the berry of the pimento tree
    B. a mixture of nutmeg, cinnamon and cloves
    C. the root of the allspice tree
    D. the bark of the cassia tree

    20._____

21. Among the following food additives, the one which is used for the purpose of enhancing the keeping quality of the food is

    A. vitamin D in milk
    B. bleaching agents in flour
    C. ascorbic acid in cider
    D. minerals and vitamins in cereals

    21._____

22. An example of the bactericidal method of food preservation is

    A. jam and jellies
    B. pickling
    C. freezing
    D. refrigeration

    22._____

23. The material which destroys the activity of biotin is

    A. the protein found in uncooked egg white
    B. fluorides in drinking water
    C. iodides in medications
    D. fluorescent substances found in milk

    23._____

24. Egg whites beat BEST if they are

    A. warm
    B. chilled thoroughly
    C. at room temperature
    D. beaten by hand

    24._____

25. The RICHEST food sources of folacin are

    A. livers and green leafy vegetables
    B. eggs and milk
    C. cereals
    D. fats

    25._____

# KEY (CORRECT ANSWERS)

| | | | |
|---|---|---|---|
| 1. | D | 11. | A |
| 2. | D | 12. | C |
| 3. | B | 13. | A |
| 4. | A | 14. | D |
| 5. | C | 15. | D |
| 6. | A | 16. | D |
| 7. | C | 17. | B |
| 8. | C | 18. | C |
| 9. | C | 19. | C |
| 10. | A | 20. | A |

21. C
22. A
23. A
24. C
25. A

# TEST 2

DIRECTIONS: Each question or incomplete statement is followed by several suggested answers or completions. Select the one that BEST answers the question or completes the statement. *PRINT THE LETTER OF THE CORRECT ANSWER IN THE SPACE AT THE RIGHT.*

1. Riboflavin is easily destroyed by  1.____
   A. alkalies and light B. acids and oxygen
   C. heat and agitation D. air and agitation

2. Cretinism is a form of idiocy due to extreme deficiency of secretion by  2.____
   A. fat-soluble vitamins in the diet
   B. B-complex vitamins in the diet
   C. thyroid gland
   D. adrenal glands

3. Nyctalopia results from a lack of  3.____
   A. vitamin A B. fluorine
   C. citric acid D. flavinoids

4. The MAJOR influence in the decline of endemic goiter in the United States is the use of  4.____
   A. saffron oil B. homogenized milk
   C. iodized salt D. enriched cereals

5. The Food Drug & Cosmetic Act of 1934 provides for  5.____
   A. retention of nutritive values
   B. fair pricing of goods
   C. purity of content
   D. accurate labeling

6. The liver is the storage depot in the body for vitamin  6.____
   A. A B. E C. C D. B

7. The anti-xerophthalmia vitamin is vitamin  7.____
   A. A B. B C. E D. K

8. The pathway of excretion of the nitrogenous end products of protein metabolism is the  8.____
   A. lungs B. skin
   C. kidneys D. large intestine

9. The term *trace elements* refers to  9.____
   A. minerals needed in very small amounts in nutrition
   B. substances which trace circulation in the body
   C. tools used in sewing
   D. potent drugs used as pain killer

10. Flavinoids which are effective in human health are

    A. biotics
    B. bioflavinoids
    C. neoflavinoids
    D. vitamins

11. Uric acid results from

    A. vitamin deficiency
    B. metabolism of purines
    C. digestion of carbohydrates
    D. injection of nicotine

12. Studies comparing the desirability of feeding to premature infants formulas warmed to body temperature and those given directly on removal from the refrigerator show

    A. no significant difference
    B. disturbed sleep following intake of cold formula
    C. regurgitation following intake of cold formula
    D. slower weight gain with cold feeding

13. Hypoglycemia is a condition of

    A. diseased eyes
    B. B, low blood sugar
    C. high blood sugar
    D. low purin content

14. The normal source of insulin in the human body is the

    A. liver
    B. thymus
    C. pancreas
    D. pineal gland

15. One of the earliest symptoms of a thiamine deficiency is

    A. polyneuritis
    B. anorexia
    C. nyctalopia
    D. conjunctivitis

16. Air is used as a leavening agent in

    A. sponge cake
    B. pound cake
    C. cookies
    D. bread

17. Cheese originates in

    A. pasteurization
    B. fermentation
    C. inversion
    D. coagulation

18. In measuring vitamin A value in foods, the International Unit is defined as the activity of

    A. 5.0 mg. calciferol
    B. 6.0 gm. tocopherol
    C. 6.0 gm. carotene
    D. 0.6 meg. betacarotene

19. In the last fifty years, the proportion of calories from milk, cheese, fruits, and vegetables in the American diet has

    A. remained the same
    B. doubled
    C. tripled
    D. quadrupled

20. Interference with absorption of vitamin A may result from 20.____

   A. a diet heavy with bulk foods
   B. overconsumption of salad oils
   C. mineral oil in salad dressings
   D. low cholesterol diet

21. Vitamin A food value is 21.____

   A. lacking in yams
   B. fairly constant in dairy products
   C. closely related to green coloring in vegetables
   D. closely related to sun available during growing time

22. The passage of digested substances into the villi for distribution through the body is called 22.____

   A. absorption               B. metabolism
   C. anabolism                D. peristalsis

23. Of the following, the RICHEST source of vitamin E is 23.____

   A. liver                    B. green leafy vegetables
   C. wheat germ oil           D. egg yolk

24. Of the following, the number of calories which MOST NEARLY approximates the daily fuel needs of a moderately active 25-year-old woman is 24.____

   A. 1500      B. 2000      C. 2500      D. 3500

25. A deficiency of riboflavin results in 25.____

   A. xerophthalmia            B. polyneuritis
   C. cutaneous lesions        D. chielosis

## KEY (CORRECT ANSWERS)

| | | | |
|---|---|---|---|
| 1. | A | 11. | B |
| 2. | C | 12. | A |
| 3. | A | 13. | B |
| 4. | C | 14. | C |
| 5. | D | 15. | B |
| 6. | A | 16. | A |
| 7. | A | 17. | B |
| 8. | C | 18. | D |
| 9. | A | 19. | B |
| 10. | B | 20. | C |

21. C
22. A
23. C
24. C
25. B

# EXAMINATION SECTION
## TEST 1

DIRECTIONS: Each question or incomplete statement is followed by several suggested answers or completions. Select the one that BEST answers the question or completes the statement. *PRINT THE LETTER OF THE CORRECT ANSWER IN THE SPACE AT THE RIGHT.*

1. The item that acts as a catalytic agent for the assimilation of calcium and phosphorus is   1._____
    A. vitamin D   B. fat   C. vitamin B   D. protein

2. Contributing MOST to the weight of the living human body is   2._____
    A. copper   B. sodium   C. calcium   D. iron

3. Before cooking, the vegetable that MUST be soaked in water is   3._____
    A. string beans   B. Brussels sprouts
    C. turnips   D. celery

4. Amino acids are absorbed MAINLY in the   4._____
    A. stomach   B. liver   C. pancreas   D. intestine

5. Little spoilage occurs in stored, sun-dried fruits because the   5._____
    A. microorganisms have been destroyed
    B. moisture content is low
    C. pectin is inactive
    D. yeasts do not flourish in the absence of light

6. In pickling, the concentrated brine   6._____
    A. softens the cellulose
    B. preserves the original color
    C. retards the growth of microorganisms
    D. increases the acid content

7. Cheese is rich in   7._____
    A. calcium   B. iron   C. sodium   D. potassium

8. Tenderized dried fruits have been   8._____
    A. sulphurized, dried, then partially cooked
    B. dried, partially cooked, then partially dried
    C. partially cooked, dried, then partially cooked
    D. dried, sulphurized, then partially cooked

9. The MOST tender cuts of beef are from the   9._____
    A. loin and rib   B. leg and rib
    C. shoulder and loin   D. rump and neck

45

10. In anabolism, the number of calories yielded by one gram of carbohydrates is

   A. two  B. four  C. six  D. eight

11. When making yeast rolls, the milk is scalded to

   A. improve the flavor of the product
   B. reduce the size of the air holes
   C. destroy the microorganisms
   D. encourage development of the yeast

12. Deterioration of dried vegetables is retarded by

   A. marinating before drying
   B. storage in metal boxes
   C. pre-cooking before drying
   D. infra-red light treatment before packaging

13. The LARGEST percentage of gluten is found in flour made from

   A. rye  B. barley  C. oats  D. wheat

14. A bed roll is a support for the patient's

   A. head  B. knees  C. back  D. feet

15. One pound of dried eggs is equivalent to _____ eggs.

   A. 50-60  B. 30-40  C. 20-25  D. 15-18

16. To store eggs at home,

   A. keep them exposed on the cupboard
   B. wash and place them in the refrigerator
   C. do not wash and place them in the refrigerator
   D. place them in a moderately cool place

17. Disease is MOST commonly spread through

   A. clothing  B. dishes  C. food  D. contact

18. For everyday use, the Fahrenheit temperature of the refrigerator should be

   A. 20°-25°  B. 35°-40°  C. 45°-50°  D. 55°-60°

19. To retard spoilage of bread, baking companies may add sodium

   A. benzoate     B. propionate
   C. sulphathionate   D. hypophosphate

20. Essential to jelly-making is

   A. proto-pectin  B. pectin
   C. pectic acid   D. pectoral liquor

# KEY (CORRECT ANSWERS)

1. A
2. C
3. B
4. D
5. B

6. C
7. A
8. B
9. A
10. B

11. D
12. C
13. D
14. B
15. B

16. C
17. D
18. B
19. B
20. B

# TEST 2

DIRECTIONS: Each question or incomplete statement is followed by several suggested answers or completions. Select the one that BEST answers the question or completes the statement. *PRINT THE LETTER OF THE CORRECT ANSWER IN THE SPACE AT THE RIGHT.*

1. A MAJOR source of riboflavin is

    A. meat
    B. whole grains
    C. fruits
    D. milk

    1.___

2. In wheat, the vitamin B complex is in the

    A. endosperm
    B. aleuron layer
    C. bran
    D. germ

    2.___

3. The duration of infectious colds has been materially diminished by dosages of vitamin

    A. A  B. $B_1$  C. $B_2$  D. E

    3.___

4. Yeast plants grow BEST at the Fahrenheit temperature of

    A. 70°-75°  B. 80°-85°  C. 90°-95°  D. 100°-105°

    4.___

5. A characteristic of riboflavin deficiency is

    A. cheilosis  B. catarrh  C. otitis  D. pellagra

    5.___

6. Anemia responds to

    A. ascorbic acid
    B. folic acid
    C. niacin
    D. carotene

    6.___

7. Legumes and nuts provide much

    A. thiamine  B. calcium  C. niacin  D. sodium

    7.___

8. Rich in thiamine is

    A. orange juice
    B. cheese
    C. polished rice
    D. brewer's yeast

    8.___

9. Carbohydrate stored in the liver is

    A. galleasss
    B. glycogen
    C. liepstarch
    D. galactose

    9.___

10. The antihemmorhagic is

    A. riboflavin
    B. vitamin A
    C. vitamin K
    D. niacin

    10.___

11. At the end of one year, the weight of an infant in relation to its birth weight should be

    A. an increase of 12 oz. monthly
    B. double
    C. 20 pounds more
    D. triple

    11.___

48

12. Pellagra indicates a deficiency of

    A. ascorbic acid      B. niacin
    C. thiamine      D. riboflavin

13. Provitamin A is

    A. ergosterol      B. carotene
    C. lysine      D. pyrodoxine

14. The nutritionally important minerals are

    A. sodium, iodine, potassium, copper
    B. iron, iodine, phosphorus, calcium
    C. iron, potassium, sulphur, copper
    D. sodium, phosphorus, sulphur, calcium

15. Root vegetables are BEST stored in atmosphere that is maintained

    A. at 36° F      B. dehumidified
    C. at 30° F      D. at 75% humidity

16. The government stamp on meats indicates

    A. date when slaughtered      B. point of origin
    C. nutritional value      D. quality

17. Whole grain products, in contrast with enriched products, possess more

    A. hydrocarbons      B. carbohydrates
    C. vitamins      D. proteins

18. In anabolism, the number of calories yielded by one gram of hydrocarbon is

    A. six      B. seven      C. eight      D. nine

19. In the digestion of starch, the intermediate product is

    A. dextrin      B. fibrinogen      C. cerine      D. maltine

20. Egg whites whip more quickly at the Fahrenheit temperature of

    A. 0°      B. 30°      C. 70°      D. 85°

## KEY (CORRECT ANSWERS)

| | | | |
|---|---|---|---|
| 1. | D | 11. | D |
| 2. | D | 12. | B |
| 3. | A | 13. | B |
| 4. | B | 14. | B |
| 5. | A | 15. | A |
| 6. | B | 16. | D |
| 7. | A | 17. | D |
| 8. | D | 18. | D |
| 9. | B | 19. | A |
| 10. | C | 20. | C |

# HEALTH SCREENING & FITNESS EVALUATION
# EXAMINATION SECTION
# TEST 1

DIRECTIONS: Each question or incomplete statement is followed by several suggested answers or completions. Select the one that BEST answers the question or completes the statement. *PRINT THE LETTER OF THE CORRECT ANSWER IN THE SPACE AT THE RIGHT.*

1. *Primary* risk factors for cardiovascular disease include all of the following EXCEPT 1.____

    A. diabetes
    B. smoking
    C. high blood pressure
    D. sedentary lifestyle

2. *Secondary* risk factors for cardiovascular disease include all of the following EXCEPT 2.____

    A. obesity
    B. high cholesterol
    C. heredity
    D. Type A behavior

3. A 40-year-old individual wishes to train at 75% Max Vo2. Using the Karvoneon method (RHR=70Bpm), this person's aerobic training heart rate is 3.____

    A. 152     B. 148     C. 116     D. 120

4. _____ may NOT be used as a cardiorespiratory testing method. 4.____

    A. Talk test
    B. Karvoneon method
    C. 1 rep max
    D. Palpation

5. Health history screening is important because it 5.____

    A. gives a person insight as to his own condition
    B. helps the trainer become aware of pre-existing chronic health problems
    C. limits liability on the trainer's part
    D. all of the above

6. The SAFEST and MOST accurate site to measure heart rate is the _____ artery. 6.____

    A. carotid     B. brachial     C. radial     D. femoral

7. If a person's RHR is 54BPM, he is 7.____

    A. in good condition
    B. out of condition
    C. training too hard
    D. of undetermined condition based on this information alone

8. The purpose of health screening is to provide 8.____

    A. protection
    B. information
    C. baseline information for appropriate programming
    D. training options

9. Health screening should include all of the following EXCEPT

   A. information regarding primary risk factors
   B. information regarding previous exercise experience
   C. information regarding pregnancy
   D. waiver of liability

10. A person with insulin-dependent diabetes

    A. must exercise below 70% intensity
    B. must exercise at a preset time and for a preset duration in relation to his insulin
    C. must consume frequent snacks while exercising
    D. can reduce his insulin if his intensity increases

11. Asthma may
    I. prevent outdoor exercising in very cold weather
    II. not be considered seriously in adults
    III. necessitate taking medications to raise heart rate
    The CORRECT answer is:

    A. I, II          B. II only          C. III only          D. II, III

12. The two MOST important components of the physical exam are

    A. flexibility and strength
    B. heart rate and percentage of body fat
    C. endurance and strength
    D. heart rate and blood pressure

13. An obese 50 year-old male would BEST be given a sub max stress test on a

    A. bicycle              B. treadmill
    C. step                 D. 1 mile walk

14. Body composition refers to

    A. lean body mass
    B. relative percentages of fat and lean body mass
    C. ideal body weight
    D. the goal of dietary limitation

15. Body composition can be determined by

    A. checking weight at regular intervals
    B. cutting down fats in the diet
    C. bioelectrical impedance
    D. clothing size relative to height

16. Skinfold measurements may be taken for both males and females at the

    A. chest                B. triceps
    C. thigh                D. suprailiac crest

17. Fitness testing should include 17.____

    A. strength testing
    B. endurance testing and recovery time
    C. flexibility
    D. all of the above

18. Exercise testing should be done prior to starting a fitness program and at frequent intervals thereafter to 18.____

    A. establish baselines
    B. help determine reasonable goals
    C. motivate
    D. all of the above

19. For men, the BEST skinfold sites for the most accurate results and least likelihood of error are 19.____

    A. chest, abdomen, and tricep
    B. abdomen, back, and thigh
    C. chest, abdomen, and thigh
    D. abdomen, tricep, and back

20. For women, the BEST skinfold sites for the most accurate results and least likelihood of error are 20.____

    A. tricep, abdomen, and thigh
    B. tricep, gluteus, and thigh
    C. tricep, suprailium, and thigh
    D. suprailium, thigh, and back

21. Girth measurement inconsistencies stem from 21.____
    I. inconsistent tape placement
    II. lack of available accurate equipment
    III. variations in the tension placed on the tape during measurement

    The CORRECT answer is:

    A. I only    B. II only    C. I, II    D. I, III

22. Trunk flexion is used to measure 22.____

    A. flexibility of the low back and hamstrings
    B. flexibility of the low back *only*
    C. flexibility of the hamstrings *only*
    D. range of motion of the quadratus lumborum

23. Trunk flexion is measured by 23.____

    A. standing and trying to touch toes
    B. sit and reach test
    C. standing and bending backwards
    D. lying on side and trying to reach toes

24. All of the following are tests for muscular strength and endurance EXCEPT the _____ test.

    A. push-up
    B. sit-up
    C. sit and reach
    D. bench press

25. The push-up test measures the strength and endurance of the

    A. triceps, anterior deltoids, and pectoralis major
    B. triceps, biceps, and deltoids
    C. pectoralis major *only*
    D. none of the above

## KEY (CORRECT ANSWERS)

| | | | |
|---|---|---|---|
| 1. | A | 11. | D |
| 2. | B | 12. | D |
| 3. | A | 13. | A |
| 4. | C | 14. | B |
| 5. | B | 15. | C |
| 6. | C | 16. | C |
| 7. | D | 17. | D |
| 8. | C | 18. | D |
| 9. | D | 19. | C |
| 10. | B | 20. | C |

| | |
|---|---|
| 21. | D |
| 22. | A |
| 23. | B |
| 24. | C |
| 25. | A |

# LEADERSHIP AND IMPLEMENTATION
# EXAMINATION SECTION
# TEST 1

DIRECTIONS: Each question or incomplete statement is followed by several suggested answers or completions. Select the one that BEST answers the question or completes the statement. *PRINT THE LETTER OF THE CORRECT ANSWER IN THE SPACE AT THE RIGHT.*

1. Adherence is defined as the

   A. intensity level of exercise performed
   B. duration of exercise performed
   C. amount of exercise performed during a specified time, compared to the amount of exercise recommended
   D. amount of exercise performed during a specified time, compared to the amount performed on the last session
   E. amount of exercise performed during a specified time, compared to the initial work-out

1.____

2. Surveys show that those MOST likely to begin an exercise program are

   A. younger men
   B. more highly educated persons
   C. non-smokers
   D. white collar
   E. all of the above

2.____

3. Personal factors found to be associated with adherence include all of the following EXCEPT

   A. perceptions of program convenience
   B. past experience with exercise
   C. actual skills
   D. all of the above
   E. none of the above

3.____

4. An assessment tool to evaluate self-motivation is

   A. Dishman inventory          B. Kasch test
   C. Michigan State test        D. Wolf's Law
   E. all of the above

4.____

5. Actual factors influencing exercise adherence include _____ factors.

   A. personal                   B. program
   C. environmental              D. all of the above
   E. none of the above

5.____

6. The qualities of an effective exercise leader include all of the following EXCEPT

   A. punctuality and dependability
   B. dedication to the exercise training endeavor

6.____

55

C. willingness to plan ahead
D. sensitivity to client's past experiences, current preferences, and current and future needs
E. none of the above

7. A method for enhancing and maintaining motivation to exercise includes reminders to set the stage, otherwise known as

   A. prompts
   B. waivers
   C. set-points
   D. overload
   E. none of the above

8. When selecting equipment, it is IMPORTANT to

   A. identify the client's needs
   B. examine the design, service, and safety of the equipment
   C. estimate a budget
   D. evaluate the available space
   E. all of the above

9. Comparable products may have lower prices due to
   I. lower profit margin by the manufacturer
   II. cheaper equipment parts
   III. better engineering allowing less costly assembly
   IV. foreign vs. domestic manufacturer

   The CORRECT answer is:

   A. I, II, IV
   B. I, IV
   C. II, III
   D. II, III, IV
   E. I, II, III, IV

10. A client would like to set up a gym in his basement. He would like both cardiovascular and strength training equipment. He has 100 sq. ft. available and can spend up to $2,000.
    The BEST recommendation for your client would be a(n)

    A. recumbent bike with one multipurpose free weight bench
    B. multistation machine, a recumbent bike, and a rower
    C. high quality treadmill, a multistation machine, a hydraulic stairclimber, and a weight bench with dumbells
    D. inexpensive treadmill and a weight bench with dumbells
    E. electronic rowing machine and a single station machine

11. The BEST recommended exercise equipment for a client who has under $500 and 20 sq. ft. of space is
    I. stationary upright bike
    II. cross-country skier
    III. electronic stairclimber
    IV. inexpensive recumbent bike

    The CORRECT answer is:

    A. I, II or IV
    B. I, II or III
    C. II, III or IV
    D. I, II, III or IV
    E. None of the above

12. The statement that describes whether a product is truly a value at its price is:  12._____

    A. You get what you pay for
    B. Bang for the buck
    C. Only the expensive is good
    D. Buy used, not abused
    E. Buy from a gym

13. In warm or hot weather, a trainer should advise his client to wear all of the following  13._____
    EXCEPT

    A. light-colored clothing          B. 100% cotton
    C. polypropylene                   D. loose-fitting clothing
    E. none of the above

14. The heart of the cushioning system is the  14._____

    A. outsole                         B. heel counter
    C. foxing and toe box              D. midsole
    E. all of the above

15. During strength training activities, lifting belts can  15._____

    A. dramatically increase intraabdominal pressure and help support the lumbar spine
    B. dramatically decrease intraabdominal pressure and help support the lumbar spine
    C. dramatically increase intraabdominal pressure and help support the cervical spine
    D. dramatically decrease intraabdominal pressure and help support the cervical spine
    E. make you look good, but really do nothing

16. When designing your aerobics class, you should consider  16._____

    A. room size, population of class, intensity, duration
    B. type of floor, music pitch, complexity of choreography
    C. population, intensity, duration, complexity
    D. all of the above
    E. none of the above

17. When creating choreography, what sources should you consider?  17._____

    A. None; you move the way music makes you
    B. Dance
    C. Borrowing from your favorite instructor
    D. All of the above
    E. None of the above

18. Modifications are important when teaching a multi-level class.  18._____
    How would you modify the following combinations?
        Jog 8 counts
        4 alternate lunges
        Twist 8 counts
        4 double ponies
        4 squats

    A. Change jog to march
    B. Change double ponies to double taps

C. Eliminate all impact movement
D. All of the above
E. None of the above

19. You have just completed evaluating an instructor's class. The footwork was not complicated, but it involved a lot of arm work. All the participants enjoyed the class, but you are concerned regarding the choreography because
    I. the participants enjoyed her class more than yours
    II. too much arm work causes an increase of shoulder joint injury
    III. increased exertion due to the pressor response
    The CORRECT answer is:

    A. I only          B. I, II          C. II, III
    D. III only        E. II only

20. When setting participant platform/step height for a step class, you should keep in mind
    A. the activity level and goals of participant
    B. the height and activity level of participants
    C. if the participant has difficulty, advise to lower the step
    D. that as long as the participant doesn't exceed 90° knee flexion, any step height is acceptable
    E. all of the above

21. A participant complains of not reaching her target heart rate during your step class. You advise the participant to
    I. increase step heights
    II. increase power moves
    III. work through full ROM and add wrist weights
    The CORRECT answer is:

    A. I               B. I, II          C. II, III
    D. I, II, III      E. II only

22. Although teaching a step class requires the same teaching techniques as a regular aerobics class, it also requires
    A. advance cuing to allow time for transitions
    B. doing the moves at half tempo
    C. demonstrating the motion while everyone watches
    D. all of the above
    E. none of the above

23. Turn step, Over the Top, V Step, and Tap up are samples of
    I. directional cuing for step class
    II. ways of changing the orientation of a combination on a step
    III. steps for a hip-hop step class
    The CORRECT answer is:

    A. I, II           B. II only        C. I, III
    D. III only        E. I only

24. When choreographing repeaters into your step routine, you should          24.____
    A. add arm movements to increase intensity
    B. do only 5 on each side
    C. make sure the heel touches on every repetition
    D. all of the above
    E. none of the above

25. The suggestions of music tempo are _____ for hi-lo, _____ calisthenics, and _____     25.____
    for step classes.
    A. 140-180; 110; 122
    B. 140-160; 118-130; 115-122
    C. 130-150; 110-120; 115-122
    D. all of the above
    E. none of the above

# KEY (CORRECT ANSWERS)

| | |
|---|---|
| 1. C | 11. A |
| 2. E | 12. B |
| 3. E | 13. C |
| 4. A | 14. D |
| 5. D | 15. A |
| 6. E | 16. D |
| 7. A | 17. D |
| 8. E | 18. D |
| 9. E | 19. C |
| 10. B | 20. E |

21. B
22. D
23. A
24. B
25. C

# PROGRAMMING FOR HEALTHY ADULTS
# EXAMINATION SECTION
# TEST 1

DIRECTIONS: Each question or incomplete statement is followed by several suggested answers or completions. Select the one that BEST answers the question or completes the statement. *PRINT THE LETTER OF THE CORRECT ANSWER IN THE SPACE AT THE RIGHT.*

1. The benefits of a proper warm-up include

   A. an increase in blood flow to active muscles
   B. a rehearsal effect
   C. reduced risk of E.I.A.
   D. all of the above

2. The recommended C.V. fitness training range is
   I. 60-80% max heart rate reserve (50-85% P.T.)
   II. 60-85% max heart rate (60-90% P.T.)
   III. 65-75% Vo2 max

   The CORRECT answer is:

   A. I, II              B. II *only*
   C. II, III            D. I, II, III

3. An example of muscular endurance is

   A. total number of sit-ups done in one minute
   B. length of time a person can hold a weight/resistance at a particular degree of flexion
   C. repeatedly being able to create a force against a resistance
   D. all of the above

4. Isometric training is contraindicated for people with

   A. arthritis          B. chondromalacia
   C. hypertension       D. all of the above

5. Muscular strength can be exhibited by
   I. dynamometer
   II. valsalva maneuver
   III. amount of pull-ups accomplished in 30 seconds

   The CORRECT answer is:

   A. I *only*           B. I, II
   C. III *only*         D. II, III

6. Which of the following could be contraindicated for a hypertensive person?

   A. I repetition max test
   B. Isometric training
   C. Repeated movements done above shoulder level
   D. All of the above

7. Ralph and Roger have identical strength capacity in their biceps muscles. However, Ralph has a longer forearm length than Roger.
   Which one (if either) has an advantage if asked to do 1 rep max bicep curl and sustain a contraction at 90% elbow flexion?

   A. Ralph - more leverage
   B. Roger - shorter lever
   C. Neither - equal strength
   D. Can't judge by this information; too many other variables involved

8. An eccentric contraction causes the affected muscle to

   A. shorten as it contracts
   B. contract without any change in muscle length
   C. lengthen as it contracts
   D. shorten at the beginning of the contraction and then relax and lengthen

9. Which type of muscle fibers are said to experience GREATER increases in size and strength (hypertrophy) with progressive resistance training?
   _____ twitch.

   A. Slow              B. Fast
   C. both A and B      D. none of the above

10. If exercise equipment is classified *dynamic constant resistance*, it means the amount of

    A. resistive force encountered will be equal to the muscle force applied
    B. resistive force encountered remains the same throughout the entire range of motion
    C. resistive force will change throughout the range of motion
    D. muscle effort remains relatively constant throughout the exercise movement

11. A plastic stretch is one that
    I. causes an elongation which is temporary and stops when the stretch is stopped
    II. is viscous
    III. causes an elongation in the tissues that will remain even after the stretch has stopped

    The CORRECT answer is:

    A. I, II             B. II *only*
    C. I, III            D. II, III

12. The _____ protects a muscle from injury by relaxing the muscle(s) if a stretch becomes too intense, causing a risk of rupture.

    A. golgi tendon organ      B. stretch reflex
    C. stabilizer muscles      D. connective tissue

13. Stretching should be encouraged

    A. prior to and following any activity
    B. when muscles are warm
    C. to stimulate an intensity to muscle spindle activity
    D. all of the above

14. Delayed onset muscle soreness is said to occur _____ after strenuous training.

    A. 2 hours
    B. 12-24 hours
    C. 24-48 hours
    D. any time soreness occurs

15. Cardiovascular health benefits include an increase in all of the following EXCEPT

    A. resting and max. stroke volume levels
    B. heart rate at rest and during sub-max. activity
    C. HDL
    D. cardiac output

16. Guidelines state that people in the *average* classification of C.R. fitness should participate in aerobic training for a duration of _____ minutes.

    A. 15-45      B. 20-30      C. 30-45      D. 15-20

17. Which type of training consists of exercising at 50-70% VO2 Max for one-three minutes each with brief rest periods of 15 seconds between stations?

    A. Anaerobic interval
    B. Fartlek training
    C. Aerobics circuit training
    D. Aerobic composite

18. Weight training is beneficial in that it can

    A. increase the size of muscle fibers
    B. increase C.V. fitness if heart rate is reached and maintained throughout session.
    C. prevent the loss of lean muscle mass that occurs with aging
    D. All of the above

19. For safe and effective strength development, a sound training recommendation involves _____ reps at _____% of maximum resistance.

    A. 6-8; 85                  B. 8-10; 80-85
    C. 8-12; 70-80              D. 12-15; 75-85

20. People just starting weight bearing aerobic activity should

    A. exercise every other day for the first 8 weeks of training
    B. have at least 36-48 hours of rest between workouts
    C. exercise at least three times a week on alternate days
    D. all of the above

21. Which type of fibers are able to produce low levels of force for long periods of time, predominately associated with aerobic/endurance training?

    A. Both fast and slow twitch fibers
    B. Fast twitch fibers
    C. Slow twitch fibers
    D. Hypertrophied muscles

22. The reason why men generally appear to be stronger than women is because

    A. the fiber-for-fiber quality of muscle is different; males' fiber is of stronger quality than women's
    B. women generally have a smaller overall percentage of muscle as opposed to men
    C. the higher level of testosterone in women negatively affects muscle mass, hence strength
    D. all of the above

23. Range of motion or joint mobility can be limited by

    A. the elasticity of connective tissue
    B. the structure of a joint
    C. hypokinesis
    D. all of the above

24. Reciprocal innervation is demonstrated as

    A. the latissimus dorsi isometrically contract during elbow flexion (bicep curl) to stabilize the shoulder
    B. ballistic stretching occurs, stimulating muscle spindle and causing reflex muscular contraction
    C. from a *reflex knee tap* as the leg extends and the quadraceps (agonists) contract and the hamstrings (antagonists) relax
    D. none of the above

25. Dysrhythmia refers to

    A. a low level of neuromuscular coordination
    B. an interruption in the normal rhythm of the heart
    C. the normal increase in the hearts b.p.m. associated with increased exercise intensity
    D. myocardial infarction

# KEY (CORRECT ANSWERS)

| | | | |
|---|---|---|---|
| 1. | D | 11. | D |
| 2. | A | 12. | A |
| 3. | D | 13. | D |
| 4. | C | 14. | C |
| 5. | A | 15. | B |
| 6. | D | 16. | A |
| 7. | B | 17. | C |
| 8. | C | 18. | D |
| 9. | B | 19. | C |
| 10. | B | 20. | D |

21. C
22. B
23. D
24. D
25. B

# TEST 2

DIRECTIONS: Each question or incomplete statement is followed by several suggested answers or completions. Select the one that BEST answers the question or completes the statement. *PRINT THE LETTER OF THE CORRECT ANSWER IN THE SPACE AT THE RIGHT.*

1. When designing an exercise program, it is important to consider

    A. muscular strength and endurance
    B. cardiovascular endurance
    C. body composition
    D. all of the above

2. Muscle strength and endurance training will help a person

    A. maintain weight control
    B. reduce risk of musculoskeletal injuries
    C. maintain a better posture
    D. assist in everyday activities

3. Training that increases the functioning capacity of the heart, lungs, and blood vessels that transport oxygenated blood to working muscles is called

    A. muscle strengthening
    B. cardiovascular training
    C. muscle toning
    D. strength training

4. An overweight person who leads a sedentary life and has smoked for 15 years should start with

    A. a high, intense aerobic program with heavy weight training
    B. high impact aerobics twice a week with light weights and much repetition
    C. moderate weight training
    D. walking or stationary bike with low weight training

5. The purpose of flexibility in a training program is to

    A. enable you to touch the toes without a problem
    B. create a balance between muscle groups
    C. reduce the risk of injury
    D. all of the above

6. Irritability, insomnia, fatigue, and depression are all signs of

    A. drug use in training
    B. elevated blood pressure
    C. over-training
    D. being overweight

7. Strength training increases muscle size by increasing the
    I. number of fibers
    II. size of the myofibrils
    III. number of cells

    The CORRECT answer is:

    A. I, II
    B. I, III
    C. III only
    D. I, II, III

8. Which has the LEAST stress to the lower back?

   A. Barbell bent over row
   B. Barbell incline press
   C. Standing dumbell press
   D. Seated dumbell press

9. Muscle tissue consists of the proteins
   I. sarcomere
   II. actin
   III. myosin

   The CORRECT answer is:

   A. I *only*
   B. I, II
   C. III *only*
   D. II, III

10. A long-distance running pattern is

    A. heel strike, pronation, toe off
    B. heel strike, supination, toe off
    C. toe strike, pronation, eversion
    D. heel strike, supination, inversion

11. To facilitate adherence to a training program, it is important to establish
    I. short-term goals
    II. long-term goals
    III. preference

    The CORRECT answer is:

    A. I *only*
    B. II *only*
    C. II, III
    D. I, III

12. Novice exercisers respond to _____ cues.

    A. specific    B. general    C. affective    D. neutral

13. Of the following, the MOST essential factor for adherence to an exercise program is

    A. progression
    B. periodization
    C. frequency
    D. intensity

14. What is valid termination of the submaximal bike test?

    A. Request to stop
    B. Heart rate above 75% max
    C. Visible fatigue
    D. Excessive sweating

15. With age,
    I. stroke volume decreases
    II. cardiac output increases
    III. BMR decreases

    The CORRECT answer is:

    A. I *only*
    B. I, II
    C. I, III
    D. II, III

16. With a given percentage of max resistance, a person with predominantly more fast twitch muscle fibers performs _____ repetitions.

    A. fewer
    B. more
    C. same
    D. none of the above are applicable

17. All of the following are factors to consider when designing and implementing the strength training component of an exercise program EXCEPT

    A. perform all exercises through a full range of motion
    B. work agonist and antagonist muscles
    C. ensure that training speed is slow and controlled
    D. none of the above

18. To accomplish progression in a strength training workout,
    I. go through the workout faster
    II. increase the amount of resistance
    III. increase the number of exercises
    The CORRECT answer is:

    A. I, II, III
    B. II only
    C. I, III
    D. II, III

19. An overweight person's program might initially consist of

    A. walking, cycle, stretching
    B. walking, jumping rope, strength training
    C. aerobic dance, calisthenics, stretching
    D. stretching, light weight training, jogging

20. The law of specificity is BEST demonstrated by

    A. cyclist cross training
    B. cyclist strength training
    C. marathon runner strength training
    D. marathon runner running

21. The MOST often overlooked or under-emphasized component of an exercise program is

    A. strength training
    B. cardiovascular training
    C. flexibility
    D. muscular endurance training

22. Stretching should be done

    A. primarily before working out to reduce chance of injury
    B. both before and after workout
    C. after workout *only*
    D. you don't have to stretch

23. Static and moving body postures are BEST judged on the basis of   23._____
    A. how well they meet the demands made upon them
    B. comparison with standardized charts
    C. muscular strength
    D. body flexibility

24. All of the following are correct principles relating to the muscular system EXCEPT:   24._____
    A. Muscles contract more rapidly following warm-up activities
    B. Muscular strength is progressively developed by the repetition of exercises of the same intensity
    C. Muscles contract more forcefully if they are first stretched, provided that they are not overstretched
    D. A muscle must be loaded beyond its customary load if strength is to be increased

25. Which of the following can result in cardiorespiratory fatigue?   25._____
    I. Hyperthermia-dehydration
    II. Progressive resistance
    III. Glycogen depletion
    The CORRECT answer is:

    A. I, II                       B. II only
    C. I, III                      D. III only

---

# KEY (CORRECT ANSWERS)

| | | | |
|---|---|---|---|
| 1. | D | 11. | D |
| 2. | B | 12. | A |
| 3. | B | 13. | C |
| 4. | D | 14. | B |
| 5. | C | 15. | C |
| 6. | C | 16. | A |
| 7. | A | 17. | D |
| 8. | B | 18. | D |
| 9. | D | 19. | A |
| 10. | A | 20. | D |

21. C
22. B
23. A
24. B
25. C

# PROGRAMMING FOR SPECIAL POPULATIONS
# EXAMINATION SECTION
# TEST 1

DIRECTIONS: Each question or incomplete statement is followed by several suggested answers or completions. Select the one that BEST answers the question or completes the statement. *PRINT THE LETTER OF THE CORRECT ANSWER IN THE SPACE AT THE RIGHT.*

1. Relaxin is a hormone associated with

    A. diabetes
    B. asthma
    C. pregnancy
    D. recovery from exercise

2. During pregnancy, physical fitness levels are said to

    A. decrease during the 1st and 2nd trimesters and increase during the third
    B. decrease during the 1st and 3rd trimesters and increase during the 2nd
    C. remain the same during the 1st trimester and decrease during the 2nd and 3rd
    D. decrease each trimester

3. Kegel exercises are

    A. advised for women who experience urinary incontinence during bouncy impact activity (running, aerobics, etc.)
    B. advised during pregnancy to increase elasticity of the muscles of the pelvic floor
    C. prescribed to speed recovery after childbirth
    D. all of the above

4. Training heart rate during pregnancy should NOT exceed _____ BPM.

    A. 120  B. 130  C. 140  D. 150

5. During pregnancy, exercising in a supine position is contraindicated

    A. after the 2nd month
    B. after the 3rd month
    C. after the 4th month
    D. only if known complications exist

6. If a diabetic client experiences low blood sugar, you should

    A. give the individual a quick carbohydrate (i.e., candy, juice)
    B. make sure he/she takes more insulin
    C. encourage the client to rest for a while and resume activity when ready
    D. all of the above

7. Rheumatoid arthritis is

    A. the more common type of arthritis
    B. caused by a degeneration of the cartilage and is associated with the aging process
    C. an autoimmune disease that causes inflammation
    D. both A and B

8. Rheumatoid arthritis

   A. is a systemic disease
   B. primarily affects weight-bearing bones
   C. causes cartilage to gradually break down
   D. both A and C

9. Which type of arthritis is said to more common among women than men?

   A. Osteoarthritis
   B. Rheumatoid
   C. Both of the above
   D. None of the above

10. When working with an arthritic client, all of the following recommendations are true EXCEPT:

    A. Time spent on warming up to improve joint mobility should be increased
    B. The intensity of the workout, rather than the duration, should be increased so that there is less repetition, hence less joint stress
    C. Range of motion exercises should be emphasized
    D. The client is expected to feel some level of discomfort in his/her joints due to the disease

11. Water workouts are great for arthritic clients. Water temperatures should range from _____.

    A. 75-78      B. 78-82      C. 83-88      D. 89-92

12. Obesity reflects a body fat percentage greater than _____% for men and _____% for women.

    A. 20; 25     B. 20; 30     C. 25; 33     D. 15; 28

13. Which of the following recommendations is appropriate for an obese individual's program?

    A. A low intensity (60-70% max heart rate reserve), long duration, low impact workout 3-5 days per week
    B. A moderate intensity (70-80% max h.r.r.), long duration, low impact workout 5-6 days per week
    C. Varying intensity levels on alternate days, with duration varying in terms of intensity, 3-5 days per week
    D. High intensity (90-90% max. h.r.r.), long duration, low impact workout 3-5 days per week

14. Chondromalacia patella

    A. is a degenerative process affecting the back surface of the knee
    B. can be irritated by isometric exercises
    C. can be irritated by exercises that require full flexion/extension
    D. A and C

15. Currently, the MOST frequent cause of activity limitation in people under 45 is

    A. obesity
    B. hypertension
    C. low back pain
    D. overweight

16. Normal blood pressure is said to be diastolic of _____ mmHg, systolic of _____ mmHg.

   A. 120; 80    B. 80; 120    C. 90; 140    D. 140; 90

17. All of the following statements about hypertension are true EXCEPT that it

   A. increases the risk of heart attack and stroke
   B. is often ideopathic in nature
   C. is a secondary risk factor for coronary heart disease
   D. requires medical clearance before a program can begin

18. A hypertensive response to exercise includes

   A. systolic pressure greater than 250 mmHg
   B. a drop in systolic pressure greater than 10 mmHg
   C. diastolic pressure greater than 110 mmHg
   D. all of the above

19. A hypertensive individual's program should

   A. stress the use of isometric activity/exercise for strength training
   B. avoid high intensity/low repetition weight training
   C. maintain a moderate to high intensity level during aerobic training (80-90% max h.r.r.)
   D. all of the above

20. Diuretics are associated with a condition known as hypokalemia, which refers to a low

   A. blood pressure           B. resting heart rate
   C. blood sugar level        D. level of potassium

# KEY (CORRECT ANSWERS)

| | |
|---|---|
| 1. C | 11. C |
| 2. B | 12. C |
| 3. D | 13. A |
| 4. C | 14. D |
| 5. C | 15. C |
| 6. A | 16. B |
| 7. C | 17. C |
| 8. A | 18. D |
| 9. B | 19. B |
| 10. B | 20. D |

# TEST 2

DIRECTIONS: Each question or incomplete statement is followed by several suggested answers or completions. Select the one that BEST answers the question or completes the statement. *PRINT THE LETTER OF THE CORRECT ANSWER IN THE SPACE AT THE RIGHT.*

1. Older adults in an aerobic training program may experience a

   A. decrease in heart rate at rest and during submax activity
   B. decrease in systolic blood pressure at rest and during submax activity
   C. delay in age-related decline in max $O_2$ capacity
   D. all of the above

2. A pregnant woman performing prolonged high intensity exercise could cause

   A. dehydration to herself
   B. lowered resting heart rate
   C. inadequate blood supply to the fetus
   D. damage to the fetal neural tube

3. In designing a program for an arthritic client, you might include
   I. extended warm-up
   II. increased use of isometric exercises
   III. water workouts
   IV. jogging

   The CORRECT answer is:

   A. I, II, III  
   C. I, II, IV  
   B. II, III, IV  
   D. All of the above

4. A 40-year-old male weighing 207 lbs. and borderline hypertensive has just finished 25 minutes of a cardiovascular workout.
   You should make sure he

   A. stops immediately and takes his pulse
   B. moves right into his weight training program without resting
   C. sits down and drinks lots of water
   D. keeps moving at a lower intensity, gradually slowing down before stopping

5. Of the following, the MOST common cause of obesity is

   A. overeating  
   C. lowered BMR  
   B. genetics  
   D. yo-yo dieting

6. A sagital curvature to the lumbar spine is known as

   A. kyphosis  
   C. lordosis  
   B. scoliosis  
   D. hailiodosis

7. The effects of caffeine include

   A. raised heart rate, increased strength, and fat mobilization
   B. fat mobilization, water loss, and raised heart rate
   C. raised heart rate, increased endurance, and speed
   D. fat mobilization, water loss, and strength

8. A hypertensive client has been cleared for exercise by his physician. He advises you he is on beta-blockers. What physiological response could you expect while this client exercises?

    A. Increase in cardiac output
    B. Increased blood pressure
    C. Slower heart rate
    D. All of the above

9. If a hypertensive client experiences a hypertensive response, the trainer should have the client

    A. increase exercise intensity
    B. increase rest periods
    C. cease exercise session
    D. lower exercise intensity

10. Signs trainers should look for in hypertensive clients that indicate termination of their exercise sessions are

    A. excess fatigue and onset of angina
    B. light-headedness, confusion, pallor, dyspnea, and nausea
    C. inappropriate drop in exercise heart rate greater than 10 bpm with increase or no change in workload
    D. all of the above

11. A client with low potassium is termed

    A. hyperglycemic
    B. hypoglycemic
    C. hypokalemic
    D. hyperkalemic

12. Which of these characteristics is TRUE of type one diabetes?

    A. Individuals are insulin dependent.
    B. Individuals are usually obese.
    C. It is the more common type of diabetes.
    D. It usually develops during adulthood.

13. Of the following exercises, the INAPPROPRIATE one for an individual with osteoarthritis would be

    A. aquasize
    B. static stretching
    C. abdominal curls
    D. hamstring curls on all fours

14. If an individual has a max MET capacity of 10 and is working at 65-80% max, he/she is working at a level of _____ METS.

    A. 1-3       B. 6.5-8       C. 8-10       D. 4.5-6

15. Calculate the training heart rate zone using the Karvonen formula: Elroy is 30 years old, has a R.H.R. of 60 BPM, and is working at an intensity of 70-80% of max. heart rate reserve.
    His training heart rate zone is between _____ BPM.

    A. 103-152   B. 121-164   C. 147-159   D. 147-178

16. Using the max heart rate formula, calculate the training heart rate for a 50 year old with a resting heart rate of 70 working at an intensity level of 60-75%.
    The training heart rate is _____ BPM.

    A. 102-118
    C. 102-127.5
    B. 107-136.5
    D. none of the above

17. Exercise intensity, according to respiratory effort, is monitored by the

    A. rating of perceived exertion
    B. dyspnea scale
    C. borg scale
    D. recovery heart rate

18. Jon weighs 100 lbs. and is exercising at a MET level of 5 for 30 minutes. Jon would require _____ calories during this activity.

    A. 119
    C. 82
    B. 247
    D. none of the above

19. The risk of heart-related problems is increased by

    A. increase in humidity
    C. pregnancy
    B. obesity
    D. all of the above

20. Generally speaking, an individual should wait _____ minutes after eating before exercise.

    A. 30   B. 90   C. 60   D. 45

## KEY (CORRECT ANSWERS)

| | | | |
|---|---|---|---|
| 1. | D | 11. | C |
| 2. | D | 12. | A |
| 3. | A | 13. | D |
| 4. | D | 14. | B |
| 5. | A | 15. | B |
| 6. | C | 16. | C |
| 7. | B | 17. | B |
| 8. | C | 18. | A |
| 9. | C | 19. | D |
| 10. | D | 20. | B |

# MUSCULOSKELETAL INJURIES
## EXAMINATION SECTION
## TEST 1

DIRECTIONS: Each question or incomplete statement is followed by several suggested answers or completions. Select the one that BEST answers the question or completes the statement. *PRINT THE LETTER OF THE CORRECT ANSWER IN THE SPACE AT THE RIGHT.*

Questions 1-2.

DIRECTIONS: Questions 1 and 2 are to be answered on the basis of the information provided in Case A.

Case A: A client you have been training for a few months starts complaining of discomfort in his right knee. He experiences pain when climbing stairs, when sitting stationary for long periods of time, and at the end of range motion.

1. As this man's personal trainer, you are concerned and advise your client to

   A. RICE, take Advil, continue exercise program, and wear a brace
   B. RICE, see a doctor, work on flexibility and strength
   C. continue exercise program, wear a brace, and work through pain
   D. all of the above

2. During an evaluation of this client, you notice that he has excessive pronation and weakness in the anterior tibialis.
   You make notes and

   A. advise him to buy an orthotic to correct pronation
   B. ask injury questions that are aggravated by excessive pronation
   C. add exercise to increase flexibility, increase strength to vastus lateralis, and advise client to see an orthopedist and begin a running program
   D. all of the above

3. After completing a step class, a participant complains of lower back pain.
   You give the following advice:

   A. RICE and get a massage
   B. RICE, see a doctor, and do stretching exercises
   C. Get a massage, stretch and strengthen abdominals
   D. All of the above

4. RICE stands for

   A. rest, ice, compression, exercise
   B. resistance, isometric, continuous exercise
   C. rest, ice, compression, elevation
   D. none of the above

5. A soft tissue injury should be treated with

   A. RICE
   B. increased strength and flexibility exercises
   C. RICE and decreased exercise to the area
   D. all of the above

6. On a hot, humid day, you advise your class to drink water _____ class.

   A. before, during, and after
   B. before and after
   C. after
   D. only up to half hour before

7. A 40-year-old male complains of chest pains after class. Your BEST action would be to

   A. call 911
   B. tell him to drive to the nearest hospital
   C. have him walk it off
   D. tell him to rest until he feels better

8. During a sub max stress test, the client's diastolic blood pressure falls. You IMMEDIATELY

   A. increase the intensity of the exercise
   B. terminate the test
   C. tell him his condition is improving
   D. slow the activity

9. A class member complains of sharp, localized tibial pain. You should

   A. insist she see a doctor before participating in your class
   B. allow her to participate but *take it easy*
   C. allow her to participate but tape her shin
   D. tell her to get new sneakers with better shock absorption

10. A participant in your aerobics class trips and hurts her ankle. She says her toes are *tingling*. You should

    A. administer RICE
    B. have her walk until the pain subsides
    C. have her sit until the pain subsides
    D. administer ice, elevate the injured ankle, and tell her to see a doctor

11. To avoid knee strain in lunges,

    A. bend the forward knee completely for a full stretch
    B. bend the forward knee no greater than 90 degrees
    C. toe out with the feet
    D. maintain straight spinal alignment

12. People with a history of low back problems should avoid all of the following EXCEPT

    A. lifting weights overhead
    B. straight leg lifts
    C. straight leg sit-ups
    D. isometric-type abdominal exercises

13. People with high blood pressure should avoid all of the following EXCEPT

    A. aerobic type exercise
    B. gripping weights
    C. high intensity strength training
    D. lifting heavy loads overhead

14. Your client complains of shin splints.
    You would NOT advise

    A. switching to non-weight bearing exercise
    B. checking exercise shoes for good shock absorbing ability
    C. staying on the ground during aerobic activity, i.e., no jumping
    D. regular hot baths

15. When your client announces she hasn't had time to eat all day but wants to do the 2 P.M. training session, you

    A. compliment her on her working on losing weight
    B. tell her not to skip meals and start the workout
    C. supply her with fruit or juice and reduce the workout intensity
    D. skip the aerobic segment and just do weights

16. The LEAST safe stretching technique is

    A. static
    B. slow sustained
    C. ballistic
    D. range of motion exercises

17. The four phases of a seizure are

    A. aura, tonic, clonic, postictal
    B. dehydration, sweating, pain, fainting
    C. dizziness, sweating, loss of balance, fainting
    D. dizziness, difficulty breathing, choking, death

18. The conditions that predispose someone to heat stroke include all of the following EXCEPT

    A. older age
    B. poor acclimatization
    C. hyperthyroidism
    D. none of the above

19. The body's ability to adapt to heat stress over time is referred to as

    A. specificity
    B. neuromuscular response
    C. acclimatization
    D. adaptation

20. Reduced skin circulation may be due to

    A. dehydration
    B. cardiovascular disease
    C. diuretics
    D. beta blockers

21. Of the following, the only one NOT recommended for the prevention of heat illnesses is:  21.____

    A. Avoid exercising in extreme heat
    B. Take salt tablets
    C. Wear sensible, porous, light-colored, loose-fitting clothing
    D. Take frequent rest periods

22. All of the following are signs of possible bone fractures EXCEPT:  22.____

    A. audible snap at time of injury
    B. abnormal motion or position of the injured limb
    C. swelling
    D. increased sports performance

23. Possible leg injuries do NOT include  23.____

    A. ACL tear                B. patellar tendinitis
    C. rotator cuff            D. achilles tendinitis

24. Patellofemoral pain syndrome is often termed  24.____

    A. ACL
    B. PFP
    C. iliotibial band syndrome
    D. chondromalacia

25. The thickened fascial structure on the outer aspect of the thigh and knee is the  25.____

    A. iliotibial band (ITB)
    B. patellar tendon
    C. anterior cruciate ligament (ACL)
    D. none of the above

## KEY (CORRECT ANSWERS)

1. B
2. B
3. B
4. C
5. D

6. A
7. A
8. B
9. A
10. D

11. B
12. D
13. A
14. D
15. C

16. C
17. A
18. D
19. C
20. C

21. B
22. D
23. C
24. D
25. A

# EXAMINATION SECTION
# TEST 1

DIRECTIONS: Each question or incomplete statement is followed by several suggested answers or completions. Select the one that BEST answers the question or completes the statement. *PRINT THE LETTER OF THE CORRECT ANSWER IN THE SPACE AT THE RIGHT.*

1. A client signs a contract stating he gives up his right to sue.
   This is an example of

   A. informed consent
   B. written contract
   C. a waiver
   D. liability insurance
   E. none of the above

2. A client decides to lead part of an exercise class with the instructor in the room. The instructor gives him permission. While leading the class, the client performs a high risk exercise and a member of the class hurts her back.
   Who is responsible for negligence?

   A. The client who taught the unsafe move
   B. The instructor for allowing the client to do it
   C. Both the instructor and the client
   D. No one; the exerciser is in class at her own risk
   E. None of the above

3. The purpose of an *informed consent* form is that the client

   A. understands inherent risks of exercise
   B. agrees to emergency medical attention if needed
   C. obtains consent for beginning an exercise program
   D. obtains liability insurance
   E. none of the above

4. An instructor who uses music in her class without having a performance license may be liable for

   A. negligence
   B. copyright infringement
   C. professional liability
   D. personal injury

5. If an instructor makes slanderous comments about another instructor to her class, it would be an example of

   A. personal injury
   B. professional liability
   C. general liability
   D. an act of omission
   E. none of the above

6. An instructor would be held legally negligent if

   A. a sexual relationship developed with a member
   B. a member did not get the results he was looking for
   C. the instructors practices and methods were below accepted standard of care
   D. the instructor never received waivers or letters of consent from his members
   E. none of the above

7. All of the following are good methods for a trainer to reduce the risk of being found legally negligent EXCEPT

    A. transferring risk through obtaining insurance policies
    B. reduction (through continuing education)
    C. retention (budgeting for minor injuries)
    D. avoidance of certain activities or equipment
    E. none of the above

8. A trainer should ONLY hook up electrodes and administer a maximum capacity test if

    A. a physician is present
    B. he has a waiver signed by the client
    C. he knows what he is doing
    D. the client has a history of heart disease
    E. none of the above

9. A trainer should not touch a client UNLESS
    I. he asks the clients permission
    II. it is essential in instruction
    III. the client is of the same sex

    The CORRECT answer is:

    A. I only          B. I, II, III       C. II only
    D. I, II           E. I, III

10. Responsibilities of a trainer include all of the following EXCEPT

    A. facilities           B. equipment
    C. supervision          D. instruction
    E. none of the above

11. If a trainer arrives at a clients home and finds a cable frayed on a piece of home equipment, he should

    A. do nothing; he is not responsible for clients equipment
    B. advise the client that the equipment needs repair, suggest that the client call the company and conduct the sessions without using the equipment until it has been repaired
    C. replace the cable
    D. tape up the cable and use it carefully
    E. none of the above

12. A trainer who is asked for recommendations about exercise equipment, clothing or shoes should
    I. not say anything and refer the client to a retail source
    II. be cautious about giving advice
    III. be knowledgeable about the advantages and disadvantages of the products
    IV. advise the client that the advice is solely based on personal experience

    The CORRECT answer is:

    A. II only         B. II, III          C. I, III
    D. II, III, IV     E. I, II, III, IV

13. Disadvantages of a corporation structure include all of the following EXCEPT

    A. complicated legal requirements
    B. high costs of formation
    C. unlimited liability
    D. extensive government regulation
    E. none of the above

14. Advantages of sole proprietorships include:
    I. They are easily formed under the law
    II. Costs of formation are low
    III. Government regulation is minimal
    The CORRECT answer is:

    A. I only          B. I, III          C. II only
    D. I, II           E. I, II, III

15. Personal trainers who declare themselves independent contractors have all of the following advantages EXCEPT

    A. choosing when and where to work
    B. charging variable fees for different situations
    C. having professional freedom in conducting work
    D. having workers compensation and unemployment insurance
    E. all of the above

16. Of the following, the element NOT necessary for a binding contract is

    A. an offer and acceptance, with mutual agreement on terms
    B. consideration - an exchange of valuable items, such as money for services
    C. legality - acceptable form under the law
    D. ability of the parties to enter into a contract with respect to age and mental capacity
    E. none of the above

17. The term *standard of care* as a legal concept for personal trainers is BEST defined as

    A. actions and practices seen as appropriate by other personal trainers
    B. first aid administered to a client
    C. a defense used by plaintiffs in court
    D. the ACSM guide book
    E. all of the above

18. If a trainer, certified in CPR, performs emergency resuscitation on a client, he

    A. may be held liable for injuries sustained
    B. may be held liable for negligence only
    C. cannot be held liable
    D. cannot be held liable only if patient makes a complete recovery
    E. none of the above

19. If a client signs a contract with the trainer in the clients house, the client may cancel the contract
    I. within three business days
    II. if no services have been performed yet
    III. at any t ime
    IV. if the client is under 18 years of age
    V. unless it has been paid
    The CORRECT answer is:

    A. II only
    B. III only
    C. IV only
    D. IV, V
    E. I, II, IV

20. Karl, a personal trainer who owns the South Shore Health Club, has sexual relations with several of his female clients. He offers to extend their memberships to his club for an additional year for free as he wants to continue to see them.
    In these circumstances, Karl
    I. is guilty of unethical behavior
    II. can lose his certification
    III. actions are illegal
    IV. may offer free memberships since it is his club
    V. should not work professionally with his sexual partners in his club
    The CORRECT answer is:

    A. I, IV
    B. I, II, III
    C. II, III, IV
    D. I, II, V
    E. III, IV, V

## KEY (CORRECT ANSWERS)

1. C
2. C
3. A
4. B
5. B

6. C
7. E
8. A
9. D
10. E

11. B
12. D
13. C
14. E
15. D

16. E
17. A
18. C
19. E
20. D

# EXAMINATION SECTION
## TEST 1

DIRECTIONS: Each question or incomplete statement is followed by several suggested answers or completions. Select the one that BEST answers the question or completes the statement. *PRINT THE LETTER OF THE CORRECT ANSWER IN THE SPACE AT THE RIGHT.*

Questions 1-9.

DIRECTIONS: In Questions 1 through 9, label the numbered structures of the human skeleton shown below.

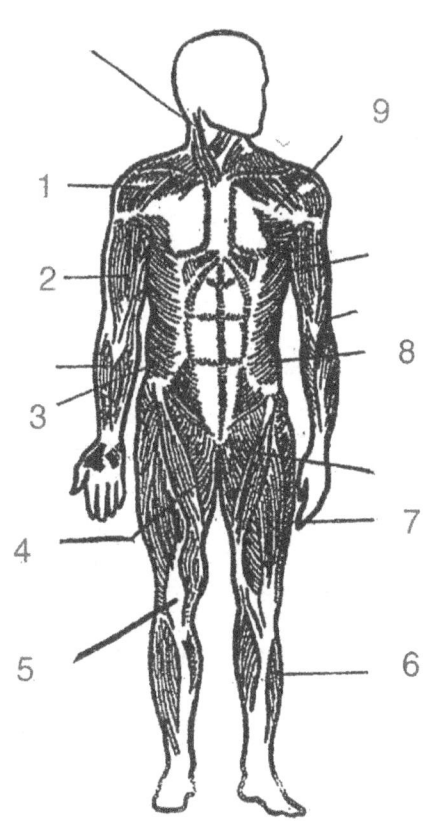

1.\_\_\_\_
2.\_\_\_\_
3.\_\_\_\_
4.\_\_\_\_
5.\_\_\_\_
6.\_\_\_\_
7.\_\_\_\_
8.\_\_\_\_
9.\_\_\_\_

10. Slow twitch fibers are characterized as having   10.\_\_\_\_

    A. many mitochondria      B. high aerobic capacity
    C. red fibers      D. all of the above

11. Which are contractile proteins?   11.\_\_\_\_
    I. Myosin
    II. Sarcomere
    III. Actin
    The CORRECT answer is:

    A. I, II      B. I, III      C. II, III      D. I, II, III

87

12. An adaptation to strength training would be

    A. increased testosterone
    B. increased oxidative enzymes
    C. hypertrophy
    D. all of the above

13. In response to strength training, _____ become stronger.

    A. muscles          B. tendons
    C. ligaments        D. all of the above

14. The fatigue which results during heavy exercise lasting from 30 seconds to about 40-60 minutes to exhaustion is due to

    A. lactic acid accumulation
    B. glycogen depletion
    C. ATP depletion
    D. heat stress

15. The stability of joints is maintained by

    A. cartilage    B. muscles    C. ligaments    D. tendons

16. Hill running, jumping rope, cycling, and toe raises with a barbell will work the

    A. anterior tibialis       B. peroneus longus
    C. peroneus brevis         D. gastrocnemius

17. Leg press, squats, and stairclimbing will work the

    A. biceps femoris          B. semitendinousus
    C. both of the above       D. none of the above

18. Bent knee curl-ups using rotation will work the

    A. erector spinae
    B. internal and external obliques
    C. rectus abdominus
    D. transverse abdominus

19. The rotator cuff is made up of

    A. subscapularis, teres minor, infraspinatus, supraspinatus
    B. serratus anterior, teres major, subscapularis, infraspinatus
    C. subclavius, infraspinatus, teres minor, supraspinatus
    D. subscapularis, infraspinatus, teres major, supraspinatus

20. The desirable range for cholesterol count is _____ mg/dl.

    A. less than 200           B. 200-239
    C. 240-260                 D. more than 246

21. The process by which carbohydrates are increased and aerobic exercise is decreased is called

    A. hypoglycemia            B. ketosis
    C. protein bulking         D. carbohydrate loading

22. A 154 lb. male needs _____ grams of protein a day.  22._____

    A. 105      B. 115      C. 95      D. 150

23. Hypertensive drugs will  23._____

    A. increase the resting heart rate
    B. decrease the exercise heart rate
    C. increase blood pressure during exercise
    D. all of the above

24. As pressure falls, the sounds heard in distinct phases are called  24._____

    A. systolic      B. diastolic
    C. korotkoff sounds      D. blood pressure

25. The force of the blood against the walls of the arteries when the heart pumps blood to the body is called  25._____

    A. systolis      B. diastolic
    C. blood pressure      D. heart rate

# KEY (CORRECT ANSWERS)

| | | | |
|---|---|---|---|
| 1. | deltoids | 11. | B |
| 2. | biceps | 12. | C |
| 3. | obliques | 13. | D |
| 4. | sartorius | 14. | A |
| 5. | patella | 15. | C |
| 6. | tibialis anterior | 16. | D |
| 7. | rectus femorus | 17. | C |
| 8. | rectus abdominis | 18. | B |
| 9. | pectoralis major | 19. | A |
| 10. | D | 20. | A |

21. D
22. A
23. B
24. C
25. C

# TEST 2

DIRECTIONS: Each question or incomplete statement is followed by several suggested answers or completions. Select the one that BEST answers the question or completes the statement. *PRINT THE LETTER OF THE CORRECT ANSWER IN THE SPACE AT THE RIGHT.*

Questions 1-13.

DIRECTIONS: In Questions 1 through 13, label the numbered structures of the human skeleton shown below.

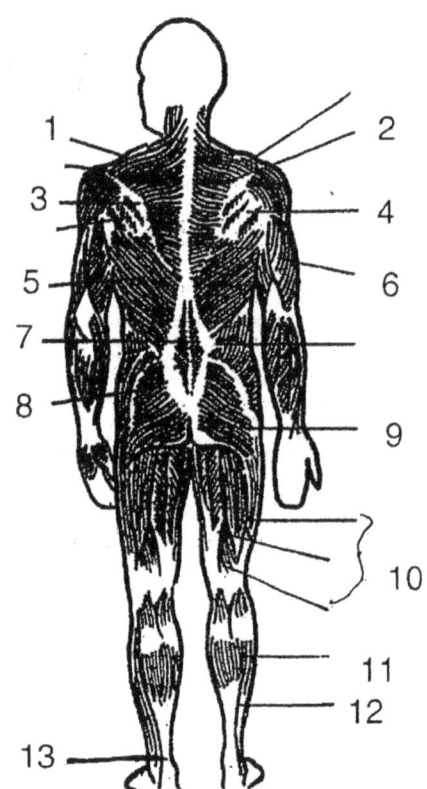

1.____
2.____
3.____
4.____
5.____
6.____
7.____
8.____
9.____
10.____
11.____
12.____
13.____

14. The *upright row* utilizes the

    A. biceps, deltoids, trapezius, levatator, scapulae
    B. triceps, deltoids, trapezius, serratus anterior
    C. biceps, latissimus dorsi, teres major, deltoids
    D. triceps, deltoids, trapezius, pectoralis major

14.____

15. The *squat* utilizes the

    A. gluts, gastrocnemius, tibialis anterior, peronius brevis
    B. gluteus maximus, rectus femoris, bicep femoris, gastrocnemius
    C. rectus femoris, biceps femoris, tibialis anterior, psoas
    D. rectus femoris, biceps femoris, gastrocnemius, psoas

15.____

16. Joan weighs 120 lbs. and has 25% body fat. If Joan were 20% body fat, she would weigh _____ lbs.

    A. 115   B. 120   C. 125   D. 112

17. The push-up test assesses

    A. endurance of chest and shoulders
    B. strength of chest and shoulders
    C. endurance with some measurement of strength of the triceps, anterior deltoid, and pectoralis major
    D. strength of the triceps, anterior deltoid, pectoralis major

18. Alan is 40 years old with an exercise intensity of 70%. His target heart rate would be

    A. 126   B. 144   C. 136   D. 156

19. Alan, now using a resting heart rate of 80 beats per minute, would have a target heart rate of

    A. 140   B. 150   C. 130   D. 160

20. The initial conditioning stage for cardiorespiratory endurance lasts

    A. 2-4 weeks
    B. 4-6 weeks
    C. 8-20 weeks
    D. 6-12 months

21. Frontal flexion of the cervical spine may be included in the warm-up

    A. if properly controlled
    B. always
    C. never
    D. but not in the cool-down

22. The definition of adduction is movement

    A. describing a 360 degree circle
    B. away from the midline of the body
    C. towards the midline of the body
    D. around the axis

23. Antagonistic muscles to the hip adductors are the

    A. quadriceps and hamstrings
    B. tensor facial latae and gluteus medius
    C. biceps femoris and vastus medialis
    D. vastus lateralis and vastus medialis

24. When performing abdominal work, which of the following BEST isolates the rectus abdominus?

    A. Curls
    B. Push-ups
    C. Elongation
    D. None of the above

25. _____ is PRIMARILY responsible for keeping a joint from moving beyond its normal range of motion.

    A. Muscle   B. Cartilage   C. Ligament   D. Tendon

# KEY (CORRECT ANSWERS)

1. upper trapezius
2. trapezius
3. rhomboideus
4. rotator cuff
5. latissimus dorsi

6. triceps
7. quatratus lumborum
8. gluteus medius
9. gluteus maximus
10. hamstrings

11. gastrocnemius
12. soleus
13. achilles tendon
14. A
15. B

16. D
17. C
18. B
19. B
20. A

21. C
22. C
23. B
24. A
25. C

# TEST 3

DIRECTIONS: Each question or incomplete statement is followed by several suggested answers or completions. Select the one that BEST answers the question or completes the statement. *PRINT THE LETTER OF THE CORRECT ANSWER IN THE SPACE AT THE RIGHT.*

1. _____ training consists of repeated intervals of exercise interspersed with intervals of relatively light exercise.  1.\_\_\_\_

    A. Interval
    B. Fartlek
    C. Continuous
    D. Aerobic composite

2. Barbells are an example of _____ equipment.  2.\_\_\_\_

    A. isokinetic
    B. dynamic variable resistance
    C. dynamic constant resistance
    D. isometric

3. The sound training recommendation for safe and effective strength development is _____ reps with _____% capacity.  3.\_\_\_\_

    A. 8; 80
    B. 10; 75
    C. 8-12; 70-80
    D. 12-20; 50-60

4. Bodybuilders typically perform _____ set(s) of _____ reps.  4.\_\_\_\_

    A. 4-6; 8-12
    B. 6-8; 2-6
    C. 1-2; 12-20
    D. 1; 8-12

5. The CORRECT spotting technique for the squat is to stand _____ the person and wrap your arms _____.  5.\_\_\_\_

    A. behind; around lower body
    B. behind; around the torso
    C. in front of; under elbows
    D. in front of; around the torso

6. The stages of the personal trainer/client relationship are  6.\_\_\_\_

    A. rapport/investigation/planning/action
    B. action/rapport/investigation/planning
    C. investigation/rapport/investigation/action
    D. planning/action/rapport/investigation

7. Which of the following are leadership qualities?  7.\_\_\_\_

    A. Punctuality
    B. Willingness to plan ahead
    C. Sensitivity to client's past experience
    D. All of the above

8. To enhance and maintain the motivation to exercise, the trainer should
   I. set high goals for the client to aspire to
   II. find out client's preferences, needs, and exercise history
   III. structure appropriate expectations at the beginning
   The CORRECT answer is:

   A. I, II            B. I, III
   C. II, III          D. I, II, III

9. The relationship between heart rate and workload is established by the _____ test.

   A. YMCA bike        B. step
   C. walk/run         D. sit and reach

10. The two PRIMARY sources of error in skinfold measurement are

    A. expensive equipment and inaccessibility
    B. improper site determination and measurement
    C. underestimating the charts and improper clothing
    D. excessive sweating and tight-fitting garments

11. An individual weighing 50 kg and at an energy level of 10 Mets would use _____ ml. of oxygen.

    A. 45    B. 1750    C. 2050    D. 175

12. If the individual's max was 10 Mets, the target zone would be _____ Mets.

    A. 5-8    B. 6-9    C. 4-6    D. 7-10

13. Delayed onset of muscle soreness can be prevented by _____ stretching.

    A. static    B. ballistic    C. PNF    D. passive

14. Which of the following are contraindicated stretches?

    A. The plough            B. Hurdlers stretch
    C. Neck hyperextension   D. All of the above

15. Flexibility is affected by

    A. age and inactivity    B. gender
    C. body type             D. all of the above

16. John weighs 150 lbs. and is 20 years old.
    How many calories should he consume a day to maintain his BMR?

    A. 1250    B. 1950    C. 1320    D. 1800

17. The LEAST effective aid in the learning process is

    A. smelling    B. touching    C. tasting    D. hearing

Questions 18-25,

DIRECTIONS: In Questions 18 through 25, match each numbered definition with the lettered term, listed in the column below, that it BEST describes.

- A. Superior
- B. Medial
- C. Posterior
- D. Inferior
- E. Distal
- F. Proximal
- G. Lateral
- H. Anterior

18. Situated below; nearer the bottom or base  18.____

19. Nearest the point of attachment  19.____

20. Situated above another, and especially another similar, part  20.____

21. Toward the dorsal or back aspect  21.____

22. Farthest from the trunk  22.____

23. Situated toward the front or the head  23.____

24. Relating to the side; to the right or left of the body's axis  24.____

25. Extending toward the middle  25.____

# KEY (CORRECT ANSWERS)

| | | | |
|---|---|---|---|
| 1. | A | 11. | B |
| 2. | C | 12. | A |
| 3. | C | 13. | A |
| 4. | A | 14. | D |
| 5. | B | 15. | D |
| 6. | A | 16. | D |
| 7. | D | 17. | C |
| 8. | C | 18. | D |
| 9. | A | 19. | F |
| 10. | B | 20. | A |

21. C
22. E
23. H
24. G
25. B

# TEST 4

DIRECTIONS: Each question or incomplete statement is followed by several suggested answers or completions. Select the one that BEST answers the question or completes the statement. *PRINT THE LETTER OF THE CORRECT ANSWER IN THE SPACE AT THE RIGHT.*

1. An antagonistic muscle to the pectoralis major is the

    A. deltoid
    B. trapezius
    C. external oblique
    D. latissimus dorsi

2. Lactic acid is a by-product of _____ metabolism.

    A. anaerobic   B. rapid   C. aerobic   D. slow

3. As the antagonist muscle contracts to move the limb, the agonist muscle stretches, providing a movement.

    A. jumpy but controlled
    B. rough and uncontrolled
    C. loose and awkward
    D. smooth and controlled

4. Hyperextension of any of the body's joints can cause

    A. postural misalignments in other body areas
    B. ligamental stress in the joint
    C. the joint to become less stable
    D. all of the above

5. When evaluating an exercise for inclusion in the class you are teaching, which of the following is NOT one of the five evaluation questions?

    A. What are you trying to accomplish with this exercise?
    B. Is the contraction eccentric or concentric?
    C. Are you able to effectively isolate the muscle you are trying to work?
    D. What is the tempo for the correct response?

6. As a person crosses his/her anaerobic threshold,

    A. target heart rate is finally achieved
    B. the body is consuming too much oxygen
    C. duration is no longer dependent upon intensity
    D. energy demands exceed aerobic energy production

7. The intensity of an aerobic workout can be increased by all of the following EXCEPT

    A. expanding the range of motion of arms and legs
    B. adding hand weights
    C. increasing the duration of the aerobic portion of the class
    D. using music with a greater number of beats per minute

8. The average healthy young adult exerciser desiring a cardiovascular training effect should perform aerobic exercise with the heart beating at _____ percent of maximum.

    A. 50-60   B. 75-85   C. 80-95   D. 85-100

9. Increased aerobic capacity refers to the body's ability to

   A. extract carbon dioxide from the bloodstream
   B. consume and process a greater volume of oxygen
   C. increase muscle size
   D. increase airway resistance

10. ATP is manufactured from the breakdown of _____ and is stored as energy within the cell.

    A. glucose
    B. protein
    C. fat
    D. none of the above

11. For every major muscle group worked, the opposing muscle group should also be worked to prevent muscular imbalance, thereby decreasing the risk of future injury. After working the quadriceps, what antagonist muscle group should be exercised?

    A. Hamstrings
    B. Gastrocalmius
    C. Gluteals
    D. Biceps

12. The GREATEST improvements in flexibility can be achieved by performing

    A. static stretches during your warm-up
    B. rhythmic limbering exercises
    C. ballistic stretches during your end of class cool-down
    D. static stretches during your end of class cool-down

13. Which of the following is NOT generally considered an aerobic exercise?

    A. Walking
    B. Swimming
    C. Sprinting
    D. Jumping rope

14. A safe and effective aerobic class format should include
    I. static stretch at the end of class
    II. stretching muscles worked immediately following stretching exercises
    III. a 3-5 minute post aerobic cool-down

    The CORRECT answer is:

    A. I, II
    B. III only
    C. I, III
    D. II, III

15. For learning retention, the technique with the HIGHEST percentage for success is

    A. hearing
    B. say and do
    C. say
    D. seeing

16. Pain around and under the patella signals a possible case of

    A. achilles tendinitis
    B. chondromalacia
    C. patellar tendinitis
    D. tears of the anterior cruciate ligament

Questions 17-25.

DIRECTIONS: In Questions 17 through 25, match each numbered definition with the lettered movement or position, listed in the column below, that it BEST describes.

      A. Flexion
      B. Pronation
      C. Rotation
      D. Adduction
      E. Supination
      F. Extension
      G. Circumduction
      H. Hyperextension
      I. Plantar flexion

17. Turning on an axis
18. Lying on the back, palms up
19. Movement into a straight position
20. Bending of the sole of the foot
21. Lying on stomach, face-down
22. The cone-shaped swinging of a limb, with the joint at the proximal end as the apex
23. Bending; movement into a bent position
24. Extreme extension
25. Movement toward the center of the body

## KEY (CORRECT ANSWERS)

| | | | |
|---|---|---|---|
| 1. | B | 11. | A |
| 2. | A | 12. | D |
| 3. | D | 13. | C |
| 4. | D | 14. | C |
| 5. | D | 15. | B |
| 6. | D | 16. | B |
| 7. | C | 17. | C |
| 8. | B | 18. | E |
| 9. | B | 19. | F |
| 10. | A | 20. | I |

21. B
22. G
23. A
24. H
25. D

# EXAMINATION SECTIOMN
# TEST 1

DIRECTIONS: Each question or incomplete statement is followed by several suggested answers or completions. Select the one that BEST answers the question or completes the statement. *PRINT THE LETTER OF THE CORRECT ANSWER IN THE SPACE AT THE RIGHT.*

1. The MAIN vessel through which oxygenated blood passes to the tissues is the

    A. pulmonary vein  B. vena cava
    C. ventricle  D. aorta

    1.____

2. Oxygenated blood from the lungs enters into the

    A. left atrium  B. right atrium
    C. left ventricle  D. right ventricle

    2.____

3. The exchange of oxygen and nutrients occurs in the

    A. arterioles  B. venules
    C. capillaries  D. arteries

    3.____

4. _____ neurons transmit impulses to the brain or spinal cord.

    A. Efferent  B. Afferent
    C. Motor  D. All of the above

    4.____

5. Which is NOT a function of the skeletal system?

    A. Factory for making glycogen
    B. Factory for making red blood cells
    C. Reservoir for minerals
    D. Provide attachments for skeletal muscles

    5.____

6. The tissues that connect one bone to another bone are called

    A. ligaments  B. cartilage
    C. tendons  D. muscles

    6.____

7. The MOST effective position for maximum work force is when the bone-muscle angle is CLOSEST to _____ degrees.

    A. 60  B. 120  C. 90  D. 30

    7.____

8. The plane that divides the body into left and right parts is the _____ plane.

    A. transverse  B. sagittal
    C. frontal  D. mediolateral

    8.____

9. An example of a ball and socket joint is the

    A. elbow  B. ankle
    C. radioulnar  D. shoulder

    9.____

10. The sternoclavicular joint is responsible for

    A. flexion-extension  B. adduction-abduction
    C. elevation-depression  D. all of the above

    10.____

11. If the arm is lifted away from the shoulder, then across the chest toward the midline of the body and then returns to a position out to the side, the movement is

    A. medial-lateral rotation
    B. flexion-extension
    C. transverse abduction-adduction
    D. none of the above

11.____

12. A functional property of muscle tissue is

    A. elasticity
    C. contractility
    B. distensibility
    D. all of the above

12.____

13. The brachioradialis is responsible for

    A. elbow flexion
    C. hip adduction
    B. hip extension
    D. all of the above

13.____

14. The muscles responsible for hip flexion are the

    A. gastrocnemius
    C. popliteus
    B. iliopsoas
    D. serratus anterior

14.____

15. What primary muscles are being used when performing a side-lying single leg lift?

    A. Tensor fuscia lata
    C. Biceps femoris
    B. Gluteus maximus
    D. None of the above

15.____

16. An exaggerated saggital curvature of the lumbar area is a condition called

    A. scoliosis
    C. kyphosis
    B. lordosis
    D. none of the above

16.____

Questions 17-20.

DIRECTIONS: The group of questions below consists of five lettered headings followed by a list of numbered phrases. For each numbered phrase, select the one heading that is MOST closely related to it.

    A. Gluteus medius
    B. Gastrocnemius
    C. Tibialis anterior
    D. Rectus femoris
    E. Serratus anterior

17. Side-lying hip abduction

17.____

18. Dorsiflexion of the ankle

18.____

19. Leg lift using frontal hip flexion

19.____

20. Seated row

20.____

21. All of the following are major minerals EXCEPT

    A. calcium
    C. iron
    B. phosphorus
    D. sodium

21.____

22. The body only needs 10 mg. of vitamin C to prevent the deficiency disease scurvy. 22._____
    The RDA for vitamin C is _____ mg.

    A. 30    B. 100    C. 150    D. 60

23. In 1977, the Senate Select Committee on Nutrition and Human Needs set new nutritional 23._____
    guidelines.
    The new percentage of total number of calories consumed in the form of complex carbohydrates became _____%.

    A. 30               B. 48
    C. 12               D. none of the above

24. An inadequate supply of _____ is thought to be one of the major contributing factors to 24._____
    osteoporosis.

    A. iron             B. niacin
    C. calcium          D. none of the above

25. According to the _____ theory, the body strives to maintain a certain level of body fat. 25._____

    A. set point        B. reversibility
    C. obesity          D. energy balance

## KEY (CORRECT ANSWERS)

| | | | |
|---|---|---|---|
| 1. | D | 11. | C |
| 2. | B | 12. | D |
| 3. | C | 13. | A |
| 4. | B | 14. | B |
| 5. | A | 15. | A |
| 6. | A | 16. | B |
| 7. | C | 17. | A |
| 8. | B | 18. | C |
| 9. | D | 19. | D |
| 10. | C | 20. | E |

21. C
22. D
23. B
24. C
25. A

# TEST 2

DIRECTIONS: Each question or incomplete statement is followed by several suggested answers or completions. Select the one that BEST answers the question or completes the statement. *PRINT THE LETTER OF THE CORRECT ANSWER IN THE SPACE AT THE RIGHT.*

1. The MOST accurate method to determine target heart rate is the

   A. met system
   B. Karvonen formula
   C. dyspnea index
   D. maximal heart rate formula

2. The target heart rate range generally accepted for MAXIMAL heart rate reserve is

   A. 50-85%    B. 60-80%    C. 40-60%    D. 60-90%

3. A 50 year-old woman has a resting heart rate of 80 and a maximal heart rate of 170. Her target heart rate at 65% intensity would be

   A. 138    B. 152    C. 160    D. 148

4. Maximal heart rate is the

   A. target training zone
   B. maximal oxygen consumption
   C. highest heart rate attained during exercise
   D. highest heart rate attained during rest

5. The BEST location to find a person's pulse is the

   A. temple    B. wrist    C. neck    D. chest

6. The _____ of the music determines the progression of exercise.

   A. rhythm    B. beats    C. measure    D. tempo

7. The essential percentage of body fat necessary for maintenance of life and reproductive function for women is _____%.

   A. 3-6    B. 8-12    C. 15-20    D. 23-25

8. The *burn* you feel in your muscles when they fatigue is caused by

   A. lactic acid           B. anaerobic glycosis
   C. aerobic glycosis      D. fatty acid oxidation

9. Fatty acid oxidation uses _____ to synthesize ATP.

   A. proteins           B. carbohydrates
   C. fats               D. all of te above

10. _____ yields unlimited ATP production and predominates during activities lasting longer than 3 minutes.

    A. Anaerobic glycolysis    B. Phosphagens
    C. Aerobic glycolysis      D. Fatty acid oxidation

11. The group MOST responsible for the growth and repair of cellular structures is

    A. carbohydrates
    B. proteins
    C. fats
    D. dairy products

12. The muscle visibly shortens and joint movement occurs during _____ muscular contraction.

    A. eccentric
    B. isometric
    C. isokinetic
    D. all of the above

13. Training adaptations will gradually decline if not regularly reinforced. This theory is called

    A. hypertrophy
    B. exercise specificity
    C. overload
    D. reversibility principle

14. The ability to repeatedly contract a muscle group against resistance is

    A. flexibility
    B. cardiovascular endurance
    C. muscular strength
    D. muscular endurance

15. Which is NOT a benefit of muscular endurance training?

    A. Muscular hypertrophy
    B. Increased vascularity
    C. Enhanced glycogen storage
    D. Improved aerobic capacity through increased oxidative enzymes

16. Ballistic stretching is characterized by
    I. jerking, bobbing, or bouncing motions
    II. typically held for 10-30 seconds
    III. invoking the stretch reflexes
    The CORRECT answer is:

    A. I, II
    B. III only
    C. I, III
    D. II, III

17. The cardiovascular respiratory system is responsible for the

    A. removal of metabolic waste products
    B. delivery of blood and oxygen to muscles
    C. extraction of oxygen from the blood
    D. all of the above

18. The function of the blood filling the heart during its resting period and the force of the contraction of the heart during its contraction is called

    A. cardiac output
    B. diastolic
    C. systolic
    D. stroke volume

19. The product of stroke volume and heart rate is

    A. maximal oxygen consumption
    B. cardiac output
    C. blood pressure
    D. none of the above

20. With cessation of exercise, the requirement for oxygen abruptly returns to initial resting level.
   This level is called

   A. oxygen debt
   B. oxygen deficit
   C. oxygen consumption
   D. homeostasis

21. Exercise intensity should be APPROXIMATELY _____ percent of maximal oxygen consumption.

   A. 60-80    B. 70-85    C. 50-85    D. 85-90

22. Benefits of aerobic exercise for healthy participants include

   A. muscular strength
   B. improved bone density
   C. all of the above
   D. none of the above

23. Which is NOT a primary objective of the warm-up phase?
   To

   A. increase the heart rate
   B. increase flexibility
   C. elevate muscle temperature
   D. develop aerobic capacity

24. Joan is 55 years old, has been sedentary and has developed arthritis.
   Her exercise program should emphasize _____ muscular strength and endurance and _____ intensity aerobics.

   A. flexibility, moderate levels of; low
   B. flexibility, no; low
   C. flexibility, no; high
   D. high levels of; low

25. Alfred is a 40 year-old male who works in construction. He has 35% body fat. His exercise program should consist of _____ intensity, _____ duration aerobic exercise _____.

   A. high; short; with a weight training program 2-3 times a week
   B. high; long; with a weight training program 3-4 times a week
   C. low; short; 2-3 times per week with no weight training
   D. low; long; 3-4 times a week

# KEY (CORRECT ANSWERS)

| | | | |
|---|---|---|---|
| 1. | B | 11. | B |
| 2. | D | 12. | C |
| 3. | A | 13. | D |
| 4. | C | 14. | D |
| 5. | B | 15. | A |
| 6. | D | 16. | C |
| 7. | B | 17. | D |
| 8. | A | 18. | D |
| 9. | C | 19. | B |
| 10. | C | 20. | A |

21. C
22. B
23. D
24. A
25. D

# TEST 3

DIRECTIONS: Each question or incomplete statement is followed by several suggested answers or completions. Select the one that BEST answers the question or completes the statement. *PRINT THE LETTER OF THE CORRECT ANSWER IN THE SPACE AT THE RIGHT.*

1. Which of the following is NOT a primary risk factor for coronary heart disease?   1.____

    A. Hypertension
    B. Abnormal blood cholesterol levels
    C. Cigarette smoking
    D. Obesity

2. Each of the following indicate that referral to a physician is absolutely necessary EXCEPT   2.____

    A. cigarette smoking
    B. hypertension
    C. past difficulty with exercise
    D. chronic illness

3. Movements in a warm-up should prepare the body for movements used in the aerobic routines.   3.____
   This concept is called

    A. transition           B. specificity
    C. progression          D. isolation

4. All of the following lower the intensity of an aerobic workout EXCEPT   4.____

    A. eliminating the arm movements of an exercise
    B. traveling less
    C. lifting the knees less
    D. reducing the duration

5. A diabetic who has taken too much insulin or has not eaten properly is at risk for   5.____

    A. hypoglycemia         B. hyperglycemia
    C. insulin shock        D. diabetic coma

6. The BEST treatment for a diabetic who has taken too much insulin is   6.____

    A. cessation of exercise
    B. increased intensity of exercise
    C. salt tablets
    D. fruit juice

7. Participants with hypertension should avoid _____ exercises.   7.____

    A. isotonic             B. isokinetic
    C. isometric            D. all of the above

8. For participants with arthritis, instructors should   8.____

A. emphasize range of motion exercises
B. increase intensity and duration of exercises
C. decrease the frequency of low impact aerobics
D. all of the above

9. Stretching involving holding a non-moving position so that the specified joint is immobilized in a position that places the desired muscles at their GREATEST possible length is called

   A. ballistic stretching
   B. stretch reflex
   C. static stretching
   D. eccentric contraction

10. Holding the breath while contracting the chest muscles is called

    A. ballistic stretching
    B. cardiac output
    C. reversibility principle
    D. valsalva maneuver

11. The MOST accurate method for determining body composition is

    A. skinfold measurement
    B. hydrostatic weighing
    C. weight scale
    D. all of the above

12. Which of the following modifications are recommended for a participant who has suffered from a cardiovascular disease?

    A. Maintain a low to moderate level of intensity during aerobics for at least 20 minutes
    B. Monitor heart rate frequently
    C. Provide thorough cool-down to prevent possible hypertension
    D. All of the above

13. During exercise, a pregnant woman should NOT let her heart rate exceed _____ BPM.

    A. 140
    B. 170
    C. 160
    D. 190

14. The pregnancy hormone that loosens the joints is called

    A. insulin
    B. relaxin
    C. beta-blocks
    D. adrenalin

15. The American College of Obstetricians and Gynecologists suggests the maximum duration for maintaining cardiovascular fitness during pregnancy is a _____ minute period _____ times per week.

    A. 15; 3-4
    B. 20-30; 2-3
    C. 20-30; 3-4
    D. 5-10; 2-3

16. All of the following are modifications for a pregnant woman participating in class EXCEPT:

    A. Reduce the frequency of each set of repetitions
    B. Breathe out with each effort to prevent the valsalva maneuver
    C. Eliminate deep squats and hyperflexion of hips, knees, and ankles
    D. Add cross body movements such as touching the opposite elbow to the knee

17. Which of the following is NOT within the general guidelines when selecting dance-exercise steps?

A. Do not repeat a movement more than four consecutive times on one leg
B. Avoid movements with forward trunk flexion
C. Avoid changing directions rapidly
D. Perform continuous movement that requires participants to remain on the balls of their feet for extended periods

18. The _____ style of teaching provides opportunities for individualization and includes practice time and private instructor feedback for each participant.

    A. command
    B. practice
    C. reciprocal
    D. self-check

19. All of the following are contraindicated exercises EXCEPT

    A. knee sitting
    B. the plough
    C. bent knee sit-ups
    D. Hurdler's stretch

20. Which of the following is an entrapment of part of an interdigital nerve that usually occurs between the third and fourth toes?

    A. Metatarsalgia
    B. Neuroma
    C. Plantar fasciitis
    D. Achilles tendinitis

21. A ligament is a band of fibers connecting one bone to another. A _____ is an injury to a ligament.

    A. sprain
    B. strain
    C. stress fracture
    D. meniscus tear

22. All of the following are procedures to follow to prevent shock EXCEPT:

    A. Establish an airway
    B. Control the bleeding and elevate the lower extremities
    C. Move the victim to a safe and quiet area
    D. Cover the victim with a blanket

23. Jagged, irregular breaks or tears in the soft tissue characterize

    A. incisions
    B. avulsions
    C. lacerations
    D. punctures

24. An instructor allows a participant to use exercise equipment without first instructing him in its safe and proper use.
    If the participant is injured, which of the following coverages applies?

    A. Personal injury liability
    B. Professional liability
    C. General liability
    D. Property insurance

25. Fibers that do not have a finely developed oxygen delivery system but are equipped with outstanding capacity for ATP and CP storage and a high capacity for anaerobic glycolysis are

    A. slow twitch fibers
    B. fast twitch fibers
    C. intermediate fibers
    D. myofibril

## KEY (CORRECT ANSWERS)

1. D
2. A
3. B
4. D
5. A

6. D
7. C
8. A
9. C
10. D

11. B
12. D
13. A
14. B
15. D

16. D
17. D
18. B
19. C
20. B

21. A
22. C
23. C
24. B
25. B

# TEST 4

DIRECTIONS: Each question or incomplete statement is followed by several suggested answers or completions. Select the one that BEST answers the question or completes the statement. *PRINT THE LETTER OF THE CORRECT ANSWER IN THE SPACE AT THE RIGHT.*

1. Which of the following is NOT a general principle specific to the enhancement of flexibility?

    A. A general warm-up should precede stretching exercises.
    B. Stretching exercises should be performed without bouncing or jerking.
    C. Attempts should be made to stretch a muscle beyond the normal range of motion.
    D. All stretching should be done gently to the extent that muscle tension is perceived but muscle pain does not occur.

2. It is important to cool down gradually after a period of vigorous exercise. Which of the following is NOT a primary objective of cool down?

    A. Aid in the prevention of blood pooling
    B. Aid in the removal of accumulated lactic acid
    C. Preventing cardiac arrhythmias
    D. Raising the heart rate

3. Health benefits of aerobic exercise include

    A. increased muscular strength
    B. improved muscular endurance
    C. improved bone density
    D. all of the above

4. The outside of a body segment is referred to as

    A. lateral            B. medial
    C. posterior          D. anterior

5. The MAIN functions of the _____ are to absorb shock and provide a frictionless surface over which the bones can move.

    A. tendons    B. cartilage    C. ligaments    D. muscles

6. _____ joints allow movement in all directions.

    A. hinge              B. saddle
    C. gliding            D. condyloid

7. The ankle, which is a hinge joint, is responsible for

    A. inversion-eversion         B. dorsi-planter flexion
    C. medial-lateral rotation    D. pronation-supination

8. Which of the following are segmental movements in the frontal plane?

    A. Elevation-depression    B. Abduction-adduction
    C. Lateral flexion         D. All of the above

9. The substances which remove cholesterol from the system, including the arterial walls, and transport it to the liver where it is reprocessed or eliminated are called

   A. low density lipoproteins
   B. high density lipoproteins
   C. beta-blockers
   D. amino acids

10. Which of the following is NOT a primary benefit of aerobic exercise for persons with diabetes?

    A. Lose body fat
    B. Reduce tension and anxiety
    C. Maintain normal blood glucose levels
    D. Increased insulin production

11. Rotation of the foot to the outside so the plantar surface tends to face away from the midline of the body is called

    A. inversion             B. eversion
    C. supination            D. pronation

12. The trapezius muscle is responsible for

    A. elevation             B. retraction
    C. depression            D. all of the above

13. Motivational strategies to improve exercise compliance include

    A. good exercise leadership
    B. periodic evaluations
    C. opportunities for having fun
    D. all of the above

14. At least _____ minutes are needed to burn enough calories and apply sufficient stimulus to improve cardiovascular fitness.

    A. 20        B. 30        C. 15        D. 40

15. To strengthen the quadriceps, an EFFECTIVE exercise would utilize which joint?
    I. Shoulder
    II. Subtaylar
    III. Knee
    IV. Hip
    The CORRECT answer is:

    A. I only                B. I, II
    C. II, IV                D. III, IV

16. Harold is a 48-year-old man who has had a sedentary lifestyle. He wants to lose weight and firm up. You would prescribe a program

    A. building muscular strength, endurance, and flexibility
    B. of high impact aerobics *only*
    C. of low impact aerobics *only*
    D. of low intensity, long duration aerobics with moderate weight training

Questions 17-20.

DIRECTIONS: The group of questions below consists of five lettered headings followed by a list of numbered phrases. For each numbered phrase, select the one heading that is MOST closely related to it.
    A. Atherosclerosis
    B. Myocardial ischemia
    C. Angina pectoris
    D. Cardiac arrest
    E. Myocardial infarctions

17. Deficiency of blood supply to the heart.     17.____

18. A feeling of pressure in the center of the chest.     18.____

19. A thickening of the walls of the arteries by deposits of cholesterol.     19.____

20. Heart attack.     20.____

Questions 21-25.

DIRECTIONS: The group of questions below consists of six lettered headings followed by a list of numbered phrases. For each numbered phrase, select the one heading that is MOST closely related to it.
    A. Flexion
    B. Extension
    C. Medial rotation
    D. Supination
    E. Protraction
    F. Transverse abduction

21. Latissimus dorsi     21.____

22. Triceps     22.____

23. Teres major     23.____

24. Pectoralis major     24.____

25. Brachioradialis     25.____

# KEY (CORRECT ANSWERS)

1. C
2. D
3. C
4. A
5. B

6. C
7. B
8. D
9. B
10. D

11. B
12. D
13. D
14. A
15. D

16. A
17. B
18. C
19. A
20. E

21. C
22. B
23. C
24. E
25. A

# EXAMINATION SECTION
# TEST 1

DIRECTIONS: Each question or incomplete statement is followed by several suggested answers or completions. Select the one that BEST answers the question or completes the statement. *PRINT THE LETTER OF THE CORRECT ANSWER IN THE SPACE AT THE RIGHT.*

1. A sprain in any part of the body PRIMARILY involves the _____ tissue.  1_____

    A. ligament    B. nerve    C. skin    D. muscle

2. A victim with a fractured neck should ALWAYS be transported lying on  2_____

    A. the stomach, face downward
    B. a stretcher
    C. his back, face upward
    D. a blanket

3. All of the following statements are correct EXCEPT:  3_____

    A. In a fracture, crepitus is usually present, but in a dislocation there is no crepitus.
    B. In a fracture, deformity may vary in extent while in a dislocation the deformity is usually marked.
    C. In a dislocation, deformity recurs after the part is placed in its normal position, while in a fracture there is no deformity after the bone is placed in normal position.
    D. In a dislocation, the head of the bone rotates with the rest of the bone, whereas in a fracture the bone moves as two bones or as a bone with a loose end.

4. All of the following are complete fractures EXCEPT a(n) _____ fracture.  4_____

    A. impacted           B. greenstick
    C. Colles'            D. Pott's

5. The CORRECT statement in regard to the first-aid care for a burn is:  5_____

    A. Burns must be treated only with moist materials
    B. Greasy substances are the best medicines for all types of burns
    C. Burns must be treated only with dry materials
    D. The depth to which the body tissues are injured determines the first aid care

6. In applying a strapping to a sprained ankle, the person applying the strapping should  6_____

    A. pull the tape tight over the bony prominence of the ankle
    B. bind the toes as well as the rest of the foot
    C. have the injured foot in a position of 90 dorsi-flexion
    D. have the injured person keep the knee of the injured leg straight

7. Hot applications should be applied  7_____

    A. in case of a sting from an insect
    B. in case of nosebleed
    C. to an ankle immediately after it is sprained
    D. none of the above

8. If a victim complains of increased pain after traction has been applied to a fractured leg, the first-aider would MOST likely conclude that

   A. the traction bands are too loose
   B. the traction bands are too tight
   C. a tourniquet must be applied
   D. the simple fracture has turned into a compound fracture

9. Care of an unconscious victim, when the cause of unconsciousness is unknown, is based upon the

   A. pulse rate
   B. odor of the breath
   C. color of the face
   D. location of the accident

10. *Starting position: one half dip position with both legs fully extended backward; count 1: bring both knees up under chest with a jumping motion; count 2: return feet to starting position with a jumping motion.*
    This exercise MAINLY

    A. stretches the hamstrings
    B. develops the back muscles
    C. is one of endurance involving the hip and thigh muscles
    D. stretches the pectorals and the latissimus dorsi

11. *Elbows completely flexed, arms in horizontal position at shoulder level; draw elbows back strongly* is an exercise to correct PRIMARILY _____ shoulders.

    A. abduction of the
    B. adduction of the
    C. uneven height of
    D. pronation of

12. In assuming a sitting position from supine position, the MOST strenuous abdominal exercise is the one that starts with

    A. both arms extended overhead
    B. one knee bent upward toward the chest
    C. both arms extended downward at sides
    D. both arms extended out to the side at shoulder height

13. All of the following statements are correct EXCEPT:

    A. In kicking a football, the rectus femoris flexes the hip and extends the knee
    B. In pitching a baseball, the triceps extends the elbow joint
    C. In putting the shot, the upper part of the pectoralis major helps to swing the arm forward and upward
    D. In push-ups, the biceps extends the elbow during the up movement

14. All of the following are muscles of the lower extremity EXCEPT the

    A. trapezius
    B. sartorius
    C. gastrocnemius
    D. quadriceps femoris

15. The secret of effortless swimming lies in the _____ of muscles.

    A. tension
    B. relaxation
    C. rhythm
    D. power

16. With regard to the amount of energy expended, the MOST efficient of the following swimming strokes is the

    A. side stroke
    B. crawl
    C. breast stroke
    D. butterfly stroke

17. Of the following, the BEST exercise for warm-up, as a rule, is a(n)

    A. odd-count exercise
    B. exercise involving eight counts
    C. four-count exercise
    D. exercise performed in uneven rhythm

18. Of the following statements regarding the teaching of a warm-up exercise, the one which has the LEAST validity is:

    A. The warm-up should be of sufficient duration and intensity so as to achieve heightened circulatory response
    B. The warm-up should aim to use those muscle groups which are going to be used in the learning of the athletic skill
    C. Warm-ups should be performed to a fast rhythm so as to speed up circulation
    D. Warm-ups should aim to stretch the flexor and extensor muscle groups

19. As a rule, in order to physiologically prepare a secondary school gymnasium class for a lesson in game skills, the pupils should be allowed to perform a four-count warm-up exercise for AT LEAST

    A. 12 counts
    B. 4 times
    C. 32 counts
    D. 20 times

20. After the teacher has set the rhythm for a four-count exercise, the BEST of the following procedures for the teacher is to

    A. have the pupils count aloud as they perform
    B. clap the counts as the pupils perform
    C. perform in rhythm with the class
    D. have the pupils perform as he observes and gives occasional cues

21. Of the following, the MOST vigorous warm-up exercise is, as a rule,

    A. double arm bending and stretching upward, outward, forward, and downward
    B. heel raising, deep knee bending and stretching, heel lowering
    C. stride standing arms at shoulder level, alternate trunk twisting
    D. jumping feet apart and together with hand clapping overhead and down to side position

22. In order to have a gymnasium class maintain the rhythm of a four-count exercise, the BEST of the following procedures is to have the teacher

    A. clap his hands to the count as the pupils perform
    B. call all the counts as the pupils perform
    C. call the first eight counts and then have the pupils continue the exercise on their own
    D. allow the pupils to call the counts

23. Of the following methods of achieving good class performance in calisthenics, the MOST effective one, as a rule, is to

    A. explain the purpose and value of each exercise
    B. practice each exercise until it is performed perfectly by the entire class
    C. increase the time devoted to calisthenics
    D. motivate the calisthenics and praise the pupils who perform with vigor and good style

24. To insure a sufficient degree of intensity in the performance of a warm-up exercise, the exercise should, as a rule, be executed for AT LEAST _____ counts.

    A. 32    B. 16    C. 8    D. 76

25. A warm-up exercise precedes strenuous physical activity in order to

    A. prepare the individual psychologically for strenuous exercise
    B. gradually increase lung capacity
    C. prevent strains
    D. replace the store of glycogen

## KEY (CORRECT ANSWERS)

1. A
2. C
3. C
4. B
5. D

6. C
7. D
8. A
9. C
10. C

11. A
12. A
13. D
14. A
15. B

16. B
17. C
18. C
19. C
20. D

21. D
22. C
23. D
24. A
25. C

# TEST 2

DIRECTIONS: Each question or incomplete statement is followed by several suggested answers or completions. Select the one that BEST answers the question or completes the statement. *PRINT THE LETTER OF THE CORRECT ANSWER IN THE SPACE AT THE RIGHT.*

1. In the teaching of rhythmic exercises, the cadence should be

    A. maintained by the teacher
    B. maintained by the pupils and the teacher
    C. set by the teacher and maintained by the pupils
    D. set and maintained by the pupils

    1\_\_\_\_

2. To insure a sufficient degree of intensity in the performance of a warm-up exercise, the exercise should, as a rule, be executed for AT LEAST _____ counts.

    A. 32     B. 16     C. 8     D. 76

    2\_\_\_\_

3. In regard to athlete's foot, there is no preventive value in

    A. keeping the feet clean and dry, especially between the toes
    B. using a foot bath before going into a swimming pool
    C. frequent airing of shoes and socks
    D. dusting a *10%* boric acid powder on the feet and between the toes after bathing

    3\_\_\_\_

4. In order to count the pulse rate, one should place the

    A. thumb on the front of the wrist and fingers on the outer side
    B. forefinger on the inner and thumb side of the wrist
    C. fingers on either or both temples
    D. thumb at the center of the inner side of the wrist

    4\_\_\_\_

5. Of the following statements, the one that BEST explains poor diets in the average American home is that the home

    A. has enough money to buy the proper foods but it does not know enough about nutrition to buy wisely
    B. is fussy and has food prejudices
    C. is too poor to buy good food
    D. won't take the time to prepare balanced meals

    5\_\_\_\_

6. All of the following associations of objections to the use of milk in the diet and means of overcoming these objects are correct EXCEPT:

    A. Presence of disease bacteria renders milk unfit for consumption - pasteurization
    B. High water content makes milk bulky and hard to keep - production of dried milks
    C. Curd formed by raw milk in the stomach disagrees with normal digestion - use of milk in cooking instead of as a beverage
    D. Milk is poor in iron and low in vitamin C - inclusion of yeast and cod liver oil in the daily diet

    6\_\_\_\_

7. Of the following, the one that is MOST important for the proper utilization of calcium and phosphorus is vitamin

    A. E     B. D     C. K     D. A

    7\_\_\_\_

119

8. Of the following, the RICHEST source of iron is 8___

    A. liver
    B. dried fruits
    C. eggs
    D. tomatoes

9. Of the following associations, the CORRECT one is 9___

    A. folic acid - vitamin B
    B. cholesterol - vitamin K
    C. ascorbic acid - vitamin D
    D. biotin - vitamin C

10. The quality of a protein food and its effectiveness in body building are determined by the 10___

    A. amount of corrective tissue it contains
    B. number and amount of the amino acids it contains
    C. acid-forming elements it contains
    D. amount of water present in the food

11. The inability of the liver to store sugar and to regulate its oxidation in the muscle is caused by the LACK of the internal secretion of the 11___

    A. pancreas
    B. kidney
    C. gall bladder
    D. pituitary

12. All of the following are found in vitamin B complex EXCEPT 12___

    A. nicotinic acid
    B. riboflavin
    C. thiamine
    D. prothrombin

13. All of the following associations are correct EXCEPT 13___

    A. sedative - quiets activity
    B. analgesic - produces insensibility to pain
    C. soporific - stimulates
    D. anodyne - relieves pain

14. A passive exercise is one in which the 14___

    A. individual moves a body part as far as he is able to move it
    B. body parts are manipulated by the instructor or by some external force without active effort on the part of the recipient
    C. individual moves in opposition to the instructor's movement
    D. movement is initiated by the individual

15. *Rotation* of vertebrae in scoliosis cases may BEST be tested by having the pupil 15_

    A. bend the trunk forward
    B. place both hands overhead, feet together
    C. sit in stride position on bench
    D. stand upright, hands'on hips

16. *Foot circling,* an exercise aimed toward the strengthening of weak arches, is COR-      16____
    RECTLY performed by

    A. circling the foot upward, outward, and downward
    B. circling the foot downward, outward, and upward
    C. circling the foot downward with toes bent, inward, and upward
    D. legs extended, toes pointed upward, circle both feet

17. *Mat treading* (knee-chest position with alternate leg extension and flexion) is a GOOD   17____
    exercise for students who are

    A. overweight           B. underweight
    C. round-shouldered     D. flat-backed

18. According to the American Red Cross, the PROPER immediate first aid care for a frost-    18____
    bitten hand is to

    A. rub the hand with snow
    B. place the part in warm water
    C. cover the hand with a woolen cloth
    D. vigorously rub the hands together

19. A four-tailed bandage is particularly useful for the                                      19____

    A. elbow and knee       B. hips and ribs
    C. ankle and wrist      D. nose and chin

20. Of the following topics in first aid, the one which usually involves the MOST extensive   20____
    study or review of anatomy is

    A. first-degree burns   B. pressure points
    C. dog bites            D. convulsions

21. According to the American Red Cross, the dislocation that a person trained in first aid   21____
    should NOT attempt to reduce is a dislocation of the

    A. lower jaw
    B. first joint of the big toe
    C. second joint of the index finger
    D. second joint of the thumb

22. Internal bleeding which is usually vomited up and has the appearance of coffee grounds   22____
    is bleeding from the

    A. bowels       B. stomach       C. liver       D. lungs

23. The symptoms of heat exhaustion are                                                       23____

    A. pale, clammy skin, low temperature, weak pulse
    B. rapid and strong pulse, dry skin, high temperature
    C. headache, red face, unconsciousness
    D. abdominal cramps, red skin, profuse sweating

24. The *back-pressure, arm-lift* method of artificial respiration is superior to other methods because it

    A. eliminates the use of the inhalator
    B. is comparable to normal respiration in regard to oxygen intake
    C. increases compression of the chest by application of rhythmic pressure of the lower ribs
    D. is similar to the action in which a person inflates his chest by taking deep breaths

24____

25. Arterial pressure points

    A. are best located by taking the pulse
    B. lie close to bones near the surface of the body
    C. are used to cut off all blood circulation
    D. are deep-seated and require great pressure

25____

## KEY (CORRECT ANSWERS)

| | | | |
|---|---|---|---|
| 1. C | | 11. A | |
| 2. A | | 12. D | |
| 3. B | | 13. C | |
| 4. B | | 14. B | |
| 5. A | | 15. A | |
| 6. D | | 16. C | |
| 7. B | | 17. A | |
| 8. A | | 18. C | |
| 9. A | | 19. D | |
| 10. B | | 20. B | |

21. D
22. B
23. A
24. D
25. B

# TEST 3

DIRECTIONS: Each question or incomplete statement is followed by several suggested answers or completions. Select the one that BEST answers the question or completes the statement. *PRINT THE LETTER OF THE CORRECT ANSWER IN THE SPACE AT THE RIGHT.*

1. Of the following, the one NOT recommended for the first aid care of burns is 1\_\_\_\_

    A. boric acid  
    B. baking soda  
    C. petrolatum ointment  
    D. Epsom salts

2. A condition in which the crystalline lens of the eye has become opaque is known as 2\_\_\_\_

    A. cataract  
    B. glaucoma  
    C. presbyopia  
    D. trachoma

3. The MAIN function of the iris of the eye is to 3\_\_\_\_

    A. carry impressions to the brain  
    B. regulate the amount of light entering the eye through the pupil  
    C. protect the delicate structures within the eyeball  
    D. clarify the details and color of impressions

4. Astigmatism is USUALLY a defect of the 4\_\_\_\_

    A. cornea  
    B. retina  
    C. eye muscles  
    D. iris

5. Of the following, the two muscles that depress the humerus are 5\_\_\_\_

    A. latissimus and teres major  
    B. deltoid and trapezius  
    C. pectoralis minor and teres minor  
    D. supraspinatus and serratus magnus

6. The two elements MOST vitally concerned with the building of red blood cells are 6\_\_\_\_

    A. calcium and potassium  
    B. iron and copper  
    C. sodium and sulfur  
    D. chlorine and phosphorous

7. In reference to the blood, all of the following statements are correct EXCEPT: 7\_\_\_\_

    A. White blood cells have no nuclei  
    B. The spleen helps in the destruction of red blood cells  
    C. Blood platelets are associated with the clotting of the blood  
    D. Red blood cells are formed in red bone marrow

8. The term identified with a condition in which one of the arteries which supply the heart with blood is suddenly closed is 8\_\_\_\_

    A. coronary thrombosis  
    B. hypertension  
    C. arteriosclerosis  
    D. cerebral hemorrhage

9. Of the following statements concerning rheumatic fever, the INCORRECT one is:

    A. Rheumatic fever occurs most frequently in childhood
    B. Rheumatic fever is contagious
    C. A person with rheumatic fever has usually had an attack of chorea
    D. One attack of rheumatic fever makes a child susceptible to further attacks

10. All of the following statements concerning tests are correct EXCEPT the one that states that a

    A. sedimentation test aids in determining the presence of an inflammatory process in the body
    B. Widal test determines the amount of hemoglobin in the blood
    C. vital capacity test determines the quantity of air a person can expel after a full inspiration
    D. basal metabolism test measures the activity of the thyroid gland

11. All of the following associations are correct EXCEPT

    A. individual immunity - power of an individual to resist infection
    B. passive immunity - transmission to the body of antibodies by injection
    C. active immunity - production by the body of antibodies brought about by an attack of the disease
    D. local immunity - resistance to disease developed in a community after a mild epidemic

12. The instrument that amplifies the sound of the heart is the

    A. electrocardiograph    B. fluoroscope
    C. stethoscope           D. sphygmomanometer

13. Of the following statements regarding ACTH, the MOST NEARLY accurate is that ACTH

    A. is carried by the bloodstream to the adrenals and stimulates the production of adrenal hormones
    B. relieves pain, but it will probably never be available for general use because of scarcity of the product
    C. attacks microbes more successfully than any of the antibiotics
    D. is a permanent cure for arthritis and asthma

14. All of the following associations are correct EXCEPT

    A. euthenics - regulation of environment
    B. genetics - heredity
    C. eugenics - selective mating
    D. geriatrics - prenatal influences

15. The lymphatic system discharges its contents into the

    A. heart    B. venous bloodstream
    C. aorta    D. arteries

16. All of the following associations are correct EXCEPT   16____

    A. apnea - superfluity of oxygen
    B. dyspnea - scarcity of oxygen
    C. eupnea - increase in depth of respiration
    D. asphyxia - deprivation of oxygen and an excessive accumulation of carbon dioxide

17. In your health guidance period, you have a pupil with a long, thin trunk.   17____
    Classifying by somatotypes, you would list this pupil as a(n)

    A. mesomorph              B. endomorph
    C. holomorph              D. ectomorph

18. All of the following associations are correct EXCEPT   18____

    A. muscle cramp - sustained involuntary contractions
    B. muscle twitch - minor irregular spasm
    C. muscle spasticity - sustained tension
    D. muscle hypertrophy - decreased size due to loss of elasticity

19. All of the following statements are correct EXCEPT: The   19____

    A. mitral valve is between the left auricle and the left ventricle
    B. tricuspid valve is between the right auricle and the right ventricle
    C. aortic-semilunar valve is between the aorta and the right auricle
    D. pulmonary semilunar valve is between the right ventricle and the pulmonary artery

20. Urea is made in the   20____

    A. kidneys                B. liver
    C. ureter                 D. urinary bladder

21. Definite sensory centers in the brain have been found for all of the following EXCEPT   21____

    A. hearing                B. pain
    C. vision                 D. equilibrium

22. Saliva is associated with all of the following glands EXCEPT the   22____

    A. submaxillary           B. parotid
    C. fundic                 D. sublingual

23. Plasma is more advantageous than whole blood in an emergency because it   23____

    A. contains more white corpuscles
    B. does not have to be typed
    C. contains more red corpuscles
    D. contains more platelets

24. In cases of lordosis, there is a marked tendency to assume a position of round shoulders   24____
    because in such cases

    A. the body compensates for the backward shifting of the body weight
    B. too much weight is thrown on the forward edges of the lumbar vertebrae
    C. the erector spinal muscles in the thoracic region are shortened
    D. the pelvis tilts backward

25. All of the following associations of conditions and causes are correct EXCEPT    25_____
    A. carbuncle - infection of a sebaceous gland
    B. wart - excessive growth of papillae of the skin
    C. mole - overdevelopment of pigment cells under the epidermis
    D. boil - infection, usually at the site of a hair follicle

## KEY (CORRECT ANSWERS)

| | | | |
|---|---|---|---|
| 1. | A | 11. | D |
| 2. | A | 12. | C |
| 3. | B | 13. | A |
| 4. | A | 14. | D |
| 5. | A | 15. | B |
| 6. | B | 16. | C |
| 7. | A | 17. | D |
| 8. | A | 18. | D |
| 9. | B | 19. | C |
| 10. | B | 20. | B |
| 21. | B | | |
| 22. | C | | |
| 23. | B | | |
| 24. | A | | |
| 25. | A | | |

# TEST 4

DIRECTIONS: Each question or incomplete statement is followed by several suggested answers or completions. Select the one that BEST answers the question or completes the statement. *PRINT THE LETTER OF TEE CORRECT ANSWER IN THE SPACE AT THE RIGHT.*

1. All of the following associations are correct EXCEPT:  1_____

   A. Peristalsis - wavelike contractions that pass along a tube
   B. Catalysis - breaking down of body cells
   C. Catharsis - purgation
   D. Metastasis - transfer of disease from a primary focus to a distant one

2. All of the following associations concerning inflammation are correct EXCEPT:  2_____

   A. Heat - calor
   B. Redness - rubor
   C. Pain - dolor
   D. Swelling - aden

3. When the term *febrile* is associated with a physical condition, it means that the condition is characterized by  3_____

   A. fibroids
   B. weakness of an organ
   C. fever
   D. decreased respiration

4. All of the following associations are correct EXCEPT:  4_____

   A. Hepatic - pertaining to the liver
   B. Herpetic - pertaining to hair
   C. Hemiplegic - pertaining to paralysis of one side of the body
   D. Hematic - pertaining to the blood

5. All of the following are important components of the visual act proper EXCEPT  5_____

   A. accommodation
   B. interpretation
   C. convergence
   D. fusion

6. Of the following, the INCORRECT association is:  6_____

   A. Sclera - white of the eye
   B. Cornea - window of the eye
   C. Lens - pupil of the eye
   D. Iris - shutter of the eye

7. All of the following statements concerning body temperature in normal, healthy persons are correct EXCEPT:  7_____

   A. During the 24-hour day, the highest temperature is registered in the late afternoon or early evening
   B. During the 24-hour day, the lowest temperature is registered between 2 and 4 M., provided the person is not working on a night job
   C. The more or less rhythmic rise and fall of body temperature is not established until adolescence
   D. In most normal people, the variations of temperature are so small that it is difficult to detect them without the use of a special thermometer

8. It has been found that, for most people, the BEST room temperature is about F with relative humidity of about _____ %.

   A. 70; 50  B. 65; 40  C. 68; 68  D. 75; 75

9. The MOST accurate of the following tuberculin tests is the

   A. Moro Test, using a tuberculin ointment
   B. Von Pirquet Test, applying tuberculin to the scratched skin
   C. Mantoux Test, injecting tuberculin preparation between the layers of the skin
   D. Patch Test, applying tuberculin ointment to the skin by gauze and adhesive plaster

10. Rheumatic fever may affect the body in all of the following ways EXCEPT by

    A. attacking the connective tissues of the body
    B. scarring the heart valves
    C. causing inflammation of the inner lining of the heart
    D. forming a clot of blood within the heart

11. All of the following terms are associated with cancer EXCEPT

    A. scotoma  B. carcinoma  C. sarcoma  D. myeloma

12. Hemolytic streptococci are associated with all of the following EXCEPT

    A. septic sore throat         B. rheumatic fever
    C. scarlet fever              D. tuberculosis

13. All of the following statements concerning viruses are correct EXCEPT:

    A. Viruses are harder to kill than ordinary bacteria
    B. Viruses depend upon living cells for food
    C. Virus cultures can be set up with surviving cells
    D. Most of the antibiotics destroy viruses

14. Of the following diseases, the one caused by protozoa is

    A. amebic dysent ery          B. trichinosis
    C. hookworm                   D. botulism

15. All of the following statements concerning epilepsy are correct EXCEPT:

    A. Seizures in about 50% of children with this condition can be controlled
    B. The correlation of epilepsy with mental retardation is relatively high
    C. The incidence of epilepsy is higher than that of polio
    D. Encephalographs have proved helpful in the diagnosis of epileptic seizures

16. A person suffering from heterophoria may find that because of his condition

    A. he is not able to walk rapidly without distress
    B. his reflexes have become slower
    C. his eyes have a tendency to turn away from the position of binocular vision
    D. he has difficulty in hearing high pitch sounds

17. Bell's palsy usually affects the

    A. abdominal area
    B. chest
    C. lower extremities
    D. facial area

18. All of the following associations are correct EXCEPT:

    A. Histology - science which deals with tissues
    B. Pathology - science which deals with the nature of disease
    C. Cytology - science which deals with cells
    D. Geomedicine - science which deals with old age and its diseases

19. All of the following are symptoms of disorders of the circulatory system EXCEPT

    A. dyspnea
    B. hypertension
    C. enteritis
    D. cyanosis

20. The grouping of types of human blood is based upon the

    A. platelets
    B. red corpuscles
    C. white corpuscles
    D. thrombocytes

21. A vaccine is introduced into the body PRIMARILY to

    A. kill the causative organism
    B. stimulate the growth of specific antibodies
    C. inhibit the growth of the causative organism
    D. produce bacteriostasis

22. All of the following advances in medicine occurred during the last fifty years EXCEPT the

    A. discovery that malignant cells can live without oxygen
    B. regulation by vitamin C of the rate at which cholesterol is formed
    C. use of typhoid fever vaccine for cases of encephalitis
    D. conversion of normal cells into cancer cells in test tubes

23. The last year was characterized by a decrease in all of the following EXCEPT

    A. poliomyelitis cases
    B. tuberculosis deaths
    C. infant and maternal deaths from childbirth
    D. heart disease and blood vessel disturbances

24. All of the following concerning heroin are correct EXCEPT it

    A. is an antispasmodic
    B. is a derivative of opium
    C. is considered a hypnotic rather than a narcotic
    D. has mild, pain-relieving powers

25. All of the following associations are correct EXCEPT:

    A. Narcotic - novocaine
    B. Barbiturate - luminal
    C. Stimulant - amphetamine
    D. Sedative - benzedrine

## KEY (CORRECT ANSWERS)

1. B
2. D
3. C
4. B
5. B

6. C
7. C
8. A
9. C
10. D

11. A
12. D
13. D
14. A
15. B

16. C
17. D
18. D
19. C
20. B

21. B
22. A
23. B
24. C
25. D

# TEST 5

DIRECTIONS: Each question or incomplete statement is followed by several suggested answers or completions. Select the one that BEST answers the question or completes the statement. *PRINT THE LETTER OF THE CORRECT ANSWER IN THE SPACE AT THE RIGHT.*

1. Alcohol supplies to the body

    A. minerals
    B. protein
    C. calories
    D. none of the above

    1_____

2. All of the following statements concerning alcohol are correct EXCEPT:

    A. The effects of alcohol upon the brain are not felt until the alcohol begins to get into the bloodstream
    B. While alcohol is absorbed quickly by the body, it is eliminated slowly
    C. The metabolism of alcohol in the body is speeded up by increased activity
    D. The stomach cannot change alcohol

    2_____

3. Tobacco has the effect of temporarily decreasing the appetite because it causes an increased concentration of blood

    A. sugar    B. protein    C. salts    D. starches

    3_____

4. The present state of research in the relationship between the incidence of lung cancer and smoking indicates the presence of a definite relationship between lung cancer and

    A. cigarette smoking
    B. pipe smoking
    C. cigar smoking
    D. all of the above

    4_____

5. Recent research indicates that the appetite center or food intake control is located in the

    A. pancreatic gland
    B. hypothalamus located at the base of the brain
    C. nerve centers that are directly controlled by the big muscles
    D. duodenum

    5_____

6. In general, all of the following act to reduce the vitamin content in any food EXCEPT

    A. storage at room temperature for long periods
    B. freezing
    C. excessive heat
    D. prolonged cooking

    6_____

7. All of the following are vitamins EXCEPT

    A. thiamine    B. niacin    C. heparin    D. biotin

    7_____

8. All of the following associations are correct EXCEPT:

    A. Sodium and potassium - normal beating of heart
    B. Iron and copper - making of hemoglobin
    C. Calcium and phosphorus - formation of bone
    D. Chlorine and sulphur - oxidative processes

    8_____

9. Dry skim milk

   A. has the same butterfat content as homogenized milk
   B. contains considerably more fat and vitamin A than whole milk
   C. has butterfat removed
   D. loses a good deal of its nutritional value when stored for several months

10. The poisonous character of carbon monoxide is due to its tendency to unite chemically with

    A. synovial fluid           B. cerebro-spinal fluid
    C. hemoglobin               D. gastric juice

11. With regard to a tourniquet, the one CORRECT first aid procedure, according to the American Red Cross, is

    A. loosening it after 20 minutes
    B. having it released only by a physician
    C. placing it on the wound
    D. having it applied only by a physician or nurse

12. For BEST all-around use, the temperature of the water in the pool should be _____ °F.

    A. 64-68       B. 65-71       C. 72-78       D. 80-86

13. A series of progressive surface dives is an imitation of a

    A. whale       B. seahorse    C. shark       D. porpoise

14. With regard to the amount of energy expended, the MOST efficient of the following strokes is the _____ stroke.

    A. side                     B. crawl
    C. breast                   D. butterfly

15. In the case of a sprained ankle, an INCORRECT procedure in first aid would be to

    A. elevate the sprained part
    B. apply cold applications
    C. massage the part to restore circulation
    D. apply a temporary support

16. Of the following, the one which is NOT a symptom of shock is

    A. cool, clammy skin        B. weak pulse
    C. flushed face             D. feeling of weakness

17. The BEST emergency measure in a case where poison has been swallowed is to

    A. give an antiseptic
    B. give an emetic
    C. put hot applications on the stomach
    D. administer a stimulant

18. Digital pressure is used

    A. to restore consciousness in cases of white unconsciousness
    B. to control arterial bleeding
    C. after a tourniquet has been applied and has failed its purpose
    D. on the wound itself in case of a compound fracture

19. The INCORRECT procedure in treating a nosebleed is to

    A. have the victim lie down immediately
    B. press the nostrils firmly together
    C. apply a large, cold, wet cloth to the nose
    D. pack the nose gently with gauze

20. A person who has fainted should be

    A. propped up on a pillow or head rest
    B. laid flat and kept quiet
    C. given a warm drink
    D. aroused as soon as possible

21. If, during a playground activity, a person loses consciousness, he is NOT suffering from heat exhaustion if his

    A. face is pale
    B. pulse is weak and rapid
    C. skin is cold and clammy
    D. face is flushed

22. A person during an epileptic seizure should be

    A. held securely so that he will not struggle
    B. left where he has fallen
    C. carried to the rest room
    D. given a stimulant

23. A sharp-edged instrument would MOST likely cause a(n) _____ wound.

    A. abraded            B. punctured
    C. lacerated          D. incised

24. The FIRST step in the treatment of a person who is injured, unconscious, and bleeding profusely is to

    A. call a doctor
    B. stop the bleeding
    C. remove the person to a hospital
    D. revive the person

25. In treating heat exhaustion, it is imperative that you FIRST

    A. treat for shock
    B. move the patient to a place where the air is as fresh and cool as possible
    C. keep the body warmly covered
    D. lay the patient with his head low

## KEY (CORRECT ANSWERS)

| | | | |
|---|---|---|---|
| 1. | C | 11. | B |
| 2. | C | 12. | C |
| 3. | A | 13. | D |
| 4. | A | 14. | B |
| 5. | B | 15. | C |
| 6. | B | 16. | C |
| 7. | C | 17. | B |
| 8. | D | 18. | B |
| 9. | C | 19. | A |
| 10. | C | 20. | B |

21. D
22. B
23. D
24. B
25. B

# EXAMINATION SECTION
## TEST 1

DIRECTIONS: Each question or incomplete statement is followed by several suggested answers or completions. Select the one that BEST answers the question or completes the statement. *PRINT THE LETTER OF THE CORRECT ANSWER IN THE SPACE AT THE RIGHT.*

1. The INCORRECT association is:  1.____

   A. Cornea - transparent part of the outer layer of the eye
   B. Lens - part of the eye where light first enters to be focused on the retina
   C. Iris - muscle which controls the size of the pupil
   D. Sclera - hard protective outer layer of the eye

2. Of the following, the CORRECT statement is:  2.____

   A. Wearing eyeglasses will always make a person's eyes stronger
   B. If a person is able to see clearly, he can be sure he doesn't need glasses
   C. Glancing occasionally at some distant object when doing close work with the eyes helps prevent eye strain
   D. Wearing sunglasses gives the eyes complete protection from the sun

3. There is evidence that all of the following disorders of the skin are caused by a viral infection EXCEPT  3.____

   A. common warts          B. shingles
   C. moles                 D. cold sores

4. In second or third degree burns, all of the following are correct first aid procedures EXCEPT  4.____

   A. applying mineral oil to the area
   B. giving fluids by mouth
   C. providing immediate first aid for shock
   D. covering the burned area with sterile dressing

5. In the execution of the back pressure-arm lift method of artificial respiration, all of the following are correct procedures EXCEPT the one in which the operator  5.____

   A. places the victim in the prone position with the face turned to one side
   B. rocks forward with bent elbows as he exerts pressure at a 70° angle
   C. draws the arms of the victim upward and toward him during the final step of the cycle
   D. repeats the cycle at a steady rate of 12 times per minute

6. When administering first aid to a pupil experiencing an epileptic attack, the teacher should FIRST  6.____

   A. loosen clothing about the neck and chest
   B. remove the victim to a room other than a classroom filled with pupils
   C. place an object between the victim's upper and lower teeth on one side of the mouth
   D. apply an ammonia ampule to the victim's nostrils

2 (#1)

7. The four types of wounds are 7.___

   A. scrapes, cuts, burns, and stabs
   B. punctures, lacerations, incisions, and abrasions
   C. friction burns, open blisters, gashes, and punctures
   D. scratches, infections, sores, and bleeding cuts

8. The group of symptoms BEST describing a case of shock is 8.___

   A. extreme thirst, skin dry, breathing deep, and pulse irregular
   B. face flushed, pulse full, pupils constricted, and nausea
   C. pulse absent, skin hot, breathing heavy, and face ashen
   D. body weakness, skin moist, pupils dilated, and breathing shallow

9. For an insect sting on the neck, the first-aider should apply to the injured part 9.___

   A. a cut in the skin at the spot to encourage bleeding in order to remove impurities
   B. suction in order to remove the injected toxin
   C. ice applications
   D. hot, wet applications

10. In regard to first aid procedures, priority in treatment should be given FIRST to cases of 10.___

    A. internal poisoning
    B. severe eye injuries
    C. stoppage of breathing
    D. severe bleeding at the neck

11. No amount of vitamin D will serve to promote normal bone development unless the diet includes, in adequate quantities, 11.___

    A. calcium and phosphorus        B. sodium and sulfur
    C. iron and magnesium            D. potassium and carbon

12. All of the following associations concerning milk are correct EXCEPT: 12.___

    A. Pasteurization - destruction of the common pathogens found in milk
    B. Homogenization - process of emulsifying milk
    C. Irradiation - sterilization of raw milk
    D. Centrifugalization - separation of cream from the milk

13. It is INCORRECT to state that cholesterol 13.___

    A. metabolism is related to atherosclerosis
    B. is a normal and essential constituent of human tissue
    C. levels in the blood are related to intake of animal fats
    D. levels in the blood are lowered by intake of saturated fats

14. Of the following, the one that is NOT an after-effect of rickets is 14.___

    A. bow-legs                      B. chicken breast
    C. knock-knees                   D. clubfoot

15. All of the following concerning amino acids are correct EXCEPT:

    A. All amino acids contain carbon, hydrogen, oxygen, and nitrogen
    B. Excess amino acids are stored in the involuntary musculature of the body
    C. Proteins are made up of amino acids
    D. Amino acids play an important role in maintaining both natural and acquired resistance to infection

16. Of the following, the CORRECT statement is:

    A. All people with rosy complexions are healthy
    B. Any food that does not smell or taste spoiled is safe to eat
    C. All children with heart murmurs will surely have heart trouble later on in life
    D. Most persons who look thin and underweight are not necessarily in poor health

17. All of the following are important in tooth development EXCEPT vitamin

    A. A  B. C  C. B  D. D

18. A sprain in any part of the body PRIMARILY involves the _____ tissue.

    A. ligament  B. nerve  C. skin  D. muscle

19. All of the following drugs are sedatives EXCEPT

    A. cocaine  B. marijuana  C. morphine  D. luminal

20. All of the following associations are correct EXCEPT:

    A. Barbiturate - produces relaxation
    B. Emollient - relieves anxiety
    C. Soporific - induces nervous stimulation
    D. Analgesic - allays pain

21. Of the following, the MOST desirable question is:

    A. Which mineral is used chiefly in the hardening of bones, calcium or iron?
    B. What one thing must we do to become healthy and strong?
    C. What about vitamins in this day and age?
    D. Why is it necessary to eat an adequate breakfast?

22. All of the following associations are correct EXCEPT:

    A. Dynamometer - measures muscle strength
    B. Manometer - measures strength of hand grip
    C. Anthropometry - measurement of the body or its various parts
    D. Ergometer - calculates work performed by a muscle or group of muscles over a specified time

23. The relationship between two consecutive administrations of a test is expressed in terms of the

    A. degree of objectivity
    B. validity coefficient
    C. reliability coefficient
    D. degree of relationship between criterion and the test

24. Vitamin A deficiency is associated with all of the following EXCEPT  24.___
    A. faulty development of the teeth
    B. impairment of vision in dim light
    C. impairment of epithelial tissue
    D. retardation in the development of bones]

25. The substances which are NOT necessary for building new tissues are  25.___
    A. water           B. carbohydrates
    C. proteins        D. minerals

---

## KEY (CORRECT ANSWERS)

1. B
2. C
3. C
4. A
5. B

6. C
7. B
8. D
9. C
10. D

11. A
12. C
13. D
14. D
15. B

16. D
17. C
18. A
19. A
20. C

21. D
22. B
23. C
24. D
25. B

---

# TEST 2

DIRECTIONS: Each question or incomplete statement is followed by several suggested answers or completions. Select the one that BEST answers the question or completes the statement. *PRINT THE LETTER OF THE CORRECT ANSWER IN THE SPACE AT THE RIGHT.*

1. A nutrient functions in any or all of the following ways EXCEPT to   1._____

    A. furnish energy
    B. provide materials for building or maintenance of body tissues
    C. help regulate body processes
    D. purify the blood

2. It is MOST important to see that reducing diets of adolescents do not lack   2._____

    A. fats
    B. proteins
    C. carbohydrates
    D. simple sugars

3. The CHIEF value of cellulose in the diet is that it   3._____

    A. is more soluble than starch
    B. gives bulk to the intestinal residues
    C. is easily digested
    D. provides an essential amino acid

4. It is CORRECT to state that enzymes   4._____

    A. are used up in chemical reactions of foods
    B. retard the process of breaking down of foods
    C. work only in acid surroundings
    D. are specific in their action

5. All of the following are important functions of fat EXCEPT that it   5._____

    A. supports and protects organs
    B. prevents the loss of heat from the body surface
    C. is used in the building and repairing of tissues
    D. serves as a reserve supply of fuel

6. All of the following concerning cheese made from whole milk are correct EXCEPT that it   6._____

    A. preserves its milk nutrients for longer periods than the liquid itself
    B. is readily digested provided it is eaten slowly and in moderation
    C. loses its fat value when cooked
    D. is a source of riboflavin

7. The sugar which can be used by the body without having to be broken down into simpler sugars is   7._____

    A. lactose    B. glucose    C. maltose    D. sucrose

8. The cells which have the property of engulfing and digesting foreign particles harmful to the body are called

   A. osteocytes
   B. phagocytes
   C. mast
   D. plasma

9. The INCORRECT association of covering and tissue is

   A. periosteum - bone
   B. perimysium - muscle
   C. peritoneum - heart
   D. perichondrium - cartilage

10. An acquired reduction in size of an organ which had previously reached mature size is called

    A. hyperotrophy
    B. atrophy
    C. necrosis
    D. calcification

11. All of the following associations are correct EXCEPT:

    A. Myocardial - pertaining to the heart muscle
    B. Myoneural - pertaining to both muscle and nerve
    C. Myogenic - having origin in the muscle
    D. Myocytic - pertaining to muscular spasm

12. All of the following are concerned with the clotting of blood EXCEPT

    A. cholesterol
    B. blood platelets
    C. vitamin K
    D. prothrombin

13. Blood plays an important role in all of the following EXCEPT in the

    A. regulation of body temperature
    B. removal of waste products
    C. maintenance of water balance
    D. production of acidity of body fluids

14. Of the following, the gland MOST closely related to muscular efficiency is the

    A. adrenal    B. gonads    C. pituitary    D. thyroid

15. The INCORRECT association of gland and location is

    A. pineal - brain cavity
    B. parotid - below and in front of the ear
    C. submaxillary - below each lower jaw
    D. thymus - at the larynx

16. A urine analysis does NOT test for the

    A. possibility of diabetes
    B. presence of albumin
    C. evidence of bladder or kidney inflammation
    D. growth of polyps in the urinary tract

17. All of the following are basic taste sensations EXCEPT _____ sensations.

    A. hot and cold
    B. sweet
    C. bitter
    D. sour

18. The accumulation of an oxygen debt by a normally healthy individual engaged in sport activity is related MOST directly to       18.____

    A. lack of endurance
    B. limited residual air
    C. strenuous exercise
    D. failure of the hemoglobin to combine with oxygen

19. The CHIEF cause of heart disease in persons under 40 years of age is       19.____

    A. heredity                B. rheumatic fever
    C. obesity                 D. elevated blood pressure

20. Normally, upon exposure to air, blood clots form within _____ minutes.       20.____

    A. 30 seconds to two       B. three to ten
    C. ten to fifteen          D. fifteen to thirty

21. The red blood cells of the body are produced in the       21.____

    A. spongy area of the long bones, in the ribs, and in the vertebrae
    B. ends of the long bones and the spleen
    C. liver and the flat bones
    D. pancreas and the liver

22. All of the following statements are correct EXCEPT:       22.____

    A. The figures used for the recording of blood pressure represent, in millimeters, the height of a column of mercury in the sphygmomanometer
    B. In high blood pressure cases, progressive damage to the blood vessels takes place, whereas hypertension is limited to harder than normal work by the heart to pump the same amount of blood around to the tissues
    C. In the recording of blood pressure, the larger figure represents the maximum pressure in the arteries with each heart beat
    D. The smaller figure in the recording of an individual's blood pressure registers the minimum pressure between heart beats

23. The physician can actually see the arteries and veins at work when he       23.____

    A. measures the pressure of the walls of the blood vessels
    B. uses the ophthalmoscope in examining a patient
    C. applies a fluoroscope in examining a patient
    D. uses the electrocardiograph

24. The blood-clotting process in the body is started by the breaking up of       24.____

    A. plasma                  B. platelets
    C. white blood cells       D. red blood cells

25. The condition that impairs the elasticity and function of the blood vessel walls and reduces the volume of blood that may pass through the afflicted arteries is       25.____

    A. hypertension            B. vascular occlusion
    C. high blood pressure     D. hardening of the arteries

## KEY (CORRECT ANSWERS)

| | | | |
|---|---|---|---|
| 1. | D | 11. | D |
| 2. | B | 12. | A |
| 3. | B | 13. | D |
| 4. | D | 14. | A |
| 5. | C | 15. | D |
| 6. | C | 16. | D |
| 7. | B | 17. | A |
| 8. | B | 18. | C |
| 9. | C | 19. | B |
| 10. | B | 20. | B |

21. A
22. B
23. B
24. B
25. D

# TEST 3

DIRECTIONS: Each question or incomplete statement is followed by several suggested answers or completions. Select the one that BEST answers the question or completes the statement. *PRINT THE LETTER OF THE CORRECT ANSWER IN THE SPACE AT THE RIGHT.*

1. All of the following statements are correct EXCEPT: 1._____

    A. There is more limited mobility of the big toe of the foot compared to that of the thumb on the hand
    B. The foot bones are held together in such a way as to form springy lengthwise and crosswise arches
    C. The much greater solidity of the big toe as compared to the fingers on the hand help the foot to support body weight
    D. The phalanges of the foot are relatively more important than those of the hand and have a greater role in the functioning of the foot than those in the hand

2. The inside of the shaft of a long bone is filled with 2._____

    A. yellow marrow          B. compact bony cells
    C. red blood cells        D. gelatinous tissue

3. Children's bones do not break so easily as those of older persons because their bones 3._____

    A. are less flexible
    B. do not carry so heavy a weight
    C. contain more cartilage
    D. receive better nutritional foods

4. All of the following associations are correct EXCEPT: 4._____

    A. Intracutaneous - within the layers of the skin
    B. Hypodermic - beneath the skin
    C. Subcutaneous - sweat glands over the entire skin surface
    D. Diaphoresis - perceptible perspiration

5. The PRIMARY purpose of melanin is to 5._____

    A. provide variation in the toughness of the skin
    B. prevent the more dangerous rays of the sun from damaging tissues
    C. convert surface skin on certain parts of the body into horny material
    D. dilate the blood vessels in the skin

6. Of the following, the SAFEST treatment for corns on toes is to 6._____

    A. apply a medicated moleskin plaster to the area
    B. wear well-fitted shoes
    C. cut off the mass of dead skin cells on the surface of the corn
    D. apply a corn remover

7. Of the following statements, the CORRECT one is:

   A. Suntan preparations enable an individual to stay in the sun longer with less risk of burning than without their use
   B. Suntan lotions increase the speed of one's natural tanning mechanism
   C. Suntan preparations shut out burning ultraviolet rays
   D. The application of suntan preparations is more effective when used during exposure to direct mid-day hours of sun rather than used on hazy, lightly overcast days

8. The MAIN objective in first aid care for a victim of poison by mouth is to

   A. first induce vomiting
   B. dilute the poison
   C. give an antidote
   D. look around for tell-tale evidence of the poison

9. With victims of shock, when medical help is not immediate, water should NOT be given to those who have

   A. suffered marked bleeding
   B. burns involving more than 10 percent of the body surface
   C. a penetrating abdominal wound
   D. a fracture of the femur

10. The INCORRECT association of first aid bandage and body area of use is:

    A. Four-tailed bandage - nose
    B. Cravat bandage - knee
    C. Triangular bandage - head
    D. Figure-eight bandage - chest

11. In the case of severe bleeding from a hand, the first-aider should IMMEDIATELY

    A. locate the pressure point above the wound and apply digital pressure at that point
    B. apply pressure directly on the wound with clean gauze or a towel
    C. apply a tourniquet in order to limit the flow of blood from the artery to the wound
    D. locate the pressure point and apply a tourniquet at that point

12. The UNIVERSAL antidote to be administered in poisoning cases if no specific antidote is known consists of

    A. several teaspoonfuls of baking soda in half a glass of water
    B. a large glass of milk diluted with an equal amount of water
    C. one part tea, two parts crumbled burnt toast, one part milk of magnesia
    D. one part milk, one part egg white, one part water

13. Of the following concerning mouth-to-mouth resuscitation, the operator can BEST be sure that no obstruction exists in the victim's air passage by following his first blowing efforts with a

    A. sharp tilt backward of the victim's head so that the chin points almost directly upward
    B. forceful opening of the victim's mouth as the victim's nostrils are held in a closed position

C. removal of his mouth by turning his head to the side in order to listen for the return rush of air from the victim's body
D. removal of mucous and foreign matter in the victim's mouth

14. If a particle is on the eyeball, one should NOT

   A. close his eyes for a few minutes in order to allow the tears to wash out the foreign matter
   B. grasp the lashes of the upper lid and draw it out and down over the lower lid in order to dislodge the particle
   C. use an eye dropper in order to flush the eye so that the particle will float out of the eye
   D. examine the eye in order to determine the location of the foreign particle and, when found, remove it from the eyeball by touching lightly with the moistened corner of a clean handkerchief

15. The LARGEST source of body heat is the _____ system.

   A. digestive    B. muscular
   C. tegumentary    D. nervous

16. The three points of support of the longitudinal arch of the foot include all of the following EXCEPT the

   A. anterior head of the first metatarsal bone
   B. anterior head of the fifth metatarsal bone
   C. anterior head of the astragalus
   D. calcaneus

17. Long bone growth is at its MAXIMUM in the _____ period.

   A. adolescent    B. pre-adolescent
   C. early childhood    D. infancy

18. The acetabulum is the anticular cup in a bone which acts as a socket for the

   A. clavicle    B. femur    C. radius    D. tibia

19. Of the following associations, the CORRECT one is:

   A. Second class lever - the forearm when it is being extended by the triceps muscle
   B. Third class lever - the foot, when rising on the toes
   C. First class lever - the head, tipping forward and backward
   D. Second class lever - the arm when it is raised sideward - upward by the deltoid muscle

20. The INCORRECT statement is:

   A. The heart of the adolescent is especially vulnerable to the stress of exercise
   B. Exercise tolerance of children is usually higher than that of adults
   C. Cardiac examinations have shown that the world's best athletic performers in the Olympics have hearts larger than normal
   D. Participation in competitive athletics should be postponed pending complete recovery after infections

21. Blood pressure is associated with all of the following EXCEPT the  21.___

    A. force of the heart beat
    B. elasticity of the walls of the blood vessels
    C. number of leucocytes present in the blood
    D. viscosity of the blood

22. In infancy, _____ is(are) more rapid than in adulthood.  22.___

    A. the heart beat
    B. the oxidation processes
    C. the respiration rate
    D. all of the above

23. All of the following are correct principles relating to the muscular system EXCEPT:  23.___

    A. Muscles contract more rapidly following warm-up activities
    B. Muscular strength is progressively developed by the repetition of exercises of the same intensity
    C. Muscles contract more forcefully if they are first stretched, provided that they are not overstretched
    D. A muscle must be loaded beyond its customary load if strength is to be increased

24. Gradations in muscular contraction are related to  24.___

    A. variations in intensity of muscular contraction
    B. the number of fibers in the muscle which contract
    C. the circulation of blood within the muscle
    D. the manufacture of lactic acid in the muscle

25. In order to determine the basal metabolic rate of an individual, all of the following conditions must be included EXCEPT that the  25.___

    A. environment temperature must be comfortably warm
    B. test must be made from 12 to 18 hours after the last meal
    C. body must be in the waking state and at complete rest
    D. test should be preceded by a ten-minute period of vigorous exercise

## KEY (CORRECT ANSWERS)

1. D
2. A
3. C
4. C
5. B

6. B
7. A
8. B
9. C
10. D

11. B
12. C
13. C
14. D
15. B

16. C
17. B
18. B
19. C
20. A

21. C
22. D
23. B
24. B
25. D

# TEST 4

DIRECTIONS: Each question or incomplete statement is followed by several suggested answers or completions. Select the one that BEST answers the question or completes the statement. *PRINT THE LETTER OF THE CORRECT ANSWER IN THE SPACE AT THE RIGHT.*

1. Static and moving body postures are BEST judged on the basis of

    A. how well they meet the demands made upon them
    B. comparison with standardized charts
    C. muscular strength
    D. body flexibility

2. All of the following increase the efficiency of lifting heavy objects from the floor EXCEPT

    A. flexing the knees
    B. bending forward from the waist
    C. holding the object as close to the body as possible
    D. keeping the feet slightly separated both laterally and anteroposteriorly

3. All of the following associations are correct EXCEPT:

    A. Dorsal flexion - bending the foot at the ankle and elevating the front of the foot and toes
    B. Supination - turning the foot outward in its relation to the leg
    C. Plantar flexion - depressing the front of the foot and toes
    D. Adduction - turning the foot inward in its relation to the leg

4. All of the following concerning the Kraus-Weber Test for muscular fitness are correct EXCEPT:

    A. Failure on any one of the subtests classifies a child as a muscular fitness failure
    B. Flexibility in this test is measured by having the child bend forward slowly and touch his fingertips to the floor without bending his knees
    C. The grip-strength test does not have much value since there is little relationship between grip strength and general body strength
    D. The test measures large muscle groups of the upper and lower back, the abdominal wall, and flexors of the hip joint

5. Of the following, the one which is designed to reveal whether a child's growth is progressing properly in terms of his own body build is the

    A. Pryor Width - Weight Tables
    B. Wetzel Grid
    C. Quinby Weight Analysis Test
    D. Rogers Strength Index of Physical Fitness Index

6. The center of gravity of an individual of average build in an erect standing position is

    A. located in the pelvis in front of the upper part of the sacrum
    B. located at the articulation of the femur and the pelvis
    C. located in the anterior wall of the pelvis
    D. lower in men than in women because of anatomical structure

7. All of the following statements concerning lateral curvatures of the spine are correct EXCEPT:

    A. Some rotation of the vertebrae always accompanies lateral flexion of the spine
    B. In a simple structural lateral curvature, the curve is confined to one region and there is no compensatory curve
    C. The shoulder on the side of a dorsal convexity is lower than the other shoulder
    D. In a functional lateral curvature of the spine, the curve disappears when the individual suspends his body by hanging from the arms

8. All of the following are necessary for proper seating EXCEPT that the pupil's

    A. lumbar region of the spine should be supported by the back of the chair
    B. feet should rest squarely on the floor
    C. hips should be pushed back in the chair as far as possible
    D. knees should be firmly supported by the forward edge of the seat

9. The cervical and lumbar spinal curves

    A. are in opposite directions to each other
    B. are inflexible
    C. are present at birth
    D. result from the efforts of the child to assume the upright position

10. Aseptic techniques in medicine are credited to

    A. Lister   B. Koch   C. Pasteur   D. Harvey

11. The disease which has caused MOST absenteeism from work is

    A. heart trouble
    C. rheumatic fever
    B. the common cold
    D. arteriosclerosis

12. All of the following concerning whooping cough are correct EXCEPT that it

    A. has caused fewer fatalities during the past 50 years than during the latter half of the 19th century
    B. can be reduced by use of a preventive vaccine
    C. is the only childhood disease that kills more boys than girls
    D. kills more babies in their first year of life than all other common infectious diseases combined

13. All of the following statements concerning rheumatic fever are correct EXCEPT:

    A. Prevention of initial attacks of rheumatic fever is accomplished through prompt treatment with penicillin
    B. A streptococcus throat infection almost always leads to rheumatic fever
    C. Recurrent attacks of rheumatic fever may be forestalled through long-term use of antibiotics or sulfa drugs
    D. Not all children who have rheumatic fever develop serious heart conditions

14. All of the following statements concerning tuberculosis are correct EXCEPT:

    A. In the United States, tuberculosis morbidity and mortality rates reach their greatest heights among young children
    B. The Mantoux test screens out people who harbor tubercular germs in their bodies
    C. One of the important factors leading to a greater decrease in deaths from tuberculosis is the control of the disease among cattle
    D. The factor no longer considered necessary in the treatment of tuberculosis is special climate

15. Of the following, the exercise BEST suited to the development of the latissimus dorsi muscles is

    A. leg raising from the standing position
    B. chinning on the horizontal bar
    C. performing push-ups from the floor
    D. standing barbell presses

16. Exercises done in the recumbent position

    A. require as much balance effort as when performed in the sitting position
    B. are less likely to fatigue the individual than when done in any other position
    C. are free from the pull of gravity
    D. should be limited to therapeutic use of musculature

17. Of the following, the one that BEST describes a passive exercise is the one in which the

    A. speed and vigor in the performance of the exercise is greatly reduced
    B. body parts are manipulated by some external force without active effort on the part of the recipient
    C. range of movement is limited within the physiological limits of a given part of the body
    D. individual moves the part to the desired position slowly because of the antagonistic muscular pull

18. In the performance of *the sit-up* exercise, the *sit-up* phase is MOST difficult if the performer

    A. crosses his arms over the chest so that each hand is on the opposite shoulder
    B. holds his arms forward at shoulder height
    C. places his hands at the back of the neck
    D. puts his hands on his hips

19. Of the following exercises, the one considered BEST for developing flexibility is the

    A. jumping jack          B. push-up
    C. running in place      D. squat thrust

20. All of the following associations of muscle and action are correct EXCEPT:

    A. Trapezius - pulls head backward
    B. Triceps - extends arm
    C. Leg adductors - moves legs apart
    D. Sterno-mastoid - moves head sideways

21. In evaluation, if all the scores made are added and divided by the number of individuals, the result obtained is the

    A. mean     B. range     C. median     D. mode

22. In regard to safe participation in sports, it is INCORRECT to state that

    A. both body and mind should be in the best possible condition in order to participate successfully in strenuous athletics
    B. many injuries are caused by an over-enthusiastic attempt on the part of the individual who lacks adequate training
    C. alertness to possible irregularities on the playing surface in the play environment can avoid needless injury
    D. many injuries occur when the individual *eases up* instead of playing hard throughout the period of physical activity

23. All of the following statements concerning isometric exercise are correct EXCEPT:

    A. An isometric contraction is one in which the subject exerts muscular force against a resistance that moves
    B. An isometric contraction can develop muscular strength at any point of stimulation throughout a range of motion
    C. An isometric exercise program should be individual rather than general in nature
    D. For best results, isometric exercises should be followed by appropriate stretching exercises

24. A program of body conditioning in preparation for participation in athletics should aim to provide for all of the following EXCEPT the

    A. accomplishment of the physical activity at peak performance without injury
    B. ability of the muscle to respond repetitively for a relatively long period of time
    C. effective use of the muscle group throughout its maximum range of motions
    D. participation in a general program of sports which in itself provides optimum benefit to the participant

25. Of the following principles associated with postural exercise, the INCORRECT one is the

    A. higher the center of gravity, the easier it is to maintain balance
    B. more sequential the movement, the more force obtainable
    C. broader the base of support, the easier the exercise is to perform
    D. slower the contraction of the muscles during the performance of an exercise, the greater the gain in strength

# KEY (CORRECT ANSWERS)

| | | | |
|---|---|---|---|
| 1. | A | 11. | B |
| 2. | B | 12. | C |
| 3. | B | 13. | B |
| 4. | C | 14. | A |
| 5. | B | 15. | B |
| 6. | A | 16. | C |
| 7. | C | 17. | D |
| 8. | D | 18. | D |
| 9. | D | 19. | A |
| 10. | A | 20. | C |

21. A
22. D
23. C
24. B
25. A

# TEST 5

DIRECTIONS: Each question or incomplete statement is followed by several suggested answers or completions. Select the one that BEST answers the question or completes the statement. *PRINT THE LETTER OF THE CORRECT ANSWER IN THE SPACE AT THE RIGHT.*

1. The body's stability will NOT be increased by    1.____

   A. *lowering* the center of gravity
   B. *decreasing* the weight of the body
   C. *increasing* the base of support
   D. *centering* the line of gravity with the base of support

2. The condition in which the coagulation time of the blood is prolonged is    2.____

   A. hematoma              B. hemolysis
   C. hemoptysis            D. hemophilia

3. Of the following, the one LEAST associated with degeneration of blood vessels is    3.____

   A. arteriosclerosis      B. thrombosis
   C. atherosclerosis       D. homeostasis

4. Normally, the pulse rate is    4.____

   A. *higher* in children than in adults
   B. *lower* in women than in men
   C. *higher* when accompanied with low blood pressure
   D. *lower* when fever is present

5. Leucocytosis almost always indicates    5.____

   A. malnutrition          B. hemorrhage
   C. anemia                D. infection in the body

6. All of the following movements are possible in the cervical region of the spinal column EXCEPT    6.____

   A. lateral flexion       B. pronation
   C. hyperextension        D. rotation

7. All of the following associations of body joints are correct EXCEPT:    7.____

   A. Gliding - wrist       B. Pivot - knee
   C. Hinge - elbow         D. Ball-and-socket - shoulder

8. Of the following, the one which is NOT absorbed by the body in the form in which it is consumed is    8.____

   A. fats                  B. mineral salts
   C. water                 D. meat extracts

9. Of the following associations of digestive fluid and enzyme activity, the INCORRECT one is    9.____

   A. intestinal juice - protein-splitting enzyme
   B. saliva - starch-splitting enzyme

153

C. pancreatic juice - fat-splitting enzyme
D. gastric juice - sugar-splitting enzyme

10. The LARGEST source of body heat is the _____ system.

    A. nervous
    B. digestive
    C. tegumentary
    D. muscular

11. The gland which plays the leading role in regulating the physiological processes of the body is the

    A. pituitary    B. adrenal    C. pancreas    D. thymus

12. All of the following concerning hyperthyroidism are correct EXCEPT that in this condition there is

    A. a tendency to gain weight
    B. an increase in the heart rate
    C. an enlargement of the thyroid gland
    D. protrusion of the eyeballs

13. It is INCORRECT to state that

    A. in many cases epileptic seizures can be controlled
    B. during an epileptic seizure, the individual is insensible to pain
    C. there is a high correlation between epilepsy and mental retardation
    D. predisposition to epilepsy may be discovered by recording the electric currents given off by the brain

14. The medulla oblongata contains all of the following centers EXCEPT the

    A. cardiac
    B. heat-regulating
    C. vasomotor
    D. respiratory

15. The use of specific drugs in treating infective diseases within the body is classified as

    A. chemotherapy
    B. gerontology
    C. immunology
    D. stereochromy

16. It is INCORRECT to state that a toxoid

    A. is made from the poison produced by the germ of a specific disease
    B. is so treated that when injected into the body it may cause discomfort but not the illness
    C. stimulates the body to develop its own antibodies
    D. brings about life-long immunization from a disease

17. Of the following, the one that represents artificial immunization against a disease is

    A. recovering from an attack of whooping cough
    B. the result of exposure to streptococcal infections
    C. vaccination against smallpox
    D. the use of antibodies which prevent mononucleosis

18. Vitamin D and phosphorus are essential for the utilization of _____ in the body.  18._____

    A. iron          B. copper         C. iodine         D. calcium

19. All of the following conditions are the result of a vitamin deficiency EXCEPT  19._____

    A. beriberi      B. pellagra       C. cretinism      D. rickets

20. All of the following statements are correct EXCEPT:  20._____

    A. Iron is relatively high in foods of low moisture content
    B. More than half of the iron in the body is in the hemoglobin of the red blood cells
    C. Iron-deficient individuals can absorb more iron from food than healthy persons
    D. When the diet's supply of iron is in excess of body needs, it is stored in the liver for later use

21. Of the following foods, the one with the LEAST number of calories is one  21._____

    A. cup of cooked spinach
    B. medium raw orange
    C. cup of popped popcorn
    D. cup of raw shredded cabbage

22. Weight reduction is BEST realized if the individual  22._____

    A. consumes his daily allotment of foods but abstains from food every other day
    B. pursues a liquid diet until desirable weight is reached
    C. follows a diet including foods high in nutrients but low in calories
    D. routinizes daily exercise with a diet low in fats

23. In bitter cold weather, regulation of the body temperature is accomplished MAINLY through the  23._____

    A. oxidation of organic foods
    B. activity of the muscles
    C. radiation from the surface of the skin
    D. increased respiratory action

24. Of the following uses of water in the body, the INCORRECT one is that it  24._____

    A. makes enzyme action possible
    B. moistens the surfaces of the lungs for gas diffusion
    C. serves as a source of energy
    D. assists in hydrolytic changes during digestion

25. If an individual takes a bitter medicine and swallows it quickly with water, he will experience more of the bitter taste if he first places it  25._____

    A. under the tongue
    B. at the tip of his tongue
    C. to the side of the mouth
    D. on the back of his tongue

## KEY (CORRECT ANSWERS)

1. B
2. D
3. D
4. A
5. D

6. B
7. B
8. A
9. D
10. D

11. A
12. A
13. C
14. B
15. A

16. D
17. C
18. D
19. C
20. C

21. D
22. C
23. B
24. C
25. D

# EXAMINATION SECTION
## TEST 1

DIRECTIONS: Each question or incomplete statement is followed by several suggested answers or completions. Select the one that BEST answers the question or completes the statement. *PRINT THE LETTER OF THE CORRECT ANSWER IN THE PACE AT THE RIGHT.*

1. Of the following body parts, one LONGEST is the

    A. trachea    B. meatus    C. cecum    D. Eustachian tube

2. All of the following are ductless glands EXCEPT the

    A. parotid    B. pineal    C. thymus    D. adrenals

3. Of the following, the tissue that has a capillary system is the

    A. dermis    B. hair    C. nails    D. outer layer of skin

4. All of the following concerning a bursa are correct EXCEPT that

    A. it is a closed sac which contains a small amount of fluid
    B. its inner lining secretes fluid
    C. it prevents friction between muscles and underlying parts
    D. arthritis is caused by inflammation of the bursa

5. In regard to body temperature, the INCORRECT statement is:

    A. Mouth temperature recording is lower than that of the rectum
    B. Since the heat-regulating center does not function well for a time after birth, new babies need to be kept somewhat warmer than adults
    C. The body temperature record obtained in the armpit is higher than that obtained from the mouth
    D. In the morning, body temperature is low because of relaxed muscles as well as lack of food

6. All of the following are effects of cigarette smoking EXCEPT a(n)

    A. increase in the heart beat
    B. constriction of the coronary arteries
    C. increase in blood pressure
    D. rise in the metabolic rate

7. All of the following statements concerning the intake of alcohol in the body are correct EXCEPT:

    A. Although alcohol has a caloric content, it is expended instead of being stored in the body
    B. A small percentage of the alcohol taken into the body is eliminated through the lungs
    C. Alcohol produces a feeling of warmth with an actual lowering of body temperature
    D. Digestive changes are necessary before alcohol can be absorbed from the stomach

8. The stimulant theobromine is found in all of the following EXCEPT

   A. cocoa  B. chocolate  C. tea  D. coffee

9. Recent research indicates that the appetite center or food intake control is located in the

   A. pancreatic gland
   B. hypothalamus located at the base of the brain
   C. nerve centers that are directly controlled by the big muscles
   D. duodenum

10. In general, all of the following act to reduce the vitamin content in any food EXCEPT

    A. storage at room temperature for long periods
    B. freezing
    C. excessive heat
    D. prolonged cooking

11. In general, when more than a half hour elapses after an accident, fluid administration should be considered for conscious victims in all of the following cases EXCEPT a

    A. fracture of the femur
    B. hemorrhage
    C. burn involving more than ten percent of the body surface
    D. penetrating abdominal wound

12. In general, NO local first aid measures are necessary in a rib fracture case if the

    A. pain is minimal
    B. swelling is hardly noticeable
    C. breathing causes discomfort
    D. deformity indicates the presence of a fracture

13. All of the following movements are possible in the cervical region of the spinal column EXCEPT

    A. lateral flexion        B. pronation
    C. hyperextension         D. rotation

14. In bitter cold weather, regulation of the body temperature is accomplished MAINLY through the

    A. oxidation of organic foods
    B. activity of the muscles
    C. radiation from the surface of the skin
    D. increased respiratory action

15. Of the following uses of water in the body, the INCORRECT one is that it

    A. makes enzyme action possible
    B. moistens the surfaces of the lungs for gas diffusion
    C. serves as a source of energy
    D. assists in hydrolytic changes during digestion

16. Of the following, the one that does NOT destroy or inhibit microorganisms is

   A. germicides  B. antiseptics
   C. disinfectants  D. prophylactics

17. Of the following foods, the one with the FEWEST number of calories is one

   A. cup of cooked spinach
   B. medium raw orange
   C. cup of popped popcorn
   D. cup of raw shredded cabbage

18. Weight reduction is BEST realized if the individual

   A. consumes his daily allotment of foods but abstains from food every other day
   B. pursues a liquid diet until desirable weight is reached
   C. follows a diet including foods high in nutrients but low in calories
   D. routinizes daily exercise with a diet low in fats

19. A group of symptoms that occur together and characterize a disease is a

   A. prognosis  B. syndrome  C. crisis  D. sequela

20. During sleep, all of the following occur EXCEPT a

   A. respiration which is slower and deeper than when awake
   B. loss of a degree of muscle tone
   C. cessation of reflexes
   D. fall in blood pressure

21. Metatarsalgia is

   A. less frequent in women than in men
   B. associated with a flat anterior arch of the foot
   C. a condition in which the second joint of the big toe is enlarged
   D. irritation of the bursa lying beneath the tendon of Achilles

22. In climbing stairs, of the following, the LEAST effective measure is to

   A. incline the body slightly forward from the ankles
   B. depend upon the extension of the knee for the lifting of the body
   C. place the forward foot flat on the next step
   D. keep the body weight over the foot on the lower step until the hip is extended

23. The lymphatic system discharges its contents into the

   A. heart  B. venous bloodstream
   C. aorta  D. arteries

24. Overexposure to sunlight is considered a MAJOR cause of

   A. premature aging of the skin
   B. arthritis
   C. brittle bones
   D. asthma

25. All of the following statements are correct EXCEPT: 25.____
    A. Iron is relatively high in foods of low moisture content
    B. More than half of the iron in the body is in the hemoglobin of the red blood cells
    C. Iron-deficient individuals can absorb more iron from food than healthy persons
    D. When the diet's supply of iron is in excess of body needs, it is stored in the liver for later use

---

## KEY (CORRECT ANSWERS)

1. A
2. A
3. A
4. D
5. C

6. B
7. D
8. D
9. B
10. B

11. D
12. A
13. B
14. B
15. C

16. D
17. D
18. C
19. B
20. C

21. B
22. D
23. B
24. A
25. C

---

# TEST 2

DIRECTIONS: Each question or incomplete statement is followed by several suggested answers or completions. Select the one that BEST answers the question or completes the statement. *PRINT THE LETTER OF THE CORRECT ANSWER IN THE SPACE AT THE RIGHT.*

1. After prolonged exercise, muscle fatigue results from   1.____

   A. an accumulation of lactic acid
   B. tired blood
   C. a lack of second wind
   D. a neuromuscular defect

2. The lengthwise plane which runs from front to back, dividing the body into right and left sides, is known as the _____ plane.   2.____

   A. coronal   B. sagittal   C. frontal   D. transverse

3. Resultant rhythm   3.____

   A. is the shifting of accents as a result of combining two unequal time values
   B. is one note against another, or melody against melody
   C. is successive additions to the original time
   D. does not have accents appearing on the regularly stressed beat

4. A PRIME purpose of warm-up exercises is to   4.____

   A. prepare the body for activity that is to follow
   B. develop physical fitness
   C. gradually increase lung capacity
   D. replace used up glycogen

5. Of the following, the one LEAST recommended for routine control of *athlete's foot* is to   5.____

   A. dry the feet carefully after bathing
   B. dust the feet with medicated powder
   C. change socks daily
   D. apply gentian violet to the feet before retiring

6. A skin disorder caused by a fungus infection is   6.____

   A. athlete's foot          B. impetigo
   C. boils                   D. eczema

7. In assuming the crouch start in track, the sprinter brings all of the following muscle groups into action EXCEPT the   7.____

   A. flexor muscles of the shoulder joint
   B. extensor muscles of the spine
   C. flexor muscles of the knee
   D. extensor muscles of the hip

161

8. In chinning the bar, LEAST use is made of the _____ muscle.

   A. biceps
   B. triceps
   C. pectorals
   D. rectus abdominis

9. When the elbow joint is in the flexed position during a *pull-up,* the forearm is in a _____ position.

   A. pronated    B. supinated    C. extended    D. abducted

10. All of the following muscle groups are in concentric contraction when pushing up from the floor to a front leaning rest EXCEPT the

    A. shoulder girdle abductors
    B. shoulder joint flexors
    C. elbow joint extensors
    D. wrist joint extensors

11. When a muscle contracts without changing its length, it is considered to be _____ contraction.

    A. isometric
    B. isotonic
    C. eccentric
    D. concentric

12. Of the following exercises, the one BEST for strengthening and increasing the tone of the abdominal muscles is

    A. sit-ups from a lying position
    B. trunk bending and stretching in the standing position
    C. push-ups from a hand-support position
    D. the jumping jack

13. All of the following concerning the standing posture are correct EXCEPT that the

    A. knees should be extended but not stiff
    B. chest should be elevated but not puffed out
    C. hips should be drawn back slightly but not protruding
    D. head should be held high but not back

14. All of the following associations of body joint and use are correct EXCEPT:

    A. Ball and socket - freedom of motion
    B. Immovable - protection
    C. Hinge - power
    D. Gliding - slight rotation in two directions

15. In the Foster Test of Physical Efficiency, all of the following are noted EXCEPT the

    A. reclining pulse rate
    B. standing pulse rate
    C. increase in pulse rate immediately after exercise
    D. return of pulse rate after exercise

16. Of the following, the test which does NOT test cardiovascular efficiency is the _____ test.

    A. Barringer
    B. Crampton
    C. Sargent
    D. Schneider

17. All of the following are muscles of the lower extremity EXCEPT the

    A. trapezius
    B. sartorius
    C. gastrochemius
    D. quadriceps femoris

18. In regard to postural defects, the INCORRECT association is:

    A. Torticollis - wry neck
    B. Kyphosis - round shoulders
    C. Lordosis - flat back
    D. Scoliosis - abnormal spinal curve

19. The INCORRECT association is:

    A. Place of muscular attachment - foramen
    B. Rounded prominence - tuberosity
    C. Long, slender bony projection - spine
    D. Depression - fossa

20. The presence of adrenalin in the blood does NOT

    A. make the heart beat faster
    B. raise the blood pressure
    C. enable the liver to provide extra sugar to the blood
    D. increase the clotting time of the blood

21. All of the following associations are correct EXCEPT:

    A. Antidermatitis - vitamin $B_6$
    B. Antihemorrhagic - vitamin K
    C. Antineuritic - vitamin $B_1$
    D. Antisterility - vitamin G

22. All of the following associations are correct EXCEPT:

    A. Sodium and potassium - normal beating of heart
    B. Iron and copper - making of hemoglobin
    C. Calcium and phosphorus - formation of bone
    D. Chlorine and sulphur - oxidative processes

23. The three muscles that form the hamstring muscles are the

    A. gluteus maximus, pectineus, and tensor
    B. sartorius, rectus femoris, and iliacus
    C. psoas, iliacus, and biceps femoris
    D. biceps femoris, semitendinosus, and semimembranosus

24. In the athlete, the process of *warming up* does all of the following EXCEPT to

    A. prepare his neuromuscular coordinating system for the impending task
    B. heighten his kinesthetic senses
    C. facilitate the biochemical reactions supplying energy for muscular contractions
    D. decrease tissue elasticity so that liability to injury is lessened

25. All of the following are vitamins EXCEPT

    A. thiamine    B. niacin    C. heparin    D. biotin

## KEY (CORRECT ANSWERS)

| | | | |
|---|---|---|---|
| 1. A | | 11. A | |
| 2. B | | 12. A | |
| 3. A | | 13. D | |
| 4. A | | 14. D | |
| 5. D | | 15. A | |
| 6. A | | 16. C | |
| 7. B | | 17. C | |
| 8. D | | 18. C | |
| 9. A | | 19. A | |
| 10. D | | 20. D | |

21. D
22. D
23. D
24. D
25. C

# TEST 3

DIRECTIONS: Each question or incomplete statement is followed by several suggested answers or completions. Select the one that BEST answers the question or completes the statement. *PRINT THE LETTER OF THE CORRECT ANSWER IN THE SPACE AT THE RIGHT.*

1. The MOST common type of *poor* posture noted in adolescent students is  1.____

    A. scoliosis  B. lordosis
    C. kyphosis  D. kypho-lordosis

2. The use of arch supports for flat feet aims to  2.____

    A. strengthen the muscles of the feet
    B. relieve pain
    C. cure the condition
    D. develop stronger arches

3. Chronic poor posture is LEAST likely to be associated with  3.____

    A. defective hearing
    B. resumption of work after recuperation from illness
    C. depressed feelings
    D. prolonged ill health

4. Of the following foods, the one that does NOT contain all of the indispensable amino acids is  4.____

    A. fish  B. gelatin  C. eggs  D. meat

5. The LARGEST source of body heat is the _____ system.  5.____

    A. nervous  B. digestive
    C. tegumentary  D. muscular

6. The gland which plays the leading role in regulating the physiological processes of the body is the  6.____

    A. pituitary  B. adrenal  C. pancreas  D. thymus

7. The medulla oblongata contains all of the following centers EXCEPT the _____ center.  7.____

    A. cardiac  B. heat-regulating
    C. vasomotor  D. respiratory

8. The term *meninges* is associated LEAST with the  8.____

    A. callus  B. dura mater
    C. pia mater  D. arachnoid

9. In determining good walking posture, all of the following are correct EXCEPT having the  9.____

    A. heel make the first contact for each step
    B. arm swing controlled within a relatively small arc
    C. balance maintained over the body base with flexion at the hips and hyperextension in the lower back
    D. big toe at the origin of the push-off at each step

10. In determining good standing posture, of the following, the parts of the body that should be situated one above the other when viewed from the side are

    A. ear lobe, point of shoulder, hip joint, rear of patella
    B. posterior end of jaw bone, crest of hip, back of knee
    C. highest point of the ear, outer end of the clavicle, crest of the hip bone
    D. nape of the neck, upper end of the femur, upper and lower ends of the fibula

11. Of the following, the BEST exercise to correct the condition of kyphosis is

    A. performing the jumping jack exercise
    B. flinging the arms vigorously sideward
    C. clasping the hands behind the body and stretching them downward past the hip area
    D. sitting with the spine pressed against the wall

12. The metatarsal arch exists

    A. for maintaining the height of the other arch of the foot
    B. only in non-weight-bearing positions
    C. for function of shock absorption
    D. primarily as a means of body support

13. Of the following, the BEST exercise to correct the condition of visceral ptosis is

    A. leg raising from a supine body position
    B. arching the back
    C. performing sit-ups
    D. bicycling

14. The esophagus is between the

    A. pharynx and the stomach
    B. epiglottis and the gullet
    C. larynx and the bronchus
    D. trachea and pylorus

15. The PRIMARY purpose of the eustachian tube is to

    A. support the tympanic membrane
    B. aid the body in maintaining its equilibrium
    C. contain the semi-circular canals
    D. allow for the equalization of air pressure in the middle ear

16. In *screening* for participation in physical activities, the examination which should PRECEDE all others is the

    A. posture and orthopedic examination
    B. height-weight-age coefficient
    C. medical appraisal
    D. motor ability test

17. It is INCORRECT to state that cholesterol                                    17._____

    A. metabolism is related to atherosclerosis
    B. is a normal and essential constituent of human tissue
    C. levels in the blood are related to intake of animal fats
    D. levels in the blood are lowered by intake of saturated fats

18. All of the following associations concerning milk are correct EXCEPT:        18._____

    A. Pasteurization - destruction of the common pathogens found in milk
    B. Homogenization - process of emulsifying milk
    C. Irradiation - sterilization of raw milk
    D. Centrifugalization - separation of cream from the milk

19. Lipase, which is necessary for the digestion of fats, is manufactured by the  19._____

    A. stomach              B. liver
    C. pancreas             D. small intestine

20. Of the following statements, the CORRECT one is that protein                 20._____

    A. is stored as glycogen
    B. releases a large quantity of energy as it is oxidized
    C. is the principal nutrient in molasses
    D. is the only nutrient which contains nitrogen

21. Food calories are                                                            21._____

    A. units that measure fuel value
    B. food nutrients
    C. fattening foods
    D. the energy in foods

22. Iron is EXTREMELY important for                                              22._____

    A. repairing body tissue
    B. carrying oxygen to various parts of the body
    C. providing nourishment to nerve tissue
    D. bringing waste materials to the liver

23. All of the following statements are correct EXCEPT:                          23._____

    A. The lack of iodine in the diet can cause goiter
    B. The majority of all digested food is absorbed in the small intestine
    C. A dietary deficiency of vitamin C can cause scurvy
    D. Pepsin is the enzyme which helps digest fats

24. The INCORRECT association of nutrient and food is:                           24._____

    A. Protein - lean meats
    B. Carbohydrates - eggs
    C. Fats - butter
    D. Mineral salts - green leafy vegetables

25. Of the following, the INCORRECT association is:

    A. Gliding joint - intercarpal
    B. Hinge joint - ankle
    C. Pivot joint - knee
    D. Ball and socket joint - hip

## KEY (CORRECT ANSWERS)

| | | | |
|---|---|---|---|
| 1. | C | 11. | C |
| 2. | B | 12. | B |
| 3. | B | 13. | C |
| 4. | B | 14. | A |
| 5. | D | 15. | D |
| 6. | A | 16. | C |
| 7. | B | 17. | D |
| 8. | A | 18. | C |
| 9. | C | 19. | C |
| 10. | A | 20. | D |
| 21. | A | | |
| 22. | B | | |
| 23. | D | | |
| 24. | B | | |
| 25. | C | | |

# TEST 4

DIRECTIONS: Each question or incomplete statement is followed by several suggested answers or completions. Select the one that BEST answers the question or completes the statement. *PRINT THE LETTER OF THE CORRECT ANSWER IN THE SPACE AT THE RIGHT.*

1. All of the following associations are correct EXCEPT: 1.____

    A. Blepharitis - inflammation of the eyelids
    B. Chalazion - tumor of the eyelid
    C. Hordeolum - infection of the eyelid near a hair follicle
    D. Otitis media - cyst on the cornea

2. Of the following, the spleen is MOST closely related to the 2.____

    A. storage of red blood corpuscles
    B. production of bile
    C. basal metabolism
    D. digestion of fats

3. The epidermis contains 3.____

    A. blood vessels            B. small nerve endings
    C. adipose tissue           D. subcutaneous tissue

4. The duct of an oil gland USUALLY empties into the 4.____

    A. blood vessel             B. hair follicle
    C. sweat pore               D. hair papilla

5. Of the following, the endocrine gland MOST closely associated with adulthood is the 5.____

    A. gonad        B. pineal        C. thymus        D. pituitary

6. All of the following statements are correct EXCEPT: 6.____

    A. Nerves reach into the interior of bones through the haversian canals
    B. The periosteum covers the surface of nearly all parts of the bone
    C. Bone marrow consists mainly of minerals and proteins
    D. The bone cells, or osteoblasts, are associated with the construction and repair of bones

7. All of the following concerning leukocytes are correct EXCEPT that they 7.____

    A. are the source of gamma globulin
    B. have ameboid movement
    C. are found only in the blood of the body
    D. vary in number according to food intake and exercise

8. The disease characterized by defective ossification of the bones and the development of various bone deformations is 8.____

    A. arthritis        B. rickets        C. apoplexy        D. clubfoot

169

9. The vitamin MOST essential for the health of the gums is vitamin

   A. C  B. B  C. A  D. K

10. Vitamin D and phosphorus are essential for the utilization of _____ in the body.

    A. iron  B. copper  C. iodine  D. calcium

11. All of the following are associated with vitamin D EXCEPT

    A. ergosterol
    B. sorbitol
    C. calciferol
    D. viosterol

12. The enzyme in the gastric juice that causes the curdling or coagulation of milk is

    A. renin  B. pepsin  C. rennin  D. lipase

13. Of the following, the one that is NOT associated with a lack of vitamins is

    A. beriberi
    B. zerophthalmia
    C. trachoma
    D. night blindness

14. All of the following associations are correct EXCEPT:

    A. Folic acid - vitamin B
    B. Tetany - parathyroids
    C. Trypsin - gastric juice
    D. Insulin - pancreas

15. All of the following associations are correct EXCEPT:

    A. Vitamin E - anti-hemorrhagic
    B. Vitamin C - anti-scorbutic
    C. Vitamin B - anti-neuritic
    D. Nicotinic acid - pellagra preventive

16. A victim of heat exhaustion will MOST likely have a

    A. high temperature
    B. flushed face
    C. moist skin
    D. strong pulse

17. In regard to overweight, it is CORRECT to state:

    A. High blood pressure is found twice as frequently in the overweight than in the underweight individual
    B. Diabetes and arthritis are somewhat more common diseases of the underweight rather than the overweight
    C. The underweight individuals are poorer surgical risks than the overweight individuals
    D. A greater number of illnesses appear to attack the overweight rather than the underweight individuals

18. If an individual really wants to lose weight, of the following, the MOST sensible way to do this is to

    A. decrease caloric intake
    B. participate in active sports
    C. follow a diet of high protein intake
    D. avoid animal fats

19. The liver is NOT associated with the

    A. storage of vitamins
    B. dispatching of sugars to the tissues for body fuel
    C. processing of iron for the blood system
    D. absorption of protein

20. All of the following associations of enzyme and digestive area are correct EXCEPT:

    A. Mouth - ptyalin
    B. Small intestine - steapsin
    C. Stomach - rennin
    D. Large intestine - pepsin

21. A comparison of the heart rate and the blood pressure in the reclining position with corresponding values in the erect position is identified as the

    A. MacCurdy's Physical Capacity Index
    B. Roger's Athletic Index
    C. Crampton Blood Ptosis Test
    D. Oppenheimer's Scale

22. All of the following statements are correct EXCEPT:

    A. The figures used for the recording of blood pressure represent, in millimeters, the height of a column of mercury in the sphygmomanometer
    B. In high blood pressure cases, progressive damage to the blood vessels takes place, whereas hypertension is limited to harder than normal work by the heart to pump the same amount of blood around to the tissues
    C. In the recording of blood pressure, the larger figure represents the maximum pressure in the arteries with each heart beat
    D. The smaller figure in the recording of an individual's blood pressure registers the minimum pressure between heart beats

23. Of the following, the one which is NOT absorbed by the body in the form in which it is consumed is

    A. fats
    B. mineral salts
    C. water
    D. meat extracts

24. The intake of excessive vitamin D is harmful to human beings because it may

    A. lead to pernicious anemia
    B. cause calcium deposits in the kidneys
    C. cause central nervous system irritability
    D. interfere with the ability to reproduce

25. Pernicious anemia is a form of anemia in which the blood does not have enough red cells and is usually treated with vitamin(s)

    A. C
    B. $B_{12}$ and folic acid
    C. E and K
    D. A

## KEY (CORRECT ANSWERS)

1. D
2. A
3. B
4. B
5. A

6. C
7. C
8. B
9. A
10. D

11. B
12. C
13. C
14. C
15. A

16. C
17. A
18. A
19. D
20. D

21. C
22. B
23. A
24. C
25. A

# EXAMINATION SECTION
# TEST 1

DIRECTIONS: Each question or incomplete statement is followed by several suggested answers or completions. Select the one that BEST answers the question or completes the statement. *PRINT THE LETTER OF THE CORRECT ANSWER IN THE SPACE AT THE RIGHT.*

1. The individual's esophagus is located between the

    A. pharynx and the stomach
    B. mouth and the larynx
    C. small and large intestines
    D. pharynx and the epiglottis

1.____

2. A physician's report indicates that a patient has injured the acromion. This injury is in the area of the

    A. ankle           B. knee
    C. elbow           D. shoulder blade

2.____

3. All of the following associations are correct EXCEPT:

    A. Bursa - cushion between the bones
    B. Cramp - an involuntary contraction of a muscle
    C. Strain - result of overuse of a muscle or group of muscles
    D. Tendon - stretchable tissue connecting bone to bone

3.____

4. The correct sitting posture does NOT include

    A. a flattened lumbar spine
    B. feet touching the floor
    C. placing the hips as far back in the seat as possible
    D. holding the head in the same position as when standing

4.____

5. All of the following associations of anatomic analysis and postural conditions are correct EXCEPT:

    A. Kyphosis - exaggerated convexity in the thoracic region of the vertebral column
    B. Scoliosis - lateral curvature in any region of the vertebral column
    C. Lordosis - exaggerated concavity in the lumbar region of the spine
    D. Kypho-lordosis - concavity in cervical and sacral regions of the spinal column

5.____

6. The *rheumatoid factor* is

    A. a substance found in normal blood which reacts quickly to drugs
    B. the poor posture over several years which aggravates the bones and cartilage of the joints
    C. a protein substance found in the blood of rheumatoid arthritics
    D. the aches and pains that come with the passing years

6.____

7. Physical therapy helps the individual with arthritic joints by all of the following EXCEPT by

7.____

2 (#1)

A. preventing the joints from locking permanently
B. improving the range of motion in the affected joint
C. relieving the inflammation of the joints
D. helping avoid atrophy of the muscles

8. Of the following diseases, the one whose inoculation has the SHORTEST duration of effectiveness is

A. measles
B. diphtheria
C. smallpox
D. whooping cough

9. Normal increase in the size of a muscle is due to an increase in the

A. number of muscle fibers
B. thickness in the fibrous sheaths
C. size of the individual muscle fibers
D. capacity to convert lactic acid to glycogen

10. All of the following are membraneous tissues covering body parts EXCEPT the

A. peritoneum
B. periosteum
C. peridiolum
D. pericardium

11. All of the following concerning muscular contractions are correct EXCEPT:

A. Uncoordinated muscular contractions involving an inconstant number of muscle groups are associated with convulsions
B. A sudden contraction of a muscle resulting from a single stimulus may be a simple muscular twitch
C. Tetanus is a sustained muscular contraction resulting from rapidly repeated stimuli
D. Muscle spasticity is incomplete muscular relaxation after repeated stimulation

12. In subdividing the volumes of air respired by the normal adult, it is CORRECT to state that the

A. tidal air is that amount of air that can be expelled after a normal expiration
B. supplemental air is the amount of air that goes in and out with normal quiet breathing
C. complemental air is the volume of air that can be taken in by the deepest inhalation after a normal inspiration
D. residual air is the volume of air that can be expelled from deepest inspiration to fullest expiration

13. In general, NO local first aid measures are necessary in a rib fracture case if

A. pain is minimal
B. swelling is hardly noticeable
C. breathing causes discomfort
D. deformity indicates the presence of a fracture

14. In spinal meningitis, the

A. nerves that carry messages to the spinal cord are injured
B. nerves that carry messages to the muscles are damaged

C. spinal cord is destroyed
D. membrane around the brain is inflamed

15. All of the following diseases are caused by the hypo-function of ductless glands EXCEPT   15.____

    A. acromegaly          B. myxedema
    C. tetany              D. Addison's disease

16. Substances which determine the various blood types are found in the   16.____

    A. white corpuscles    B. platelets
    C. red corpuscles      D. plasma

17. All of the following substances are needed in blood clotting EXCEPT   17.____

    A. fibrinogen          B. lymph
    C. prothrombin         D. calcium

18. All of the following associations are correct EXCEPT:   18.____

    A. Blood group O - universal donor
    B. Blood group AB - universal recipient
    C. RH factor - agglutinin
    D. Coagulant - heparin

19. The larynx is between the   19.____

    A. pharynx and the nasal passages
    B. esophagus and the thyroid
    C. nose and the thyroid cartilage
    D. trachea and the pharynx

20. All of the following associations of types of joints are correct EXCEPT:   20.____

    A. Ball and socket - hip       B. Gliding - toes
    C. Pivot - head and neck       D. Hinge - elbow

21. The eight small bones that form the wrists are called the   21.____

    A. carpals             B. metatarsals
    C. tarsals             D. phalanges

22. The condition in which the ankles deviate inward, throwing a great portion of body weight on the plantar ligaments and causing the medial portion of the foot to contact the ground is called   22.____

    A. pes planus          B. pes cavus
    C. talipes varus       D. talipes calcaneus

23. Of the following, the MOST important muscle in maintaining the longitudinal arch of the foot during weight bearing is the   23.____

    A. flexor hallucis longus    B. flexor digitorum longus
    C. tibialis posterior        D. peroneus longus

24. An absence of nicotinic acid in the diet results in a(n)   24._____

    A. condition characterized by an enlargement of the thyroid gland
    B. condition identified as gastric hypoacidity
    C. inflammation and cracking of the lips and the corners of the mouth
    D. disease of the skin and digestive tract

25. Liver is valuable in one's diet because it contains large amounts of   25._____

    A. phosphorus      B. vitamin D
    C. iron      D. calcium

---

# KEY (CORRECT ANSWERS)

| | | | |
|---|---|---|---|
| 1. | A | 11. | D |
| 2. | D | 12. | C |
| 3. | D | 13. | A |
| 4. | A | 14. | D |
| 5. | D | 15. | A |
| 6. | C | 16. | C |
| 7. | C | 17. | B |
| 8. | A | 18. | D |
| 9. | C | 19. | D |
| 10. | C | 20. | B |

21. A
22. A
23. C
24. D
25. C

# TEST 2

DIRECTIONS: Each question or incomplete statement is followed by several suggested answers or completions. Select the one that BEST answers the question or completes the statement. *PRINT THE LETTER OF THE CORRECT ANSWER IN THE SPACE AT THE RIGHT.*

1. All of the following enzymes aid in the digestion of proteins EXCEPT  1.____

    A. ptyalin  B. pepsin  C. rennin  D. trypsin

2. Minerals in the daily diet are used by the body to  2.____

    A. balance high calorific foods
    B. provide body heat and energy
    C. stimulate and increase the appetite
    D. regulate body processes

3. The pair of diseases that result from diet deficiencies is  3.____

    A. pellagra and hookworm
    B. scurvy and botulism
    C. rickets and cheilosis
    D. tularemia and typhoid

4. In a metabolism test,  4.____

    A. a graph is made of the patient's heart action
    B. the red and white corpuscles in a patient's blood are counted
    C. both the otoscope and the opthalmoscope are employed
    D. the amount of oxygen inhaled for a given period of time is determined

5. The swelling associated with a wrenched joint is caused by  5.____

    A. an unusual flow of synovial fluid
    B. decreased elasticity of the tendons
    C. poor muscle tone
    D. the effect of the wrench on the blood vessels

6. When a dislocation occurs, there is  6.____

    A. a bone out of place at a joint
    B. always a surface wound to be treated
    C. seldom, if any, pain
    D. less deformity than when a joint is sprained

7. A colles fracture is one which may affect the movement of the _____ joint.  7.____

    A. knee  B. shoulder  C. hip  D. wrist

8. The malpighian cells of the skin are found in  8.____

    A. outer surface of the epidermis
    B. dermis
    C. papillae
    D. deeper growing layer of the epidermis

9. All of the following are correct EXCEPT:

   A. When taking an individual's pulse, count the pulse beats for one full minute, then check the rate by counting for another full minute
   B. If there is any marked rise or drop in a patient's temperature, check the thermometer reading by taking the temperature again
   C. When taking an individual's respiration rate, count for one full minute each rise of the chest
   D. When taking the temperature at the armpit, the thermometer must be kept in position for five minutes before taking a reading

10. All of the following measure cardiovascular efficiency EXCEPT the _____ test.

    A. Foster    B. Holmgren    C. Schneider    D. Crampton

11. When the feet are functioning as a support for the body, the MOST characteristic point about weak feet is

    A. their abducted position
    B. the degree of rigidity
    C. the depressed transverse arches
    D. the flexion of the toes

12. In attempting to correct a condition of weak feet, the individual should AVOID

    A. toeing out when walking
    B. walking on a balance beam
    C. *pencil writing* with the toes
    D. gripping marbles with the toes

13. All of the following will affect the relation of the line of gravity to an individual's base of support EXCEPT carrying a

    A. heavy suitcase in the right hand
    B. tray in both hands in front of the chest
    C. basketball in a dribble position
    D. moderately heavy basket on the head

14. A condition in which a series of vertebrae remains constantly deviated from the normal spinal axis accompanied by a degree of rotation of the vertebrae is known as

    A. kypholordosis           B. structural scoliosis
    C. mobile sclerosis        D. functional scoliosis

15. The gland which has the GREATEST influence on the rate of oxygen consumption is the

    A. thyroid    B. pineal    C. adrenal    D. buccal

16. Training of the muscular system brings about all of the following EXCEPT an increase in the

    A. strength of the muscles        B. endurance of the muscles
    C. number of muscle fibers        D. size of the muscles

17. All of the following concerning joints are correct EXCEPT the                                17._____

    A. synovial fluid lubricates the joint
    B. capsule determines the degree of movement in the joint
    C. ligaments help hold the ends of the bones at the joint in place
    D. cartilage decreases friction between the two bones

18. The MAIN sources of body heat are the                                                         18._____

    A. lungs and pancreas
    B. muscles and the liver
    C. skin and large intestine
    D. intestines and the stomach

19. For an adult with a normal skin, the temperature of the hot water bottle should be            19._____
    between _____ °F.

    A. 120-130      B. 100-110      C. 140-150      D. 160-170

20. The food which is acid-forming is                                                             20._____

    A. fruits                       B. vegetables
    C. meat                         D. nuts

21. The LEAST desirable method of preparing vegetables is by                                      21._____

    A. adding baking soda to preserve the color
    B. steaming
    C. boiling for a short time in a small amount of water
    D. baking

22. A low-calorie diet should NOT be low in _____ content.                                        22._____

    A. fat                          B. fluid
    C. carbohydrate                 D. protein

23. Skim milk is rich in all of the following EXCEPT                                              23._____

    A. calcium                      B. riboflavin
    C. vitamin A                    D. protein

24. As alcohol is oxidized in the body tissues, the energy it contains is                         24._____

    A. used up in muscular activity
    B. used in accelerated activity of the nervous system
    C. stored in the body
    D. given off as heat

25. A stimulant for the respiratory center is                                                     25._____

    A. carbon dioxide               B. ethyl chloride
    C. oxygen                       D. nitrous oxide

# KEY (CORRECT ANSWERS)

| | | | |
|---|---|---|---|
| 1. | A | 11. | A |
| 2. | D | 12. | A |
| 3. | C | 13. | D |
| 4. | D | 14. | B |
| 5. | A | 15. | A |
| 6. | A | 16. | C |
| 7. | D | 17. | B |
| 8. | D | 18. | B |
| 9. | D | 19. | A |
| 10. | B | 20. | C |

21. A
22. D
23. C
24. A
25. A

# TEST 3

DIRECTIONS: Each question or incomplete statement is followed by several suggested answers or completions. Select the one that BEST answers the question or completes the statement. *PRINT THE LETTER OF THE CORRECT ANSWER IN THE SPACE AT THE RIGHT.*

1. The parts of the nervous system stimulated by strychnine are the   1._____

    A. hepatic and renal nerves
    B. brain and spinal cord
    C. automatic ganglia and sciatic nerves
    D. coronary and pulmonary nerves

2. Natural resistance to infection is LOWERED by   2._____

    A. fatigue
    B. reducing diets
    C. cold weather
    D. lack of immunization

3. MOST economic for protein reinforcement of the diet is   3._____

    A. egg yolk
    B. ice cream
    C. cream cheese
    D. skim milk powder

4. The CHIEF value of cellulose in the diet is that it   4._____

    A. provides an essential amino acid
    B. is easily digested
    C. gives bulk to the intestinal residues
    D. is more soluble than starch

5. Of the following, the one considered the MAJOR cause of obesity is   5._____

    A. too little exercise
    B. emotional disturbance
    C. excessive eating
    D. inheritance

6. The mineral that is essential to the process of oxidation by helping to carry oxygen to every cell is   6._____

    A. iodine    B. sodium    C. magnesium    D. iron

7. In the body, the interchange of food, oxygen, and waste takes place in the   7._____

    A. capillaries
    B. plasma
    C. red blood cells
    D. lymph

8. In nutrition, the utilization of absorbed products is called   8._____

    A. osmosis
    B. metabolism
    C. anabolism
    D. catabolism

9. It is CORRECT to state that the *immediate* effect of alcohol on the body is to   9._____

    A. constrict surface blood vessels
    B. decrease the rate of the heart beat
    C. increase blood pressure
    D. decrease body temperature

10. Poor diet influences MOST the occurrence of

   A. metabolic diseases
   B. cancer
   C. nephritis
   D. hypertension

11. In proper handwashing, be sure to use

   A. cold water
   B. soap, water, and adequate friction
   C. liquid soap
   D. very hot water

12. Of the following symptoms, the one which would be LEAST likely to cause a person to consult a physician for chest examination is

   A. continuous loss of weight
   B. a cough lasting longer than three weeks
   C. a slight elevation of temperature in the afternoon
   D. fresh blood in the stools

13. The _____ gland is known to regulate body metabolism.

   A. thymus     B. pineal     C. thyroid     D. parotid

14. The system of healing that is based upon the manipulation of the spine is

   A. chiropractic
   B. naturopathy
   C. osteoptics
   D. ophthalmology

15. Arterial bleeding can usually be stopped by applying pressure at a spot between the wound and the heart where the artery crosses a

   A. gland     B. muscle     C. vein     D. bone

16. With respect to obesity and diet, the LEAST acceptable statement of the following is that

   A. obesity constitutes a public health problem of importance since obese persons are more apt to develop diabetes and degenerative diseases
   B. obesity usually results from an habitual intake of more food than the energy output requires
   C. the treatment of obesity should involve re-education of the appetite
   D. the recommended intake for an obese person is 3000 calories daily since the diet should be adequate in respect to all essential nutrients

17. A lateral curvature of the spine is known as

   A. scoliosis
   B. lordosis
   C. kyphosis
   D. trichinosis

18. Cerebral palsy can BEST be described as a

   A. nerve infection which causes the incoordination of the muscles
   B. muscular deformity chiefly affecting the upper extremities
   C. neuro-muscular disability caused by injury to the motor centers of the brain
   D. muscular disfunction caused by injury to the spinal column

19. Vitamin A is stored in the                                                                                                        19.____

    A. skeletal muscles            B. liver
    C. thyroid                     D. brain

20. The MOST important single item of the diet is                                                                                     20.____

    A. carbohydrates               B. water
    C. milk                        D. protein

21. Obesity may be caused by                                                                                                          21.____

    A. lack of vitamins            B. excessive calorie intake
    C. gastronomy                  D. high protein diet

22. A compound fracture is one in which                                                                                               22.____

    A. a bone is broken in two or more places
    B. the broken end of a bone pierces the skin
    C. a bone is both broken and out of place at a joint
    D. there is both a broken bone and a sprained muscle

23. Calorie is a                                                                                                                      23.____

    A. unit of measurement
    B. term used for digestibility
    C. need for nutrients
    D. catalytic agent

24. A SUBSTANTIAL source of iron is found in                                                                                          24.____

    A. apricots        B. almonds        C. potatoes        D. cheese

25. Pasteurized milk is valuable in the diet because it is a GOOD source of                                                           25.____

    A. vitamin K                   B. amino acids
    C. vitamin B                   D. rutin

## KEY (CORRECT ANSWERS)

| | | | |
|---|---|---|---|
| 1. | B | 11. | B |
| 2. | A | 12. | D |
| 3. | D | 13. | C |
| 4. | C | 14. | A |
| 5. | C | 15. | D |
| 6. | D | 16. | D |
| 7. | A | 17. | A |
| 8. | C | 18. | C |
| 9. | B | 19. | B |
| 10. | A | 20. | B |

21. B
22. B
23. A
24. A
25. B

———

# TEST 4

DIRECTIONS: Each question or incomplete statement is followed by several suggested answers or completions. Select the one that BEST answers the question or completes the statement. *PRINT THE LETTER OF THE CORRECT ANSWER IN THE SPACE AT THE RIGHT.*

1. Vitamin A helps to prevent    1.____

   A. night blindness
   B. hemorrhage in newborn infants
   C. scurvy
   D. destruction of connective tissue

2. Swelling, heat, and redness occur in an inflamed area because the capillaries become    2.____

   A. constricted         B. dilated
   C. ruptured            D. fenestrated

3. Bone owes its hardness CHIEFLY to the mineral salt    3.____

   A. calcium phosphorus    B. potassium iodide
   C. sodium carbonate      D. stearic acid

4. The number of vertebrae of the spinal column of a human is    4.____

   A. 33      B. 42      C. 28      D. 21

5. Sebaceous glands    5.____

   A. aid digestion
   B. have ducts
   C. are attached to the muscles of the eyes
   D. increase blood pressure

6. Ringworm is caused by    6.____

   A. fungi
   B. pediculi
   C. infection of the intestines
   D. impetigo

7. Bones and teeth are strengthened by foods rich in    7.____

   A. potassium and iodine     B. potassium and iron
   C. calcium and phosphorus   D. calcium and chlorine

8. A person with a non-functioning gall bladder will have difficulty digesting    8.____

   A. fats      B. sugars      C. starches      D. proteins

9. Minerals in the daily diet should be stressed because they    9.____

   A. balance high calorific foods
   B. promote growth and maintain body tissues
   C. stimulate and increase the appetite
   D. supply fuel for energy and cushion body organs

10. When treating a victim of simple fainting, the first aider should

   A. give the victim coffee to drink
   B. place the victim on his back in a recumbent position
   C. rub the victim's wrists
   D. hold a gauze pad sprinkled with ammonia over the victim's nostrils

10.____

11. In respiration,

   A. expiration is slower than inspiration
   B. receptors of the skin respond
   C. the hypothalmus is expanded
   D. enzymes are rendered inert

11.____

12. Metabolism

   A. expresses the fact that nerve fibres give only one kind of reaction
   B. summarizes the activities each living cell must carry on
   C. possesses the properties of irritability and conductivity
   D. describes the membrane theory

12.____

13. The heat of the body is maintained by

   A. oxidation   B. vertigo   C. gravity   D. hyperpnea

13.____

14. The vitamin MOST essential for the health of the gums is vitamin

   A. C   B. B   C. A   D. K

14.____

15. Vitamin D and phosphorus are essential for the utilization of _____ in the body.

   A. iron   B. copper   C. iodine   D. calcium

15.____

16. The heart rate

   A. varies in individuals
   B. increases from birth to old age
   C. increases during first hours of sleep
   D. decreases in hemorrhage

16.____

17. A neuron consists of

   A. fluid in the semicircular canals
   B. conjugated protein which yields globin and hemin
   C. a cell body and processes
   D. a band of spectrum colors ranging from red to violet

17.____

18. Of the following, the BEST source of natural vitamin D is

   A. tomatoes         B. salmon
   C. eggs             D. green vegetables

18.____

19. A movement in the ankle is accomplished with the aid of a _____ joint.

   A. hinged           B. pivot
   C. gliding          D. ball and socket

19.____

20. Carbon dioxide and oxygen are exchanged in the air sacs by　　　　20.____
   A. infusion　　　　　　　　　　　B. diffusion
   C. reaction　　　　　　　　　　　 D. filtration

21. The absorption of water through the intestinal wall is by　　　　　21.____
   A. filtration　　　　　　　　　　　B. osmosis
   C. infiltration　　　　　　　　　　D. fusion

22. The body organ controlling the water content and osmotic pressure of the blood is the　　22.____
   A. pancreas　　　B. kidneys　　　C. lungs　　　D. stomach

23. The lowering of the head, when a person feels faint, will increase the blood supply to the head by　　23.____
   A. suction　　　　　　　　　　　　B. gravity
   C. siphonage　　　　　　　　　　 D. centripetal force

24. The ventricles of the heart act like a　　　　　　　　　　　　　　24.____
   A. lever　　　　B. pump　　　　C. siphon　　　　D. barometer

25. A rubber hot water bottle transfers heat to the skin CHIEFLY by　　25.____
   A. conduction　　　　　　　　　　B. convection
   C. radiation　　　　　　　　　　　D. oxidation

---

# KEY (CORRECT ANSWERS)

1. A        11. A
2. B        12. B
3. A        13. A
4. A        14. A
5. B        15. D

6. A        16. A
7. C        17. C
8. A        18. B
9. B        19. A
10. B       20. B

21. B
22. B
23. B
24. B
25. A

# EXAMINATION SECTION
# TEST 1

DIRECTIONS: Each question or incomplete statement is followed by several suggested answers or completions. Select the one that BEST answers the question or completes the statement. *PRINT THE LETTER OF THE CORRECT ANSWER IN THE SPACE AT THE RIGHT.*

1. All of the following are associated with movement of the femur at the hip joint EXCEPT: 1.____

   A. Flexion - outward rotation
   B. Inversion - supination
   C. Inward rotation - circumduction
   D. Extension - abduction

2. Of the following, the one necessary for the formation of thyroxin, which controls the metabolic rate, is 2.____

   A. phosphorus             B. sodium chloride
   C. iodine                 D. calcium

3. Excluding the coronary circulation, the average time for the complete circulation of the blood through all the circuits of the adult human body is APPROXIMATELY 3.____

   A. 23 seconds             B. 5 minutes
   C. 1 minute, 15 seconds   D. 10 minutes

4. Of the following, the substance necessary for the clotting of blood is 4.____

   A. ptyalin                B. prothrombin
   C. gastrin                D. rennin

5. Of the following, the ones which CANNOT be converted into heat or other forms of energy are 5.____

   A. fats                   B. proteins
   C. minerals               D. carbohydrates

6. Of the following suggestions for reducing weight, the one MOST likely to be given by doctors to their otherwise healthy patients is to 6.____

   A. omit all desserts and bread
   B. increase the protein intake, to omit duplication in starches at each meal, and to eat low calorie desserts
   C. omit potatoes, bread, and all desserts except fruit for the main meal
   D. follow a diet made up entirely of protein, fruit, and vegetables

7. Blood sugar is low 7.____

   A. in untreated diabetes mellitus
   B. during emotional stress
   C. after meals
   D. during severe and prolonged muscular exertion

8. The substances which are NOT necessary for building new tissues are 8.____

   A. water                  B. carbohydrates
   C. proteins               D. minerals

9. A nutrient functions in any or all of the following ways EXCEPT to

   A. furnish energy
   B. provide materials for building or maintenance of body tissues
   C. help regulate body processes
   D. purify the blood

10. It is most important to see that reducing diets of adolescents do NOT lack

    A. fats
    B. proteins
    C. carbohydrates
    D. simple sugars

11. The CHIEF value of cellulose in the diet is that it

    A. is more soluble than starch
    B. gives bulk to the intestinal residues
    C. is easily digested
    D. provides an essential amino acid

12. It is CORRECT to state that enzymes

    A. are used up in chemical reactions of foods
    B. retard the process of breaking down of foods
    C. work only in acid surroundings
    D. are specific in their action

13. The acetabulum is the articular cup in a bone which acts as a socket for the

    A. clavicle    B. femur    C. radius    D. tibia

14. Of the following associations, the CORRECT one is:

    A. Second class lever - the forearm when it is being extended by the triceps muscle
    B. Third class lever - the foot, when rising on the toes
    C. First class lever - the head, tipping forward and backward
    D. Second class lever - the arm when it is raised sideward-upward by the deltoid muscle

15. All of the following are correct principles relating to the muscular system EXCEPT:

    A. Muscles contract more rapidly following warm-up activities
    B. Muscular strength is progressively developed by the repetition of exercises of the same intensity
    C. Muscles contract more forcefully if they are first stretched, provided that they are not overstretched
    D. A muscle must be loaded beyond its customary load if strength is to be increased

16. Gradations in muscular contraction are related to

    A. variations in intensity of muscular contraction
    B. the number of fibers in the muscle which contract
    C. the circulation of blood within the muscle
    D. the manufacture of lactic acid in the muscle

17. In order to determine the basal metabolic rate of an individual, all of the following conditions must be included EXCEPT that the

    A. environment temperature must be comfortably warm
    B. test must be made from 12 to 18 hours after the last meal
    C. body must be in the waking state and at complete rest
    D. test should be preceded by a ten-minute period of vigorous exercise

18. The center of gravity of an individual of average build in an erect standing position is

    A. located in the pelvis in front of the upper part of the sacrum
    B. located at the articulation of the femur and the pelvis
    C. located in the anterior wall of the pelvis
    D. lower in men than in women because of anatomical structure

19. All of the following statements concerning lateral curvatures of the spine are correct EXCEPT:

    A. Some rotation of the vertebrae always accompanies lateral flexion of the spine
    B. In a simple structural lateral curvature, the curve is confined to one region and there is no compensatory curve
    C. The shoulder on the side of a dorsal convexity is lower than the other shoulder
    D. In a functional lateral curvature of the spine, the curve disappears when the individual suspends his body by hanging from the arms

20. When taking the wrist pulse rate, one should AVOID

    A. taking the pulse with the thumb
    B. counting the pulse beats for 1 minute, then checking the rate by counting for another minute
    C. having the patient support his arm and hand in a relaxed position
    D. taking the pulse on the thumb side of the wrist between the tendon and the wrist bone

21. Ringworm is caused by a microscopic

    A. mold    B. worm    C. yeast    D. virus

22. All of the following associations of suffixes found in technical terms on a health record and meanings are correct EXCEPT:

    A. Osis - swelling
    B. Emia - blood
    C. Itis - inflammation
    D. Algia - pain

23. All of the following statements are correct EXCEPT:

    A. The presence of a sufficient quantity of fats in the diet does away with the necessity of using protein for fuel.
    B. Any considerable amount of fat in food eaten will slow down the digestion of the whole meal.
    C. The digestion of fats begins in the stomach.
    D. Layers of fat under the skin help to keep the body temperature constant.

24. The body's CHIEF means of increasing heat production is by 24.____

   A. perspiring
   B. dilating the blood vessels
   C. shivering
   D. none of the above

25. All of the following concerning the feet are correct EXCEPT: 25.____

   A. The height of the arch is an indication of the strength of the foot
   B. Arch supports are temporary expedients for the relief of foot pain
   C. Neglected, weak feet become flexible, flat feet
   D. Rigid flat feet show depressed arches when the weight is not borne on the feet

---

## KEY (CORRECT ANSWERS)

| | | | |
|---|---|---|---|
| 1. B | | 11. B | |
| 2. C | | 12. D | |
| 3. A | | 13. B | |
| 4. B | | 14. C | |
| 5. C | | 15. B | |
| 6. B | | 16. B | |
| 7. D | | 17. D | |
| 8. B | | 18. A | |
| 9. D | | 19. C | |
| 10. B | | 20. A | |

21. A
22. A
23. C
24. C
25. A

# TEST 2

DIRECTIONS: Each question or incomplete statement is followed by several suggested answers or completions. Select the one that BEST answers the question or completes the statement. *PRINT THE LETTER OF THE CORRECT ANSWER IN THE SPACE AT THE RIGHT.*

1. The INCORRECT association is:

    A. Endomorph - soft, round, tendency to lay on fat
    B. Somatomorph - tall, athletic, broad-shouldered
    C. Ectomorph - linear, fragile, delicate
    D. Mesomorph - square, rugged, hard

2. All of the following statements concerning protein are correct EXCEPT:

    A. Protein is a source of energy
    B. Protein is required for tissue building and repair
    C. Vegetable proteins are generally as satisfactory as meat proteins in meeting body requirements
    D. Cheese contains important animal proteins

3. Foods rich in calcium and protein are also the BEST sources of

    A. iodine
    B. phosphorus
    C. copper
    D. fluorine

4. With regard to nutrition, the CORRECT statement is:

    A. Malnutrition is found only in low-income families
    B. Obesity is generally due to faulty glands
    C. Nutrition is affected by rest, recreation, and general mental health
    D. Adolescents should take additional vitamin preparations in order to insure adequate vitamin intake

5. In order to improve the muscular state of the nation, it would be desirable to do all of the following for our youth EXCEPT to

    A. encourage participation in daily calisthenics
    B. promote participation in swimming
    C. popularize soccer as a game for school children
    D. emphasize competitive sports

6. The grating of the broken pieces of a bone in a simple fracture is called

    A. crepitus
    B. contusion
    C. chorisis
    D. comminution

7. All of the following associations of pressure points and bleeding points are correct EXCEPT:

    A. Brachial artery - bleeding from the wrist
    B. Carotid artery - bleeding from the shoulder joint
    C. Subclavian artery - bleeding from the arm
    D. Femoral artery - bleeding from the lower leg

193

8. Of the following associations of fractures and distinguishing characteristics, the CORRECT one is

   A. Colles' fracture - radial bone
   B. compound fracture - point of fracture in contact with the external surface of the body
   C. Pott's fracture - tibiofibular joint
   D. Greenstick fracture - broken ends of the bone are interlocked

9. Foods which provide for growth and body repair must be rich in

   A. carbohydrates
   B. fats
   C. minerals
   D. proteins

10. Of the following, the one which is the BEST source of iron is

    A. milk
    B. liver
    C. prunes
    D. cheese

11. Of the following, the BEST source of vitamins is

    A. injections
    B. capsules
    C. tablets
    D. foods

12. The two elements MOST vitally concerned with the building of red blood cells are

    A. calcium and potassium
    B. iron and copper
    C. sodium and sulfur
    D. chlorine and phosphorous

13. Two minerals present in combined form in the bones and teeth are

    A. calcium and phosphorous
    B. iron and chlorine
    C. sodium and iron
    D. potassium and magnesium

14. Yeast contains all of the following EXCEPT

    A. ascorbic acid
    B. riboflavin
    C. thiamin
    D. niacin

15. Carotene is changed to vitamin A CHIEFLY in the

    A. liver
    B. pancreas
    C. small intestine
    D. large intestine

16. Foods which ordinarily will NOT start the process of dental decay are

    A. cakes
    B. carbonated beverages
    C. meats
    D. preserves

17. The term *trace elements* is applied to

    A. the use of patch tests to determine allergies
    B. minerals present in foods in very small amounts
    C. hereditary factors
    D. symptomatic indications of illnesses

18. The exchange of oxygen and carbon dioxide between inspired air and the blood takes place in the

    A. bronchioles
    B. alveoli
    C. arterioles
    D. villi

19. Of the following associations of the number of vertebrae and area of the spinal column, the INCORRECT one is:

    A. Cervical - 7
    B. Thoracic - 10
    C. Lumbar - 5
    D. Sacrum - 5

20. A carbuncle is a(n)

    A. collection of boils in one spot
    B. ringworm infection due to a fungus
    C. infection of a hair follicle
    D. inflammation of the oil glands

21. A deviated septum is NOT associated with

    A. impaired breathing
    B. hoarseness
    C. post-nasal drip
    D. malocclusion

22. The cervical and lumbar spinal curves

    A. are in opposite directions to each other
    B. are inflexible
    C. are present at birth
    D. result from the efforts of the child to assume the upright position

23. All of the following are necessary for proper seating EXCEPT that the student's

    A. lumbar region of the spine should be supported by the back of the chair
    B. feet should rest squarely on the floor
    C. hips should be pushed back in the chair as far as possible
    D. knees should be firmly supported by the forward edge of the seat

24. All of the following conditions are considered to be deviations of the spine EXCEPT

    A. scoliosis
    B. keratosis
    C. lordosis
    D. kyphosis

25. All of the following associations are correct EXCEPT:

    A. Ankle - hinge joint
    B. Wrist - biaxial joint
    C. Hip - ball-and-socket joint
    D. Knee - pivot joint

## KEY (CORRECT ANSWERS)

| | | | |
|---|---|---|---|
| 1. | B | 11. | D |
| 2. | C | 12. | B |
| 3. | B | 13. | A |
| 4. | C | 14. | A |
| 5. | D | 15. | A |
| 6. | A | 16. | C |
| 7. | B | 17. | B |
| 8. | D | 18. | B |
| 9. | D | 19. | B |
| 10. | B | 20. | A |

21. D
22. D
23. D
24. B
25. D

# TEST 3

DIRECTIONS: Each question or incomplete statement is followed by several suggested answers or completions. Select the one that BEST answers the question or completes the statement. *PRINT THE LETTER OF THE CORRECT ANSWER IN THE SPACE AT THE RIGHT.*

1. The gland that maintains harmony among the body functions by its control and coordination of the other endocrine glands is the
   A. thyroid    B. pituitary    C. adrenals    D. pineal

   1.____

2. The maintenance of body balance is MOST closely associated with the
   A. eustachian tube          B. ear drum
   C. semi-circular canals     D. stapes

   2.____

3. The terms endomorph, mesomorph, and ectomorph relate to
   A. extreme varieties of human physique
   B. digestive organs
   C. muscular system
   D. subcutaneous tissues

   3.____

4. Even if an individual has lost the use of the pectoralis major, he is able to perform all of the following actions EXCEPT to
   A. employ power in forward and downward movements of the arm
   B. raise his hand to any position in front of the trunk
   C. fold his arms
   D. place the hand on the opposite shoulder

   4.____

5. The muscle which depresses the humerus, draws it backward, and rotates it inward is the
   A. deltoid           B. trapezius
   C. latissimus dorsi  D. biceps

   5.____

6. All of the following statements are correct EXCEPT:
   A. Striated voluntary cells are found in muscles of the arm
   B. Smooth involuntary cells are found in the walls of the alimentary canal
   C. Smooth voluntary cells are found in muscles of the eye
   D. Striated involuntary cells are found in the heart muscle

   6.____

7. An example of a vestigial structure in the human body is
   A. a sweat gland      B. the appendix
   C. the pineal gland   D. a kidney

   7.____

8. An example of an anti-peristaltic movement is
   A. blushing    B. swallowing
   C. relaxing    D. vomiting

   8.____

9. The vision by which a baseball player stealing second base can see not only the player covering the base but others indirectly approaching the base is called _____ vision.

    A. tunnel
    B. barrel
    C. peripheral
    D. functional

10. For an individual with weak posture, the recumbent position for exercise is easier than the standing position because of all of the following reasons EXCEPT that, in the recumbent position, the

    A. effort in maintaining balance is relatively less
    B. gravity assists the body to be more at rest
    C. individual is less likely to fatigue
    D. heart and respiratory rates are increased, thus creating a better physiological approach to muscle action

11. All of the following are types of faulty posture occurring in the anteroposterior plane EXCEPT

    A. stoop shoulders
    B. round back
    C. high right shoulder
    D. hollow back

12. Sedentary occupations are MOST frequently associated with

    A. overdeveloped trapezius muscles
    B. strong rhomboid muscles
    C. increased tone and strength of the pectoral muscles
    D. powerful erector spinal muscles

13. When treating wounds, it is IMPORTANT to remember that

    A. puncture wounds can cause tetanus
    B. lacerations and punctures are the most serious
    C. the danger of tetanus is possible in all wounds
    D. wounds which bleed are more serious than those which don't bleed

14. Fractures of bones may be classified as

    A. comminuted, simple, and closed
    B. compound, simple, and comminuted
    C. comminuted, contaminated, and open
    D. simple, compound, and closed

15. When a product is advertised as having many curative powers, it is called a

    A. placebo
    B. panacea
    C. nostrum
    D. proprietary medicine

16. The MOST serious danger associated with quackery in the treatment of health problems is that it

    A. may delay medical treatment until it is too late
    B. leads to incompetent persons obtaining money falsely
    C. leads to false hope by the patient
    D. involves many innocent people who are *used* by the quack

17. A state program of medical assistance to needy persons which is financed by state and federal governments is

    A. Medicare
    B. Medicaid
    C. Blue Cross-Blue Shield
    D. Health Insurance Plan

18. *Nader's Raiders* activities brought about much-needed reforms in the

    A. Federal Trade Commission
    B. Food and Drug Administration
    C. Department of Health, Education, and Welfare
    D. Hazardous Substances Act

19. The system of healing that is based on the manipulation of the spine is

    A. chiropractic
    B. naturopathy
    C. osteoptics
    D. ophthalmology

20. More leisure time, labor saving devices, spectator sports, and automation have increased the incidence of the medical problem of

    A. obesity
    B. diabetes
    C. high blood pressure
    D. strokes

21. Man does NOT contract most animal diseases because he has

    A. acquired immunity
    B. passive immunity
    C. immune serum
    D. natural immunity

22. Bones and teeth of children are strengthened by foods rich in

    A. potassium and iodine
    B. potassium and iron
    C. calcium and phosphorus
    D. calcium and chlorine

23. A student with a non-functioning gall bladder will have difficulty digesting

    A. fats   B. sugars   C. starches   D. proteins

24. During the digestive process, amino acids are produced primarily from

    A. fats
    B. carbohydrates
    C. vitamins
    D. proteins

25. The chemical element MOST often found to be deficient in both city and country diets is

    A. iron   B. calcium   C. iodine   D. sodium

## KEY (CORRECT ANSWERS)

1. B
2. C
3. A
4. A
5. C

6. C
7. B
8. D
9. C
10. D

11. C
12. C
13. A
14. D
15. B

16. A
17. B
18. A
19. A
20. A

21. D
22. C
23. A
24. D
25. A

# TEST 4

DIRECTIONS: Each question or incomplete statement is followed by several suggested answers or completions. Select the one that BEST answers the question or completes the statement. *PRINT THE LETTER OF THE CORRECT ANSWER IN THE SPACE AT THE RIGHT.*

1. The sources of saturated fats are  1.____
   - A. meats and cereals
   - B. fish and vegetable oils
   - C. vegetables and meats
   - D. meats and dairy products

2. The energy required for the body to maintain its internal life process is called  2.____
   - A. basal metabolism
   - B. metabolic rate
   - C. nutritional requirement
   - D. caloric balance

3. In the exercise of *double leg lifting* while in a supine position, the abdominal muscles act as  3.____
   - A. stabilizers
   - B. prime movers
   - C. neutralizers
   - D. assistant movers

4. The vastus medialis and the popliteus are muscles primarily involved with movement of the  4.____
   - A. elbow
   - B. knee
   - C. neck
   - D. hip

5. The CORRECT association is:  5.____
   - A. sartorius - chest
   - B. gastrocnemius - leg
   - C. trapezius - foot
   - D. pectoralis minor - back

6. Exercises for those with chronic heart conditions should  6.____
   - A. consist of isometrics
   - B. be completely eliminated
   - C. consist of simple, light movements
   - D. be mildly competitive

7. The amount of water eliminated daily through perspiration by the average person is APPROXIMATELY _____ quart(s).  7.____
   - A. 2 to 3
   - B. 4 to 5
   - C. $\frac{1}{2}$ to 1
   - D. none of the above

8. Floor or scuff *burns* are examples of _____ wounds.  8.____
   - A. abrasion
   - B. puncture
   - C. laceration
   - D. incision

9. When applying an arm sling in cases of injury to the hand or lower forearm, the sling should be adjusted so that the hand is  9.____

A. completely covered
B. four inches above the level of the elbow
C. on the same level as the elbow
D. six inches below the level of the elbow

10. The first aid procedure for strains is to

    A. massage the affected part vigorously
    B. apply warm, moist applications
    C. immediately immobilize the affected part
    D. bandage tightly to restrict movement

11. In all fracture cases, the IMMEDIATE objective of the first aider is to

    A. try to set the bone
    B. move the victim to a more comfortable position
    C. prevent further damage
    D. take the victim to a doctor or hospital

12. When fluid accumulates between the epidermis and dermis following irritation of a local area, a _____ has formed.

    A. callous        B. boil        C. corn        D. blister

13. Of the following, the food HIGHEST in calorie value per pound is

    A. lamb        B. chocolate        C. butter        D. sugar

14. Of the following foods, the one contributing MOST to growth and repair of tissue is

    A. bread              B. honey
    C. string beans       D. cheese

15. Of the following types of wounds, the one considered MOST dangerous from the point of view of infection is the

    A. laceration    B. abrasion
    C. puncture      D. incision

16. Of the following, the MOST characteristic symptom of a third degree burn is

    A. the skin is blistered
    B. there is deep destruction of tissue
    C. the skin is reddened
    D. the skin is charred

17. The medical term for *hardening of the arteries* is

    A. carcinoma     B. arthritis
    C. thrombosis    D. arteriosclerosis

18. The process of destroying micro-organisms which cause disease or infection is called

    A. contamination    B. immunization
    C. inoculation      D. sterilization

19. Carpus, ethmoid, and coccyx are

    A. arteries    B. bones    C. enzymes    D. ligaments

20. The quality of a protein food and its effectiveness in body building are determined by the

    A. amount of corrective tissue it contains
    B. number and amount of the amino acids it contains
    C. acid-forming elements it contains
    D. amount of water present in the food

21. All of the following are found in vitamin B complex EXCEPT

    A. nicotinic acid          B. riboflavin
    C. thiamine                D. prothrombin

22. All of the following associations are correct EXCEPT:

    A. Sedative - quiets activity
    B. Analgesic - produces insensibility to pain
    C. Soporific - stimulates
    D. Anodyne - relieves pain

23. Sickle cell anemia is a blood disease MOST commonly found in children whose parents are

    A. Caucasian               B. interracial
    C. black or Latin American D. oriental

24. In order to determine the basal metabolic rate of an individual, all of the following conditions must be included EXCEPT that the

    A. environment temperature must be comfortably warm
    B. test must be made from 12 to 18 hours after the last meal
    C. body must be in the waking state and at complete rest
    D. test should be preceded by a ten-minute period of vigorous exercise

25. The accumulation of an oxygen debt by a normally healthy individual engaged in sport activity is related MOST directly to

    A. lack of endurance
    B. limited residual air
    C. strenuous exercise
    D. failure of the hemoglobin to combine with oxygen

# KEY (CORRECT ANSWERS)

1. D
2. A
3. A
4. B
5. B

6. C
7. A
8. A
9. B
10. B

11. C
12. D
13. C
14. D
15. C

16. B
17. D
18. D
19. B
20. B

21. D
22. C
23. C
24. D
25. C

# BASIC FUNDAMENTALS OF ANATOMY AND PHYSIOLOGY

## CONTENTS

| | | Page |
|---|---|---|
| SECTION I. | Basic Concepts | 1 |
| SECTION II. | Anatomical and Medical Terminology | 5 |
| SECTION III. | The Skeletal System | 9 |
| SECTION IV. | The. Skeletal Muscular System | 19 |
| SECTION V. | The Skin | 23 |
| SECTION VI. | The Circulatory System | 25 |
| SECTION VII. | The Respiratory System | 35 |
| SECTION VIII. | The Digestive System | 37 |
| SECTION IX. | The Urinary System | 42 |
| SECTION X. | The Nervous System | 44 |
| SECTION XI. | The Endocrine System | 54 |
| SECTION XII. | The Reproductive System | 56 |

# BASIC FUNDAMENTALS OF ANATOMY AND PHYSIOLOGY

## Section I. BASIC CONCEPTS

### 1. General

The science of anatomy is the study of the structure of the body, its organs, and the relation of its parts. There are many subdivisions or branches of this science. Physiology is the study of the functions and activities of the parts of the body. This science also has many subdivisions. In this chapter both anatomy and physiology will be presented in the discussion of the structure and function of the various systems of the human body, all of which are closely interrelated and interdependent.

### 2. Cells

The cell is the basic functioning unit in the composition of the human body, as well as in all other living organisms. The human body is composed of billions of cells which vary in shape and size. Cells are microscopic in size, however, the largest being only about 1/1000 of an inch. Because of this, a special unit of measurement, the micron, is used to determine cell dimensions. (One micron equals 1/1000 millimeter or about 1/25,000 of an inch.) A group of the same type of cells is called a tissue and performs a particular function. The human body is composed of many groups of cells performing a variety of functions.

*a.* Cells reproduce to replace wornout cells, to build new tissues, and to bring about the growth of the body as a whole. Cells reproduce themselves or increase by dividing, maturing, and dividing again. This process is known as growth by division. It results in a mass of apparently identical cells; however, as cell division continues, differences begin to appear in various groups of cells as they develop the characteristics necessary for them to perform their roles in the development and functions of the body. This development of special characteristics is called *cell differentiation.*

*b.* Cells are composed of a substance called protoplasm. A typical animal cell (fig. 2-1) is made up of a cell membrane and two main parts—the *nucleus* and the *cytoplasm,* which are types of protoplasm. The *nucleus* controls all activities of the cell, including growth and reproduction. *Cytoplasm* is the matter surrounding the nucleus and is responsible for most of the work done by the cell. The cell membrane incloses the protoplasm and permits the passage of fluid into and out of the cell. This permeable cell membrane is an important structural feature of the cell. It is through the cell membrane that all materials essential to metabolism are received and all products of metabolism are disposed of. The bloodstream and tissue fluid which constantly circulate around the cell transports the materials to and from cells.

(1) *Metabolism* is the ability to carry on all the chemical activities required for cell function. It includes using food and oxygen, producing and eliminating wastes, and manufacturing new materials for growth, repair, and use by other cells.

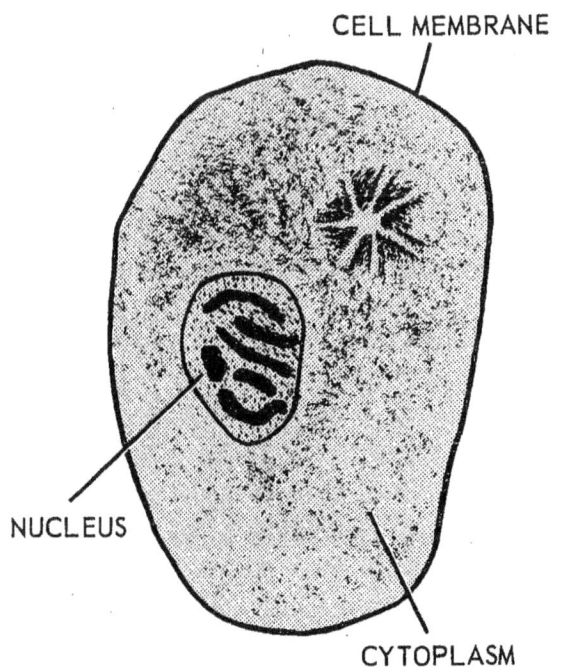

*Figure 2-1. Simple cell.*

(2) *Tissue fluid* is the body fluid that lies outside blood vessels and outside cells and is therefore also called *extravascular* (outside blood vessels) or *extracellular* (outside cells) fluid. Living body cells contain large amounts of water and must be bathed continuously in a watery solution in order to survive and carry on their functions. The colorless and slightly salty tissue fluid is derived from the circulating blood.

### 3. Tissues

A tissue is a part of the body made up of similarly specialized cells which work together to perform particular body functions. There are four main types of tissues, each of which has a particular function (fig. 2–2).

*a. Epithelial.* Epithelial tissue forms the outer layer of skin for the protection of the body. It is also a lining tissue. As *mucous membrane*, it lines the nasal cavity, mouth, larynx, pharynx, trachea, stomach, and intestines. As *serous membrane*, it lines the abdominal, chest, and heart cavities and covers the organs that lie in these cavities. As *endothelium*, it lines the heart and blood vessels. It lines respiratory and digestive organs for the functions of protection and absorption. It helps form organs concerned with the excretion of body wastes, certain glands for the purpose of secretion, and certain sensory organs for the reception of stimuli. Based on the shape of the cells, there are 3 types of epithelial tissue (fig. 2–2Ⓐ). As illustrated, squamous (flat) epithelial cells in a single layer compose such structures as the microscopic air sacs of the lungs; in other places as in the skin, squamous epithelium is in several layers or stratified (not illustrated). Columnar epithelium cells are more important in the formation of ducts.

*b. Connective.* Connective tissue is distributed throughout the body to form the supporting framework of the body and to bind together and support other tissues. It binds organs to other organs, muscles to bones, and bones to other bones. There are five principal types of connective tissue—

(1) Areolar tissue is a fibrous connective tissue which forms the subcutaneous layer of tissue. It fills many of the small spaces on the body, and it helps to hold organs in place.

(2) Adipose tissue (fig. 2–2Ⓑ) is a fatty connective tissue which is found under the skin and in many other regions of the body. It serves as a padding around and between organs. It insulates the body, reducing heat loss, and it serves as a food reserve in emergencies.

(3) Reticular tissue is a fibrous connective tissue which forms the supporting framework of lymph glands, liver, spleen, bone marrow, and lungs.

(4) Elastic tissue is a fibrous connective tissue composed of elastic fibers and is found in the walls of blood vessels, in the lungs, and in certain ligaments.

(5) Cartilage (fig. 2–2Ⓑ) is a tough, resilient connective tissue found at the ends of the bones, between bones, and in the nose, throat, and ears.

*c. Muscular.* Muscular tissue is composed of long, slender cells held together by connective tissue. There are three kinds of muscle tissues: striated, smooth, and cardiac (heart muscle). Muscle tissue has the ability to contract (shorten) and, by so doing, to produce movement.

(1) Striated muscle has striations (its fibers are divided by transverse bands) (fig. 2–2Ⓒ) when viewed through a microscope. Because most striated muscle attaches to bones, it is often referred to as skeletal muscle. Skeletal muscle contraction is stimulated by impulses from nerves and, in theory, the nerve impulses can be controlled by voluntary or conscious effort. Skeletal muscle tissue is therefore referred to as striated, voluntary muscle tissue.

(2) Smooth muscle which has no striations when viewed through a microscope (fig. 2–2 Ⓒ), is found in the walls of internal organs (viscera), blood vessels, and internal passages. Contraction of smooth muscle helps propel the contents of internal structures along. Smooth muscle contractions are stimulated by nerve impulses not under conscious control. Smooth muscle is therefore referred to as visceral, nonstriated, involuntary muscle.

(3) Cardiac muscle (fig. 2–2Ⓒ) is found only in the walls of the heart; i.e., myocardium is heart muscle.

*d. Nervous.* Nervous tissue is composed of cells highly specialized to receive and transmit impulses (messages). These nerve cells, which are called neurons (fig. 2–2Ⓓ), are bound together by a special structure called neuroglia.

### 4. Organs

An organ is a group of tissues which has combined to perform a specific function. The body is

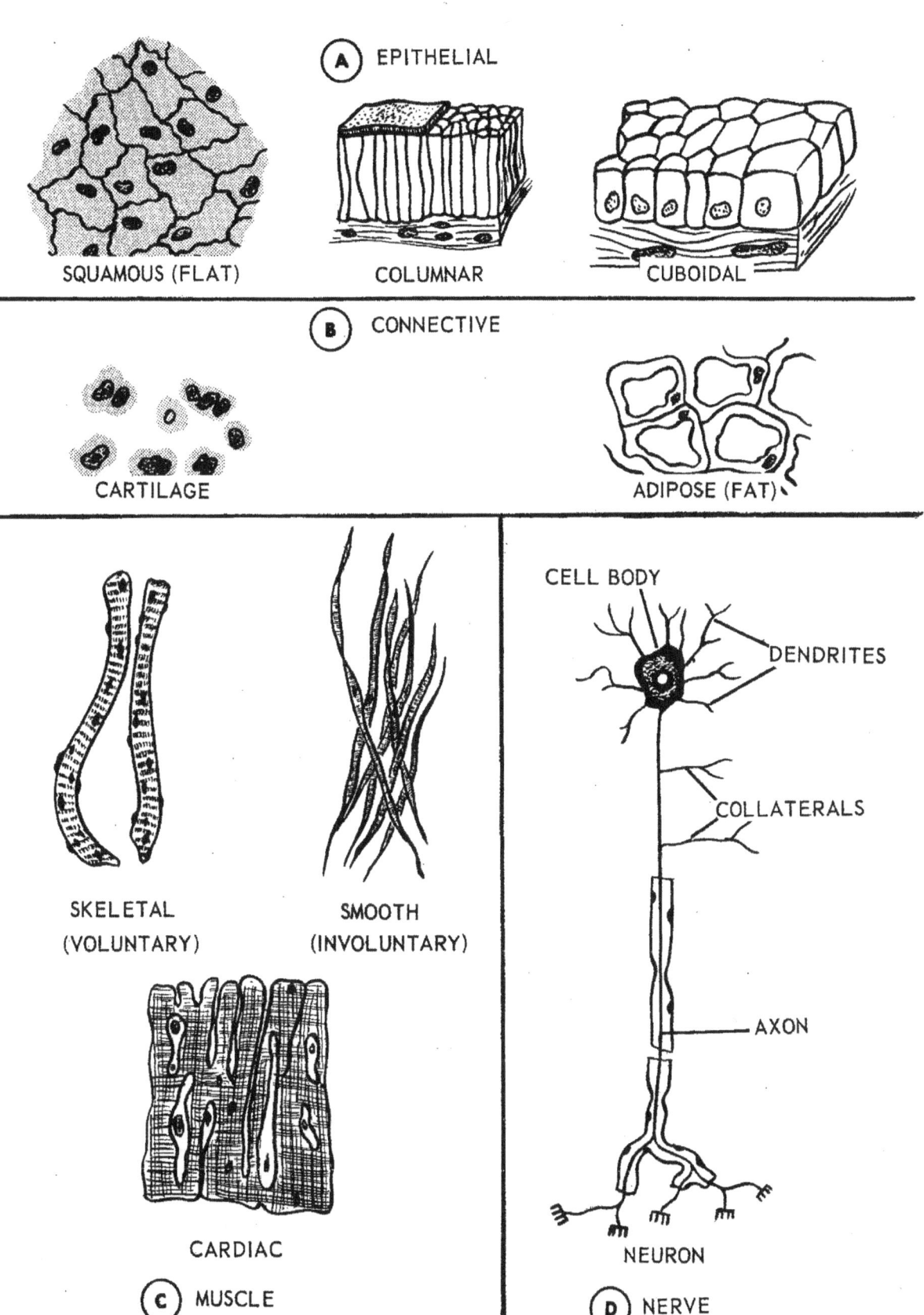

Figure 2-2. Types of tissues.

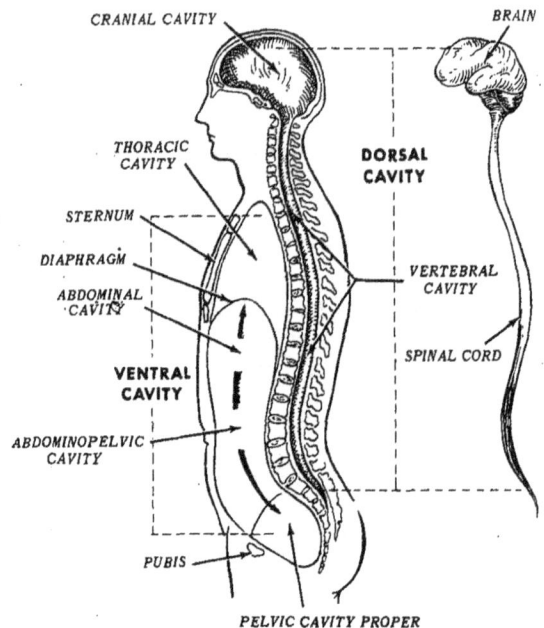

*Figure 2-3. Main body cavities.*

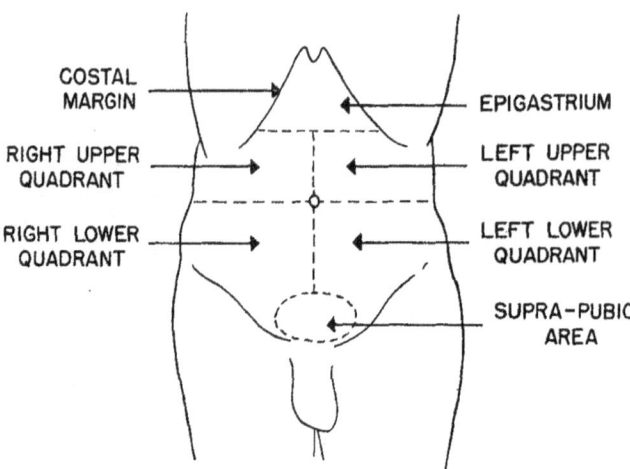

*Figure 2-4. Areas of the abdomen.*

composed of many organs, each with its own specialized function.

## 5. Body Cavities

The organs of the body are located in certain cavities, the major ones of which are the dorsal cavity (toward the back part of the body) and the ventral cavity (toward the front part of the body) (fig. 2-3).

*a. Dorsal Cavity.* The dorsal cavity has a cranial area, which contains the brain, and a vertebral area, which contains the spinal cord. These areas are continuous.

*b. Ventral Cavity.* The ventral cavity has a thoracic cavity and an abdomino pelvic cavity. These areas are separated by the diaphragm.

(1) In the thoracic cavity are two pleural cavities, each containing a lung. In the space between the pleural cavities is the pericardial cavity, which contains the heart, and the mediastinal region, in which are contained the trachea, esophagus, thymus gland, large blood and lymphatic vessels, lymph nodes, and nerves.

(2) In the upper part of the abdomino pelvic cavity are the stomach, small intestine, liver, gallbladder, pancreas, spleen, kidneys, adrenal glands, and ureters. The lower part of the cavity (pelvic cavity) contains the urinary bladder, the end of the large intestine (rectum), and parts of the reproductive system.

*c. Anterior Abdominal Surface Area.* The large anterior area of the abdomino pelvic cavity is divided into four parts or quadrants (fig. 2-4). Initials that identify quadrants are LUQ (left upper), RUQ (right upper), LLQ (left lower), and RLQ (right lower). These initials are often used to indicate the approximate location of an organ, pain, a wound, or a surgical incision. In addition to identification by quadrants, the upper central abdominal region is referred to as epigastric (over the stomach), and the lower central region as suprapubic (above the pubis). The rib area is called costal.

## 6. Membranes

Certain membranes are combined layers of tissue that form partitions, linings, envelopes, or capsules. They reinforce and support body organs and cavities. Others are a combination of connective tissues only (*examples:* mucous, pleural, pericardial, and peritoneal membranes). Connective tissue membranes are combinations of connective tissue only (*examples:* meninges, fascia, periosteum, and synovia). Different kinds of membranes are associated with different body systems (*examples:* pleural membranes with the respiratory system; pericardial membranes with the circulatory system; peritoneal membranes with the digestive system; meningeal membranes with the nervous system; fascial membranes with the muscular system; and periosteal and synovial membranes with the skeletal system).

## 7. Body Systems

The organs of the human body are arranged into major systems, each of which has its specific function to perform and all of which are interdependent. The body systems and their overall functions are—

*a. Skeletal.* This system provides the body framework, supports and protects body organs, and furnishes a place of attachment for muscles.

*b. Muscular.* This system moves and propels the body.

*c. Skin.* The integumentary system, or skin, covers and protects the entire body surface from injury and infection, has functions of sensation (heat, cold, touch, and pain) and assists in regulation of body temperature and excretion of wastes.

*d. Circulatory.* This system transports oxygen and nutrient material in the blood to all parts of the body and carries away the waste products formed by the cells.

*e. Respiratory.* This system takes in air, delivers oxygen from the air to the blood, and removes the waste (carbon dioxide) from the blood.

*f. Digestive.* This system receives, digests, and absorbs food substances and eliminates waste products.

*g. Urinary.* This system filters waste products from blood and excretes waste products in urine.

*h. Nervous.* This system gives the body awareness of its environment, enables it to react to stimuli from the environment, and makes the body work together as a unit.

*i. Endocrine.* This system controls many body activities by the manufacture of hormones which are secreted into the blood.

*j. Reproductive.* This system produces and transports reproductive (sex) cells.

## Section II. ANATOMICAL AND MEDICAL TERMINOLOGY

### 8. Anatomical Terminology

Terms of position, direction, and location that are used in reference to the body and its parts include the following:

*a. Terms of Position.*

(1) Anatomical position—the body standing erect, arms at side, palms of hands facing forward. The anatomical position is the position of reference when terms of direction and location are used.

(2) Supine position—the body lying face up.

(3) Prone position—the body lying face down.

(4) Lateral recumbent—the body lying on the left or right side.

*b. Terms of Direction and Location.*

(1) Superior—toward the head (cranial).

(2) Inferior—toward the feet (caudal).

(3) Anterior—toward the front (ventral—the belly side).

(4) Posterior—toward the back (dorsal—the backbone side).

(5) Medial—toward the midline.

(6) Lateral—to right or left of midline.

(7) Proximal—near point of reference.

(8) Distal—far away from point of reference.

*c. Body Regions.* Terms of location in relation to body regions are shown in figure 2–5 Ⓐ and Ⓑ.

*d. Anatomical Planes.* Imaginary straight line divisions of the body are called planes. Medical illustrations and diagrams that indicate internal body structure relationships are labeled to indicate the plane division as—

(1) Sagittal—a lengthwise division, producing right and left sections.

(2) Transverse—a crosswise division, producing top and bottom sections.

(3) Frontal—a side-to-side division, producing front and back sections.

### 9. Medical Terminology

To understand most medical words, all that is necessary is to break the words into their parts and to know the meaning of these parts. Many medical words contain a stem or root to which is affixed either a prefix, a suffix, or both. A prefix is a group of letters combined with the beginning of a word to modify its meaning. A suffix is a group of letters added to the end of a word to modify its meaning. *For example,* the word "myocarditis"

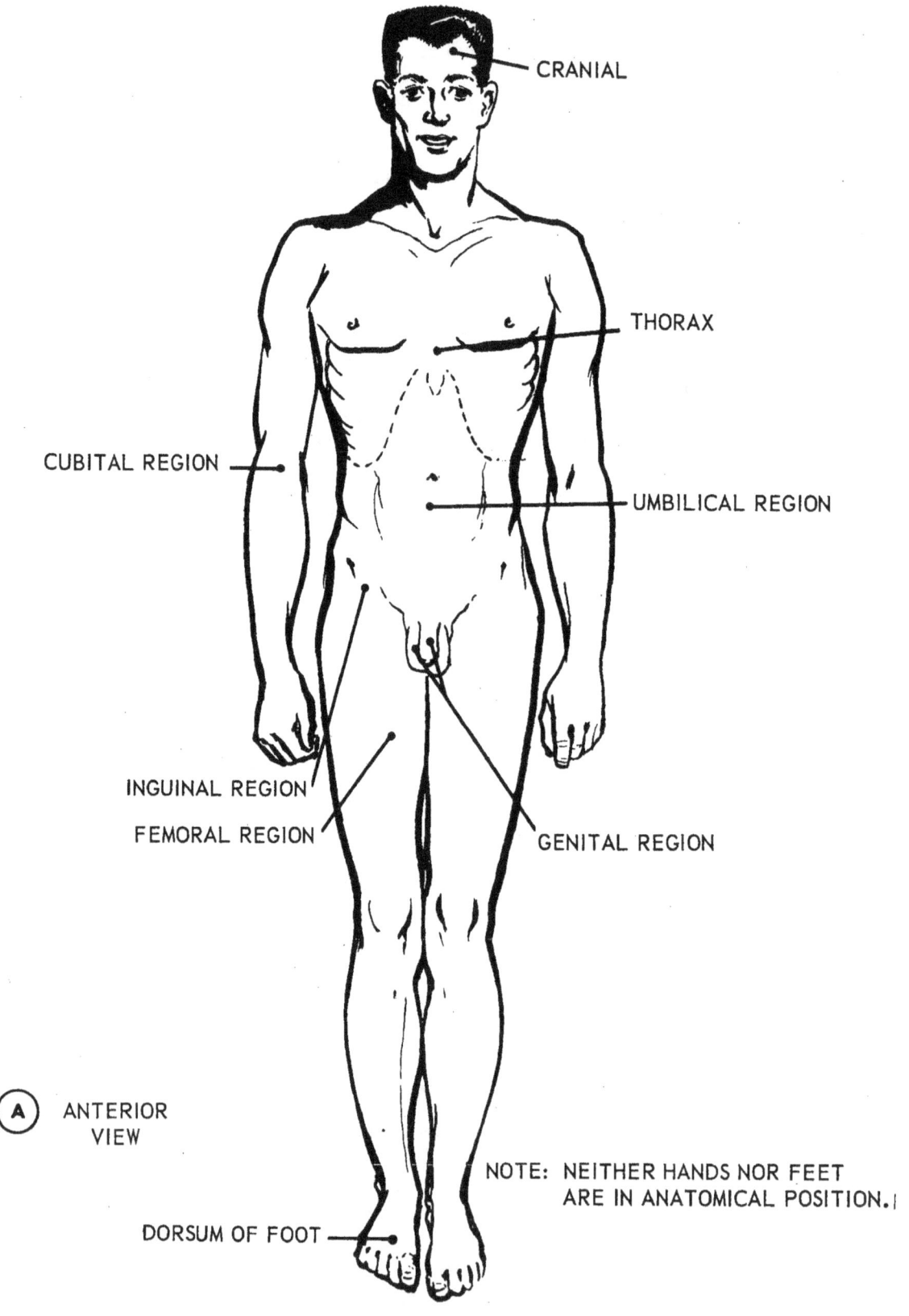

Figure 2-5. Names of body regions.

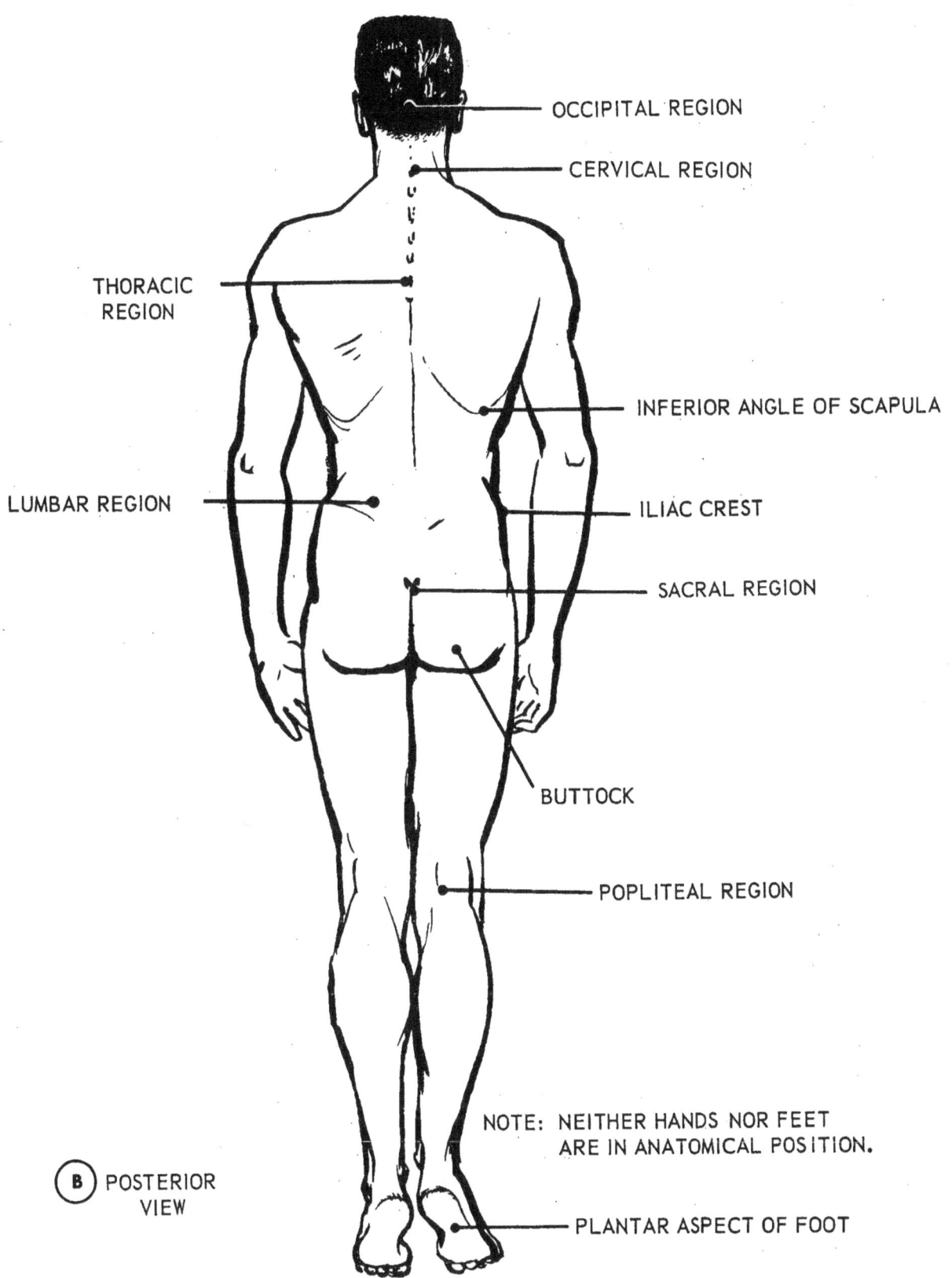

Figure 2-5—Continued.

consists of the prefix "myo," the stem "card," and the suffix "itis." Myo means "muscle." Card means "cardiac" or "heart." Itis means "inflammation." Thus, myocarditis means inflammation of muscles of the heart. Table 2–1 gives combining forms that are commonly used in medical terminology. These must be learned to understand medical references that will occur from now on.

Table 2-1. Medical Terminology

| STEM WORDS | MEANING | PREFIX | MEANING | EXAMPLE OF USE IN MEDICINE | DEFINITION OF EXAMPLE | SUFFIX | MEANING | EXAMPLE OF USE IN MEDICINE | DEFINITION OF EXAMPLE |
|---|---|---|---|---|---|---|---|---|---|
| adeno | gland | a-, an- | absence of, deficiency | atrophy | shrinking, wasting away | -algia | pain | otalgia | ear ache |
| arthro | joint | endo- | inner, inside | endocardial | inside the heart | -ectomy | surgical removal | nephrectomy | surgical removal of a kidney |
| cardio | heart | | | | | | | | |
| cephalo | head | epi- | upon, on the outside | epidermis | outside layer of skin | -emia | a condition of the blood | septicemia | blood poisoning |
| cysto | bladder | hyper- | more than normal, over | hypertrophy | enlargement | -itis | inflammation | hepatitis | inflammation of the liver |
| cyto | cell | hypo- | less than normal, under | hypotension | low blood pressure | -oma | a tumor, a swelling | adenoma | a glandular tissue tumor |
| dermo | skin | | | | | -plasty | surgical repair | thoracoplasty | surgical repair of the chest wall |
| entero | intestine | inter- | between | interneural | between nerves | | | | |
| gastro | stomach | intra- | inside | intraocular | inside the eye | -scopy | looking into or through an instrument | cystoscopy | examination of the urinary bladder through a cystoscope |
| hemo | blood | peri- | surrounding | periosteum | membrane surrounding bone | | | | |
| hepato | liver | | | | | | | | |
| myelo | *spinal cord | | | | | -stomy | surgical opening creating a hole | gastrostomy | artificial opening into the stomach through the abdomen |
| myo | muscle | | | | | -tomy | surgical incision | arthrotomy | incision into a joint |
| nephro | kidney | | | | | | | | |
| neuro | nerve | | | | | | | | |
| oculo | eye | | | | | | | | |
| osteo | bone | | | | | | | | |
| oto | ear | | | | | | | | |
| procto | rectum | | | | | | | | |
| thoraco | chest | | | | | | | | |
| | *or bone marrow | | | | | | | | |

## Section III. THE SKELETAL SYSTEM

### 10. Functions and Divisions
(fig. 2-6 Ⓐ and Ⓑ)

The skeletal system includes the bones and the joints (articulations), where separate bones come together. The skeletal system has several important functions, in addition to providing the bony framework of the body.

*a. Skeletal System Function.*

(1) To give support and shape the body.
(2) To protect internal organs.
(3) To provide movement when acted upon by muscles.
(4) To manufacture blood cells.
(5) To store mineral salts.

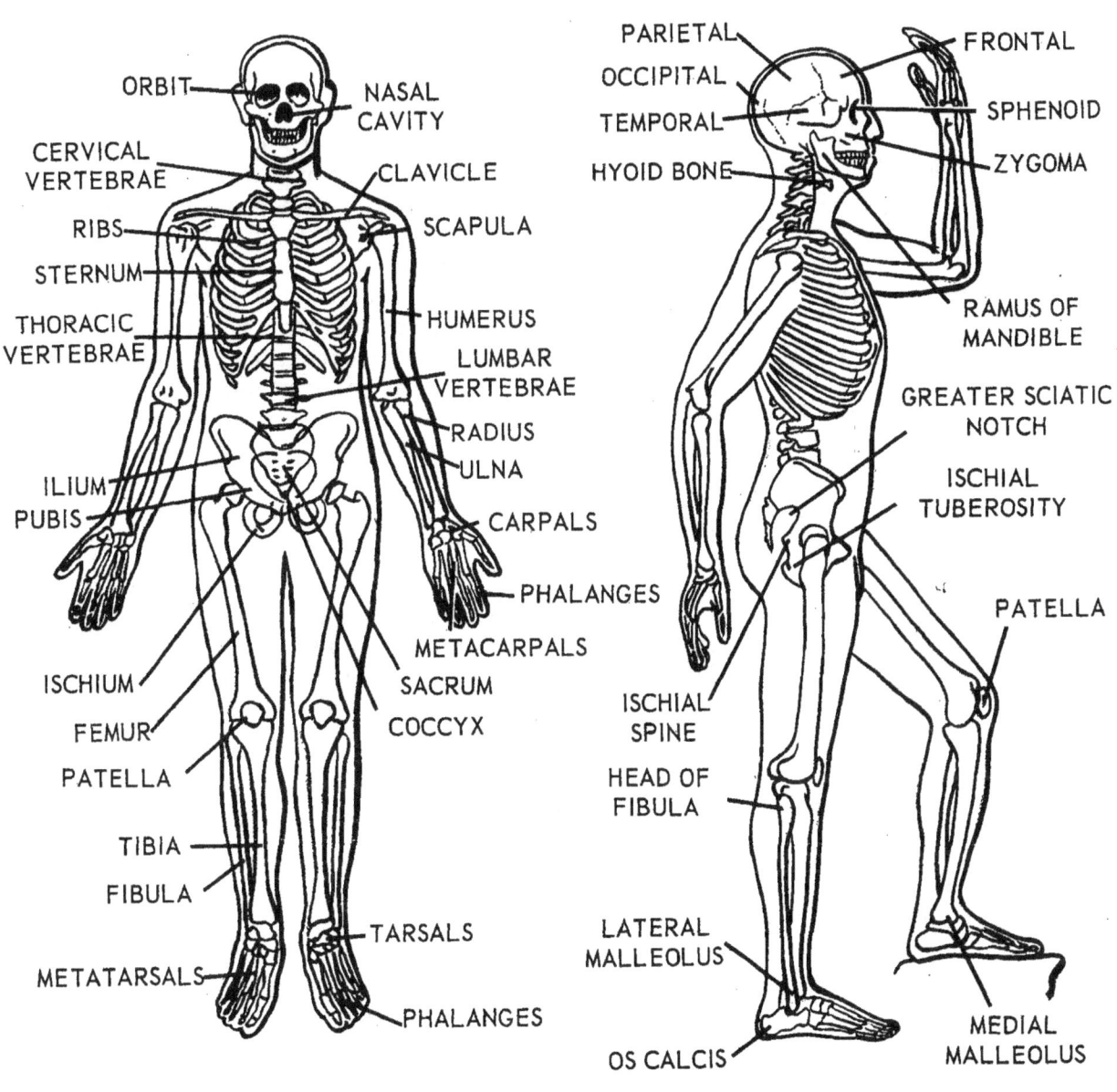

*Figure 2-6. Human skeleton.*

b. *Divisions of the Skeleton.* For study purposes, the 206 bones of the adult are divided into the bones of the axial skeleton (80 bones) and the appendicular skeleton (126 bones). The axial skeleton includes the skull, vertebral column, ribs, and sternum. The appendicular skeleton includes bones of the shoulder girdle, upper limb, the pelvic girdle, and lower limb.

## 11. Bone Structure and Shape of Bones

a. Bone is living tissue, containing blood vessels and nerves within the hard bone structures. The living cells that form bones are osteocytes. Bone cells have the ability to select calcium and other minerals from blood and tissue fluid and to deposit the calcium in the connective tissue fibers between cells. With increasing age, from childhood to adulthood, bones become harder; in old age, bones become brittle because there are higher proportions of minerals and fewer active cells. Periosteum, the membrane covering bone surfaces, carries blood vessels and nerves to the bone cells. Bone-producing cells in periosteum are active during growth and repair of injuries. Two kinds of bone are formed by the bone cells—compact and cancellous. Compact bone is hard and dense, while cancellous bone has a porous structure. The combination of compact and cancellous bone cells produces maximum strength with minimum weight.

b. Bones are classified by their shape as long, short, flat, and irregular. Long bones are in the extremities and act as levers to produce motion when acted on by muscles. Short bones, strong and compact, are in the wrist and ankle. Flat bones form protective plates and provide broad surfaces for muscle attachments; *for example,* the shoulder blades. Irregular bones have many surfaces and fit into many locations; *for example,* the facial bones, vertebral, and pelvic bones. A long bone is used as an example of bone structure (fig. 2–7).

(1) Long bones have a shaft (the diaphysis) and two extremities (the epiphyses). The shaft is a heavy cylinder of compact bone with a central medullary (marrow) cavity. This cavity contains bone marrow, blood vessels, and nerves. Cancellous bone is located toward the epiphyses and is covered by a protecting layer of compact bone.

(2) Articular cartilage covers the joint surfaces at the ends of a long bone. The cartilage provides a smooth contact surface in joint formation and gives some resilience for shock absorption.

(3) Periosteum, the membrane covering the bone surface, is anchored to the bone by connective tissue fibers. It is essential for bone nourishment and repair. In severe bone injuries, the periosteum may be torn away or damaged, inhibiting repair of the bone.

## 12. Bone Marrow

Two kinds of marrow, yellow and red, are found in the marrow cavities of bones. Red bone marrow is active blood cell manufacturing material, producing red blood cells and many of the white blood cells. Deposits of red bone marrow in an adult are in cancellous portions of some bones—the skull, ribs, and sternum, for example. Yellow bone marrow is mostly fat and is found in marrow cavities of mature long bones. The examination of red marrow deposits is important for diagnostic tests when the condition of developing blood cells must be determined. For microscopic examination, the doctor obtains a small amount through a special needle puncture, usually in the sternum.

## 13. Bone Landmarks

The special markings and projections on bones are used as points of reference. Each marking has a function; *for example,* in joint formation, for muscle attachments, or as passageways for blood vessels and nerves. Terms used to refer to bone markings include—

a. Foramen—an opening, a hole.

b. Sinus—an air space.

c. Head—a rounded ball end.

d. Neck—a constricted portion.

e. Condyle—a projection fitting into a joint.

f. Fossa—a socket.

g. Crest—a ridge.

h. Spine—a sharp projection.

## 14. The Skull

The skull forms the framework of the head. It has 29 bones—8 cranial, 14 facial, 6 ossicles (3 tiny bones in each ear), and 1 hyoid (a single bone between the skull and neck area).

a. *Cranial Bones.* The cranial bones support and protect the brain. They fuse together after birth in firmly united joints called sutures. The eight

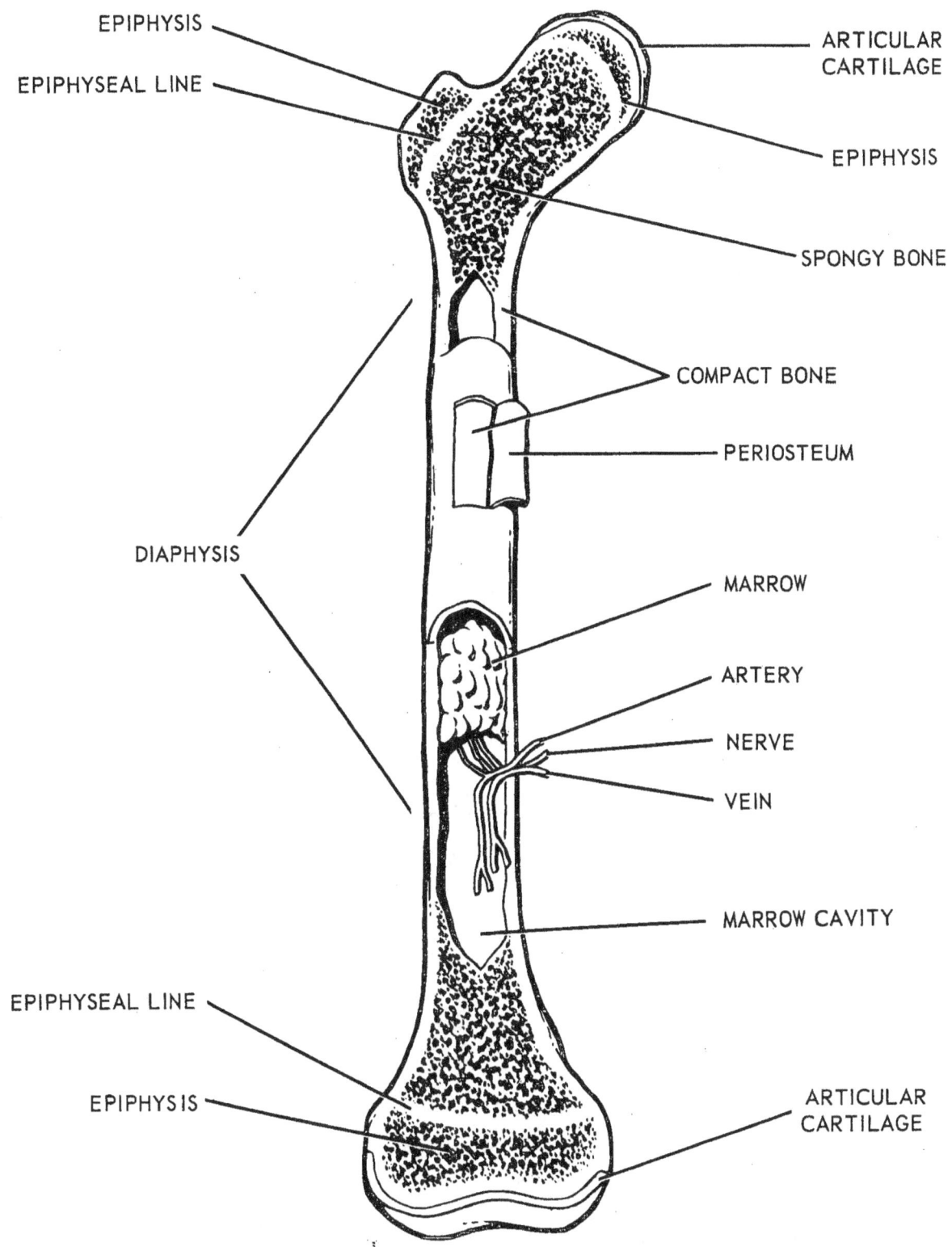

*Figure 2-7. A long bone (femur).*

cranial bones include one frontal, two parietal, one occipital, two temporal, one ethmoid, and one sphenoid (fig. 2-8 Ⓐ). The frontal bone forms the forehead, part of the eye socket, and part of the nose. The parietal bones form the dome of the skull and the upper side walls. The occipital bone forms the back and base of the skull. (The foramen magnum, the large hole in the lower part of the occipital bone, is the passageway for the spinal cord.) The temporal bones form the lower part of each side of the skull and contain the essential organs of hearing and of balance in the middle and

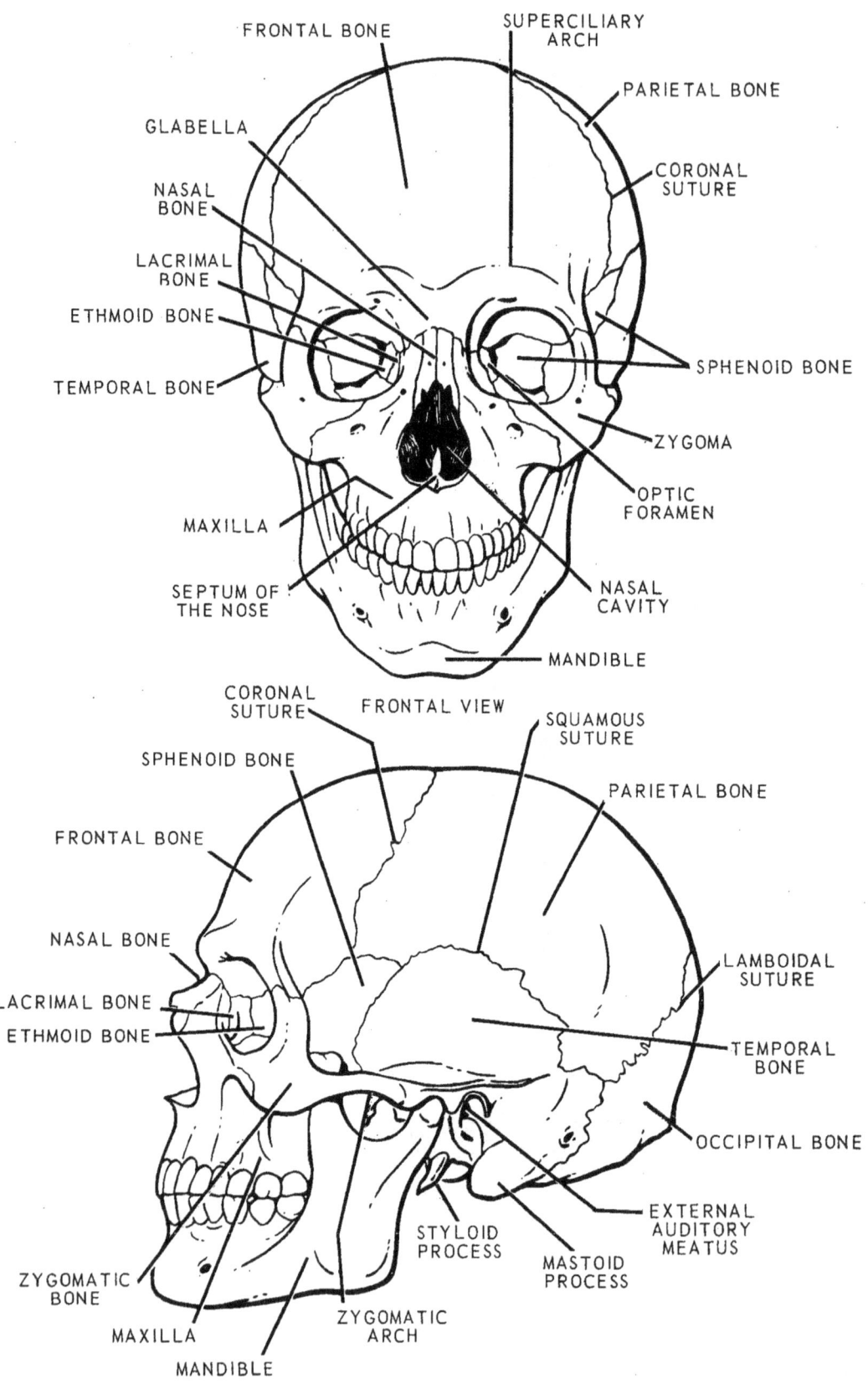

Figure 2-8. The skull.

inner parts of the ear. The ethmoid and sphenoid bones complete the floor of the cranium, the ethmoid toward the front and the sphenoid toward the center. The air spaces in the frontal, ethmoid, and sphenoid bones are sinuses.

  b. *Facial Bones.* The 14 facial bones fit together like a very complicated jigsaw puzzle; for example, part of 7 different cranial and facial bones form each eye socket; 2 maxillary bones, the upper jaw; 2 zygomatic, the upper cheeks; and 1 mandible, the lower jaw (fig. 2-8 Ⓑ). The maxillary bones support the upper teeth, and the mandible supports the lower teeth. The joints formed by the mandible and temporal bones permit jaw movement. Nine smaller facial bones complete the nose and roof of the mouth (two nasal, two turbinate, one vomer, two lacrimal, and two maxilla).

## 15. The Vertebral Column
(fig. 2-9)

The 26 bones of the vertebral column form a flexible structure, supporting the head, thorax, and the upper extremities. The arrangement of the vertebrae provides a protected passageway for the spinal cord. Vertebral bones are classified into four regions—cervical (neck); thoracic (chest); lumbar (lower back); and sacral-coccygeal (pelvic).

  a. *Vertebral Structure.*

  (1) A typical vertebra has an anterior portion, the body, and a posterior portion, the arch (fig. 2-10). The body and the arch encircle the spinal canal, the opening through which the spinal cord passes. Between vertebral bodies are the intervertebral discs, which are fibrocartilage structures that serve as shock-absorbing connections between vertebrae. The irregular projections from the arches are spinous processes posteriorly (these are the projections you feel when you run your fingers along the midline of the back) and transverse processes laterally. Intervertebral foramena are openings on either side of the arches for passage of spinal nerves to and from the spinal cord.

  (2) The movement of casualties suspected of having a spinal injury is always potentially hazardous. Careless movement increases the possibility of damage to the spinal cord. At least three persons are needed to move such a casualty. It is particularly important that the individual directing the movement understand the anatomy and physiology of the vertebral column and its relationship with the spinal cord and nerves.

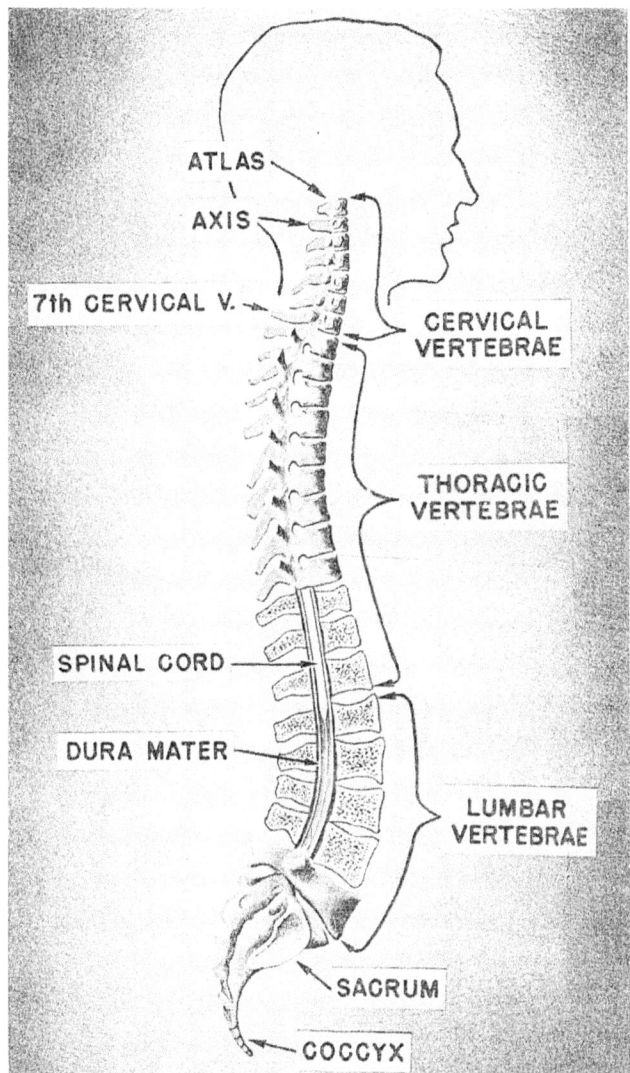

*Figure 2-9. Vertebral column.*

  b. *Vertebral Curves.* The vertebral column has four normal curves for strength and balance—cervical and lumbar curves are concave, curving inward; thoracic and sacral curves are convex, curving outward. Abnormal, exaggerated spinal curvatures can be disabling.

  c. *Classification of Vertebrae.* Seven cervical vertebrae are in the neck region. The first cervical vertebra is called the atlas, the second vertebra, the axis. These are the only named vertebrae. All other vertebrae are numbered according to region. The prominent knob at the base of the neck is formed by the spinous process of the 7th cervical vertebra. Twelve thoracic vertebrae form the posterior wall of the chest, and each thoracic vertebra articulates with one pair of ribs. The five lumbar vertebrae are in the lower back and support the posterior abdominal wall. The sacrum, a

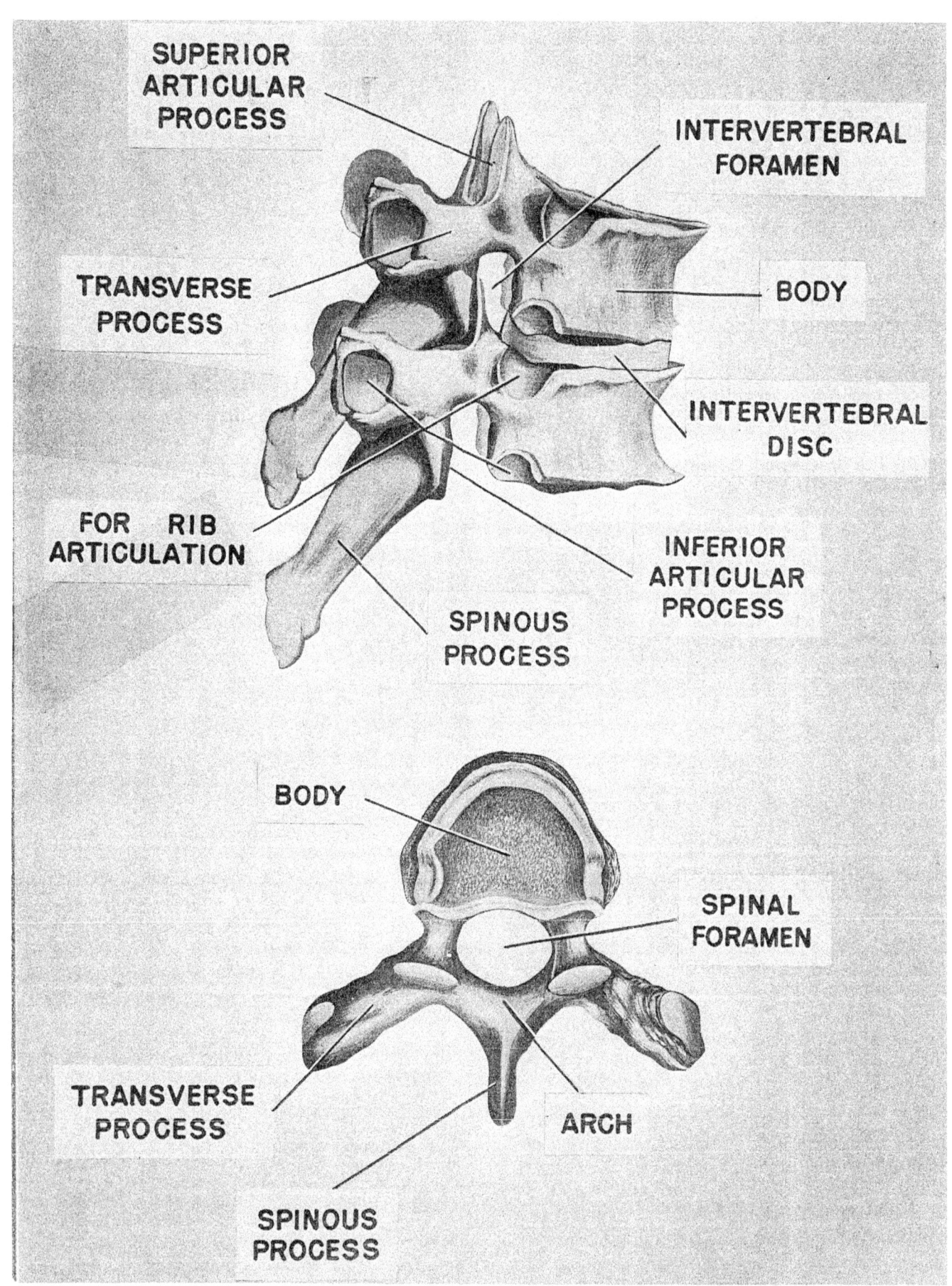

Figure 2-10. Typical vertebrae.

flat, spade-shaped bone, forms the posterior part of the pelvic girdle. The coccyx is the "tail bone," the thin, curving end of the vertebral column. In the adult, five sacral bones have fused to form one sacrum, and four coccygeal bones have fused to form one coccyx.

### 16. The Thorax

The thorax, or chest cage, is formed by 25 bones: 12 thoracic vertebrae, 2 pairs of ribs, and 1 sternum. Rib cartilages (costal cartilages) complete the chest cage. The thorax contains and protects the heart, lungs, and related structures of circulation and respiration. The ribs curve outward, forward, and downward from their posterior attachments to the vertebrae. The first seven pairs of ribs are joined directly to the sternum by their costal cartilages. The next three pairs (numbered 8, 9, 10), are attached to the sternum indirectly—each cartilage attaches to the one above—while the last two pairs, "the floating ribs," are not attached to the sternum. The sternum is the anterior flat breastbone and the ribs form the expandable chest cage wall.

### 17. The Shoulder Girdle and Upper Limbs

(fig. 2–11)

The shoulder girdle is a flexible yoke that suspends and supports the arms. Held in place by muscles, it has only one point of attachment to the axial skeleton—the joint between the clavicle and sternum. The shoulder girdle is formed by two scapulae posteriorly and two clavicles anteriorly. The bones of the shoulder and upper limb include the scapula (shoulder blade); clavicle (collar bone); humerus (arm bone); radius and ulna (forearm bones); carpals (wristbones); metacarpals (hand bones); and phalanges (finger bones).

*a.* The scapula is a large triangular bone extending from the second to the seventh or eighth ribs, posteriorly. The heavy ridge extending across the upper surface of the scapula ends in a process called the acromion, which forms the tip of the shoulder and the joint with the clavicle, anteriorly. A socket for the head of the humerus is on the lateral surface of the scapula. Strong muscles attach to the scapula for shoulder and arm movement.

*b.* The clavicle is a slender, S-curved bone lying horizontally above the first rib. The lateral end of the clavicle forms a joint with the scapula (acromio-clavicular joint). The medial end of the clavicle forms a joint with the sternum at the sterno-clavicular joint, which can be felt as the knob on either side of the notch at the base of the throat. The clavicle acts as a shoulder brace, holding the shoulder up and back. When the clavicle is fractured, the shoulder slumps forward.

*c.* The humerus is a heavy long bone in the arm that extends from the shoulder to the elbow. The rounded proximal end fits into the scapula in a socket, the glenoid fossa. The distal end of the humerus forms the elbow joint, articulating with the ulna and part of the radius. Strong muscles reinforce the shoulder joint and attach to the humerus, protecting the large blood vessels and nerves that extend along the bone.

*d.* The radius and ulna (fig. 2–12) are the bones of the forearm. The ulna, on the little finger side, forms the major part of the elbow joint with the humerus. A projection of the ulna, the olecranon, is the "funny bone" at the point of the elbow. The radius, on the thumb side, forms the major part of the wrist joint. The action of the radius about the ulna permits hand turning.

*e.* The wrist (fig. 2–12) has eight small bones (carpal bones) arranged in two rows of four each. They articulate with each other and with the bones of the hand and forearm. Articulating with the carpals are five metacarpals which form the bony structure of the palm of the hand. The metacarpal of the thumb is particularly important—its muscular attachment permits the thumb to meet the other fingers of the hand, an action called opposing. (This opposing thumb enables the human hand to manipulate articles with great dexterity.) The 14 phalanges in each hand are the finger bones, 3 in each finger and 2 in each thumb. The nerves, blood vessels, and tendons in the hand and wrist are close to the surface and, when injured, can cause serious disability. Injuries to the hand require special evaluation and painstaking treatment to prevent deformities and crippling of finger movements.

### 18. The Pelvis and Lower Limbs

The two hip bones form the pelvic girdle, which provides articulation for the lower limbs. The pelvis, jointed by the hip bones, sacrum, and coccyx, forms a strong bony basin which supports the trunk and protects the contents of the abdomino pelvic cavity. When the upright body is in proper alinement, the pelvis distributes the weight evenly to both lower extremities. The bones of the pelvis

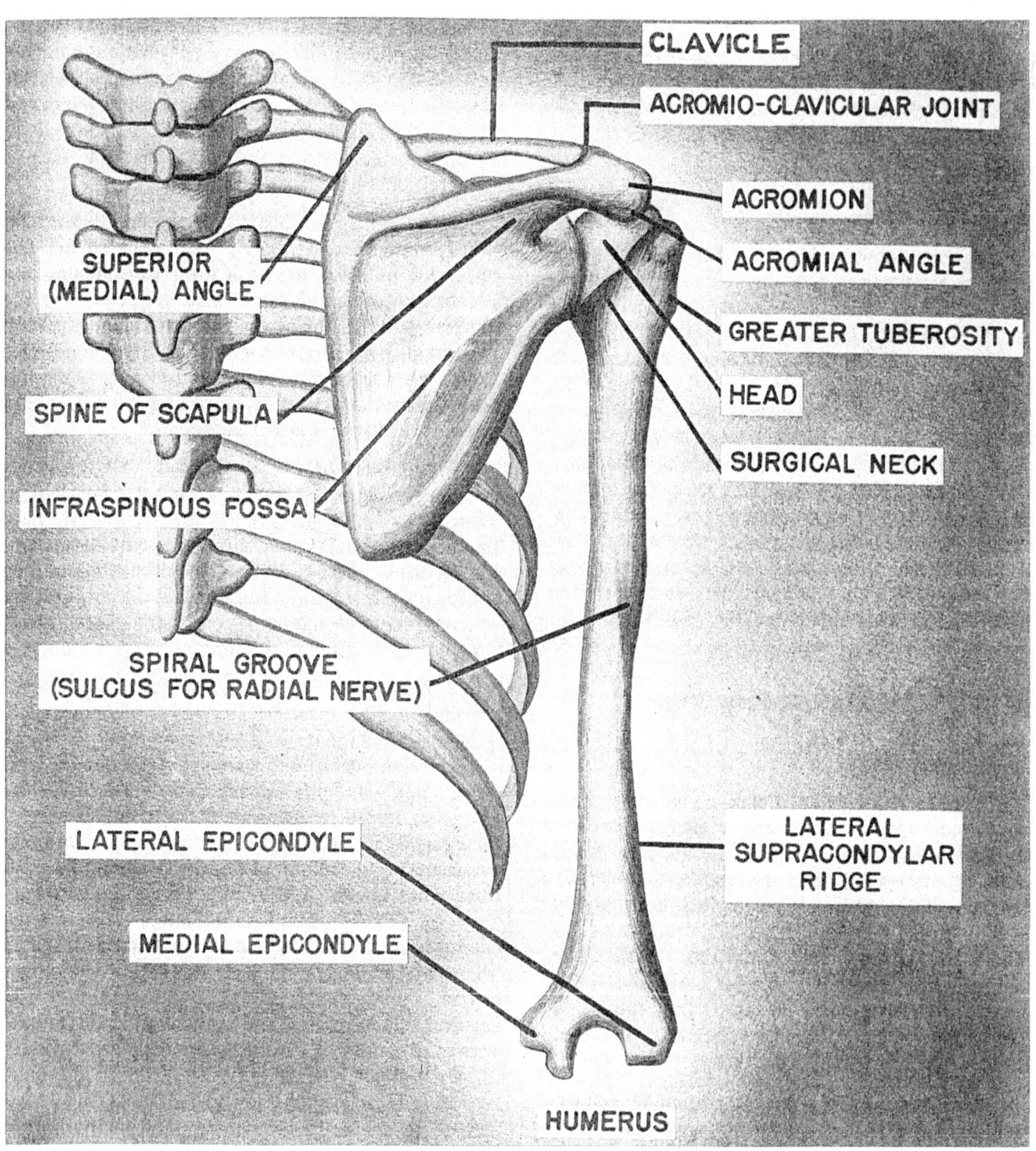

*Figure 2-11. Shoulder girdle.*

and lower extremity are the os coxa (hip bone), femur (thigh bone), patella (knee cap), tibia and fibula (leg bones), tarsals (ankle bones), metatarsals (foot bones), and phalanges (toe bones) (fig. 2-6). In contrast to the shoulder girdle, the pelvic girdle is inflexible and very strong (for weight bearing).

a. The hip bone is formed by the fusion of three bones into one massive, irregular bone, the os coxa. The two hip bones are joined together anteriorly in the symphysis pubis. Posteriorly, the hip bones are fused to the sacrum. Each hip bone has three distinctive parts—the ilium, ischium and pubis (fig. 2-13). The ilium is the broad, flaring

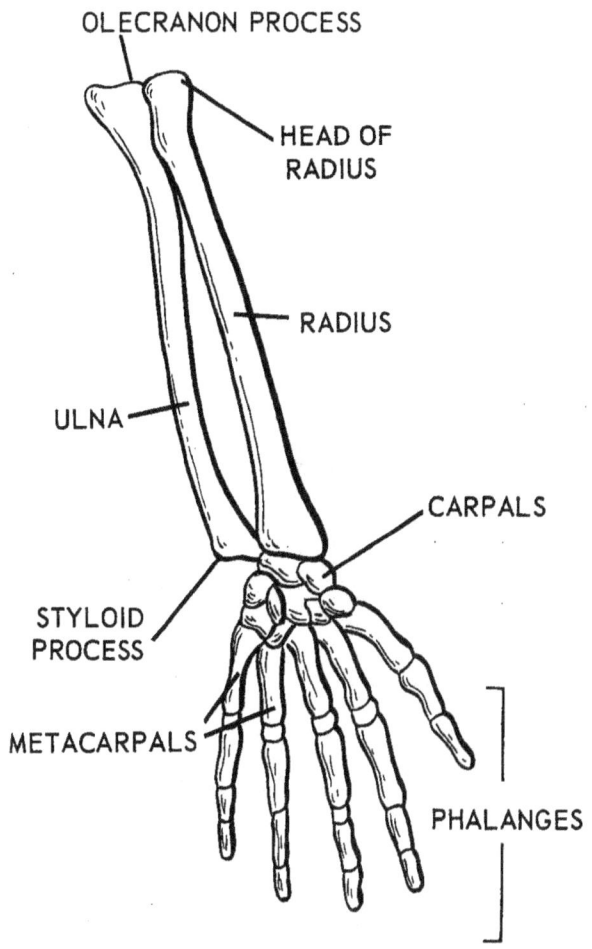

*Figure 2-12. Forearm and hand.*

that extends from the strong anterior thigh muscles. The patella has an oval shape in cross section and is classified as a sesamoid bone (bone embedded in tendons).

*d.* The tibia and fibula are the two bones in the leg. The tibia, which is thicker and stronger, is the shin bone. It supports body weight and articulates with the femur in the knee joint. The projection at its lower end is the medial malleolus, the inner ankle bone. The fibula, the lateral leg bone, is joined to the tibia at its proximal end, but not to the femur. The projection at the distal end of the fibula is the lateral malleolus, the outer ankle bone.

*e.* The skeleton of the foot consists of the tarsals, metatarsals, and the phalanges. Seven tarsals form the ankle, heel, and posterior half of the instep. The talus is the largest ankle bone, and the calcaneus is the heel bone. Five metatarsals form the anterior half of the instep. The tarsals and metatarsals together form the arch of the foot, a structure important in weight distribution to the foot. Tendons and ligaments hold the tarsals and metatarsals in their arched position, and when this support is weak, the foot is flat. The 14 phalanges of the toes are similar to finger bones but are less important for foot function than fingers are for hand function.

## 19. Joints (Articulations)

A joint is a structure which holds together separate bones. Joints are classified according to the amount of movement they permit—immovable, slightly movable, and freely movable (fig. 2-14).

*a.* Immovable joints have bone surfaces fused together to prevent motion. At one time during skeletal development, these joints had some movement but as the bones matured they grew together for stability. The pelvic girdle, sacral and coccygeal vertebrae, and skull bones are examples of immovable joints.

*b.* Slightly movable joints have cartilage discs between bones and are held in place by strong ligaments. The cartilage permits some give, and ligaments prevent bone separation. Vertebral bodies and the symphysis pubis are examples of slightly movable joints.

*c.* Freely movable joints permit maximum motion. These joints have a more complex arrangement since they have joint cavities. The several parts of a joint cavity include the joint capsule, the capsule lining (synovial membrane), and some lubricating fluid within the cavity. Ligaments are

upper part of the hip. The iliac crests, the upper ridges of the ilium, are important landmarks. The ischium is the lower, posterior portion on which one sits. The pubis is the anterior portion of the hip. A deep, cup-shaped socket, the acetabulum, is located on the lower lateral surface of each hip bone. The cup shape of the acetabulum fits the head of the femur to form the hip joint.

*b.* The femur or thigh bone (fig. 2-7) is the longest, strongest bone in the body. The head of the femur fits into the acetabulum of the hip bone. The neck of the femur, just below the head, is the part most frequently fractured, particularly by elderly individuals. The distal end of the femur articulates with the tibia, to form the knee joint. A large prominent projection at the junction of the shaft and neck of the femur is the trochanter, which is an important attachment for strong thigh muscles.

*c.* The patella, or knee cap, is the bone protecting the front of the knee joint. It is a special kind of bone embedded within the powerful tendon

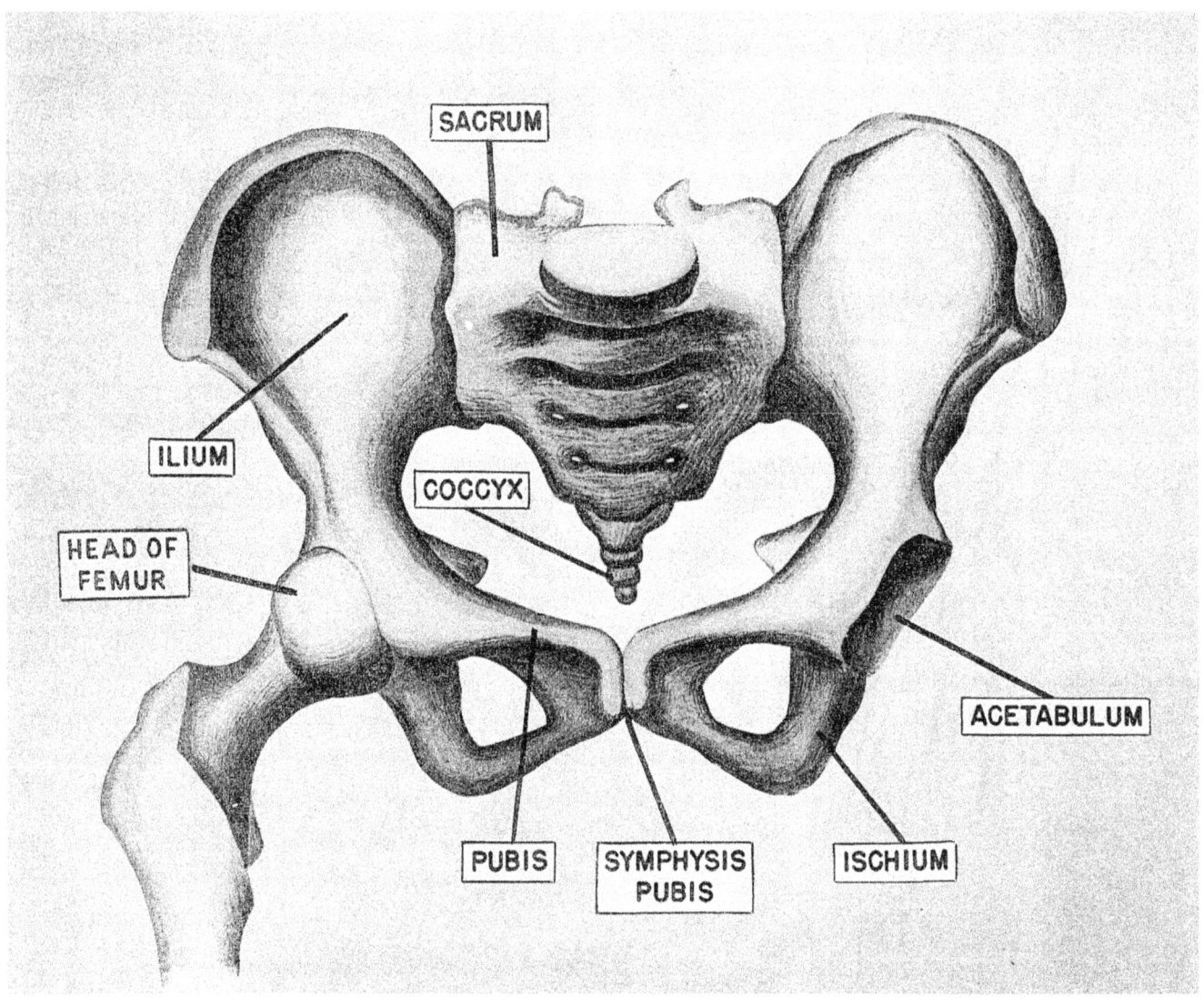

*Figure 2-13. Pelvis.*

strong fibrous connective tissue bands that hold the bones together at the joint. In some joints, the ligaments enclose the joint, forming the joint capsule.

*d.* Some joint disorders are mechanical—the parts of the joint are displaced or dislocated. Another term for a type of dislocation is "subluxation," a partial displacement of one bone surface within the joint. When the ligaments holding the joint together are partially torn, but the joint is not displaced, the injury is called a sprain.

**20. Joint Movements**

*a.* Movable joints allow change of position and motion. Examples of joint movement (app. B) are flexion (bending), extension (straightening), abduction (movement away from the midline), and adduction (movement toward the midline), pronation (turning the forearm so that the palm of the hand is down), and supination (turning the forearm so that the palm of the hand is up).

*b.* Attempts to force joints to move beyond their normal limitations can be disastrous. The structure of the joint determines the kind of movement that is possible, since the bone ends reciprocate, or fit into each other, at the joint. Examples of joint structure that permit certain kinds of joint movement include:

(1) Ball and socket joints, as in the shoulder and hip. These joints permit the widest range of motion—flexion, extension, abduction, adduction, and rotation.

(2) Hinge joints, as in the elbow and knee. Hinge joints permit flexion and extension. Elbow joints have forward movement—the anterior bone surfaces approach each other. Knee joints have

backward movement—the posterior bone surfaces approach each other.

(3) Pivot joints, as at the head and neck, at the first and second cervical vertebrae. The distal ends of the radius and ulna also form a pivot joint for rotation of the wrist.

### 21. Joints and Bursae

At some joint locations, the tendon connecting muscle to bone passes over a joint; *for example*, at the shoulder, elbow, knee, and heel. To reduce pressure, small sacs containing fluid are formed over and around the tendon. The sac is a bursa, and an irritated bursa is bursitis. The knee has four bursae, over and around the patella. When domestic chores included scrubbing floors on hands and knees, inflammation of the knee bursae was called "housemaid's knee." Bursitis can be very painful, and normal movement may be impossible.

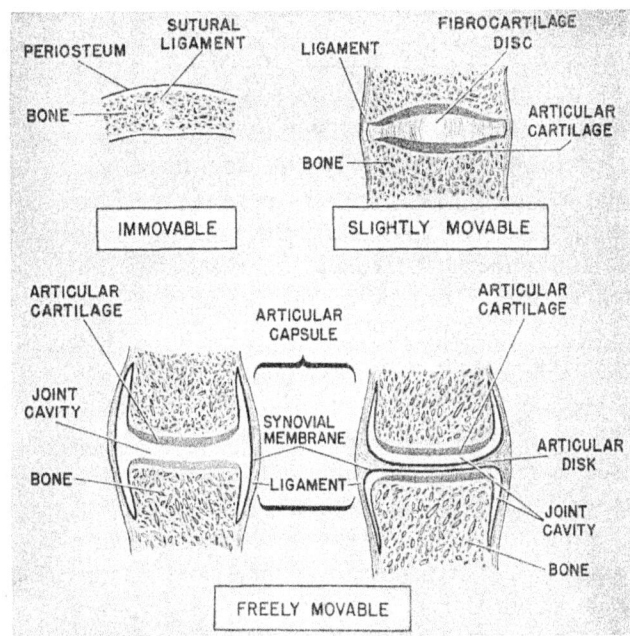

*Figure 2-14. Types of joints.*

## Section IV. THE SKELETAL MUSCULAR SYSTEM

### 22. Muscles

The muscles of the body include the smooth muscle in the walls of internal organs, the cardiac muscle in the walls of the heart, and the skeletal muscle attached to and causing movements of bones. Muscles have the ability to contract, and it is this power of muscle contraction that produces body movements. The skeletal muscles and their action and movements on bones and joints will be discussed in this section.

### 23. Skeletal Muscles

Although skeletal muscles are called voluntary muscles, they require a functioning nerve supply and something to pull against for normal contraction. It is important to think of skeletal muscles as one part of a three-part, neuro-muscular-skeletal unit. *For example*, a functioning nerve supply (a motor nerve from the central nervous system) is needed to stimulate muscle contraction; the muscle itself must be able to contract and to relax; and the power of the muscle contraction must be transmitted to a bone, or other attachment, to produce the desired movement. When any one part of this three-part unit cannot function normally, the other two parts also lose their ability to function normally. When all three parts— nerve, muscle, and bone—are intact, the many movements associated with skeletal muscles are possible. Skeletal muscle movements include locomotion, or moving from place to place; rhythmic breathing movements; blinking of eyelids; position changes; chewing and swallowing; coughing; and changes in facial expression. Many of these movements are essential for survival.

### 24. Muscle Structure and Muscle Movements

Long, slender muscle cells form fibers; muscle fibers are grouped together into bundles; and muscle bundles are grouped together to form an individual skeletal muscle. Each skeletal muscle is wrapped in a connective tissue sheath, a form of fascia. This muscle sheath incloses the blood vessels and nerves that stimulate and nourish the muscle cells. The connective tissue parts are opaque, or whitish, in color, while the muscle bundles are the lean, red-meat part of muscles. Individual muscles differ considerably in size, shape, and arrangement of muscle fibers. The fiber arrangement determines the line of pull of an individual muscle.

*a. Muscle Attachments.* Extensions of muscle sheath become continuous with tough connective tissue attachments such as tendons or aponeuroses that bind muscles to bones or to adjacent muscles. Tendons are cordlike attachments of connective tissue that unite with the periosteum of bone. Aponeuroses are broad, sheetlike attachments which can unite with muscle sheaths of adjacent muscles. At the midline of the abdomen, where there are no bones for muscles to attach to, abdominal muscles to the left and right of the midline are attached to central aponeuroses.

*b. Muscle Movements.* When muscle fibers are stimulated to contract by an impulse received from a motor nerve, the muscle shortens and pulls against its connective tissue attachment. One attachment is sometimes a fixed joint or anchor, and the direction of motion is then toward it. The power of the muscle contraction is transmitted to the bone or to an adjacent muscle, and movement occurs.

*c. Muscle Tone.* Healthy muscle is characterized by active contraction in response to the reaction of the nervous system to the environment. This readiness to act (resulting in firing of motor units) as stimuli from the environment impinge upon the nervous system is called muscle tone. Muscles that have lost their tone through lack of exercise, through primary muscle disease, or through nerve damage become flabby (flaccid). The tone of muscles is due to the constant, steady contraction and relaxation of different muscle fibers in individual muscles, which helps to maintain the "chemical engine" of the muscle cells. Even minor exercise movements help maintain tone by renewing blood supply to muscle cells. Wriggling the toes, flexing and extending the fingers, changing the depth of respirations, turning and repositioning the body are examples of exercises that help restore and maintain muscle tone.

*d. Muscle Activity.* Muscle contraction consumes food and oxygen and produces acids and heat. Muscle activity is the major source of the body's heat. Acids accumulating as a result of continued activity cause fatigue, which occurs most rapidly when contractions are frequent. It occurs slowly if rest periods are taken between contractions. Exercise causes muscles to become larger, stronger, and better developed. An increase in muscle size is hypertrophy; wasting away of muscles due to inactivity is atrophy. Physical exercise is necessary to keep muscles in good condition.

### 25. Principles of Skeletal Muscle Action

A few general principles about skeletal muscle action should be understood. The three principles listed will help associate muscle actions with normal body movements and patient care activities.

*a.* Muscles produce movements by pulling on bones. Since bones move at joints, most muscles attach to bones above and below a joint. One bone is stabilized while the other bone moves.

*b.* Muscles moving a part usually lie proximal to the part moved. *For example,* muscles moving the humerus are in the shoulder, chest, and back; muscles moving the femur are in the lumbar and pelvic region.

*c.* Muscles almost always act in groups rather than singly. The coordinated action of several muscles produces movement—while one group contracts, the other group relaxes, and vice versa. The muscle whose contraction produces the movement is the prime mover. The muscle which relaxes is the antagonist. In bending (flexing) and stretching (extending) the forearm, the biceps and triceps in the upper arm are, alternately, prime movers and antagonists.

### 26. Principal Groups of Skeletal Muscles

Since there are more than 400 individually named skeletal muscles, only a few will be discussed in this manual. In figure 2–15, both Ⓐ and Ⓑ illustrate the general location of the muscles discussed. Muscles are usually named for one or more features such as their location, action, shape, or points of attachment.

*a. Head and Face.* Muscles of the head and face act in movements of the eye, facial expressions, talking, chewing, and swallowing. The orbicularis oculi closes the eyelid; the orbicularis oris closes the lips; the masseter closes the jaw and clamps the back teeth together.

*b. Neck.* The muscles of the neck move the head from side to side, forward and backward, and rotate it. Some also assist in respiration, speaking, and swallowing. The sternocleidomastoid bends the head forward and helps turn it to either side.

*c. Chest.* The strong chest muscles move the arm, brace the shoulder, and compress the chest for effective coughing. The diaphragm, the major muscle of respiration, separates the thoracic and abdominal cavities. (It is not shown in the diagram of superficial skeletal muscles.) The pectoralis major draws the upper arm forward across the chest. The latimus dorsi and trapezius are major muscles of the posterior thorax.

*d. Arm.* Among the muscles which cause movement of the arms are the deltoid, biceps, and triceps. (The extensors and flexors cause hand and finger movements.)

(1) The deltoid is a triangular-shaped muscle, capping the shoulder and upper arm. The deltoid lifts the arm forward, sideways, and to the rear.

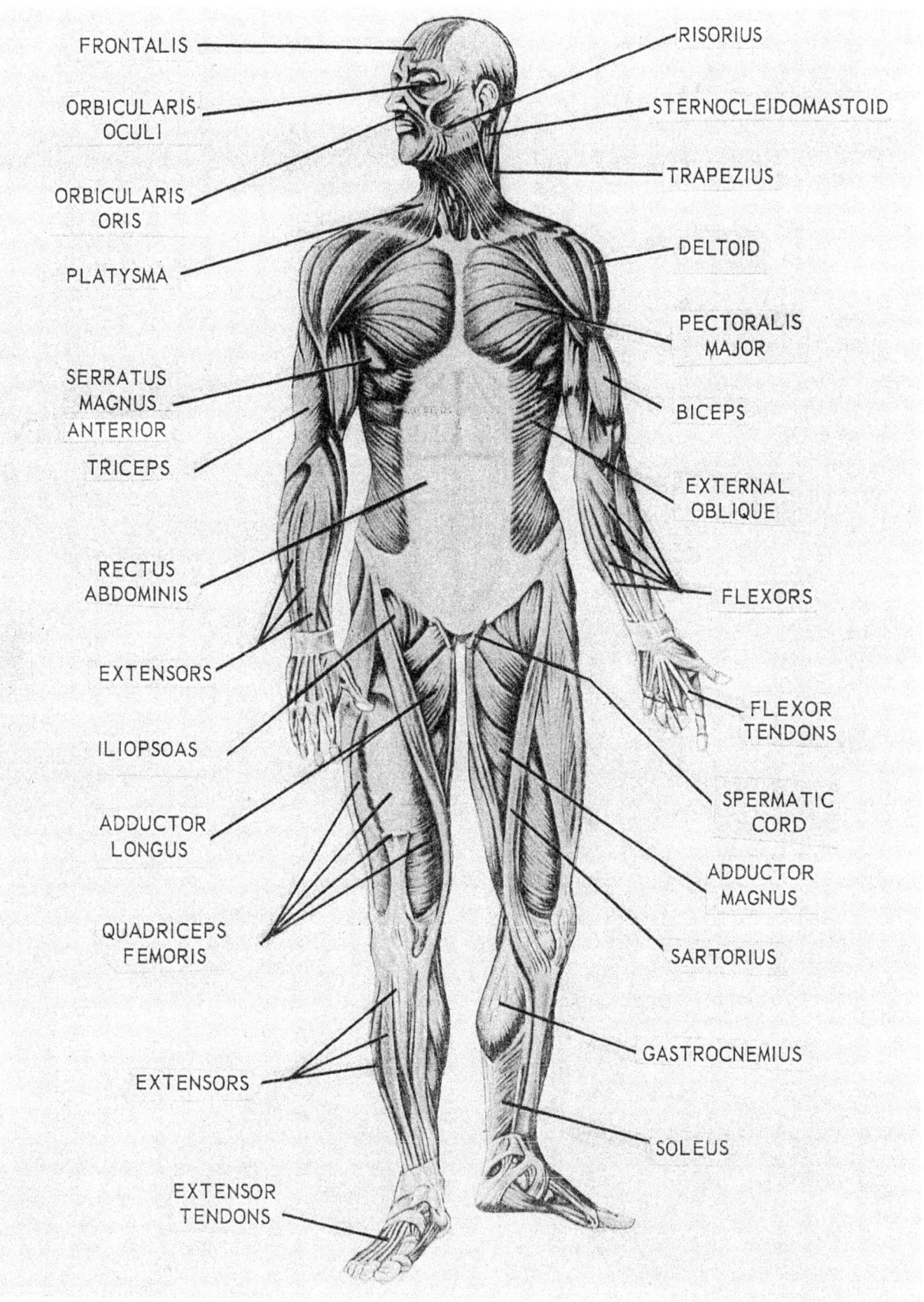

Figure 2-15. Superficial muscles.

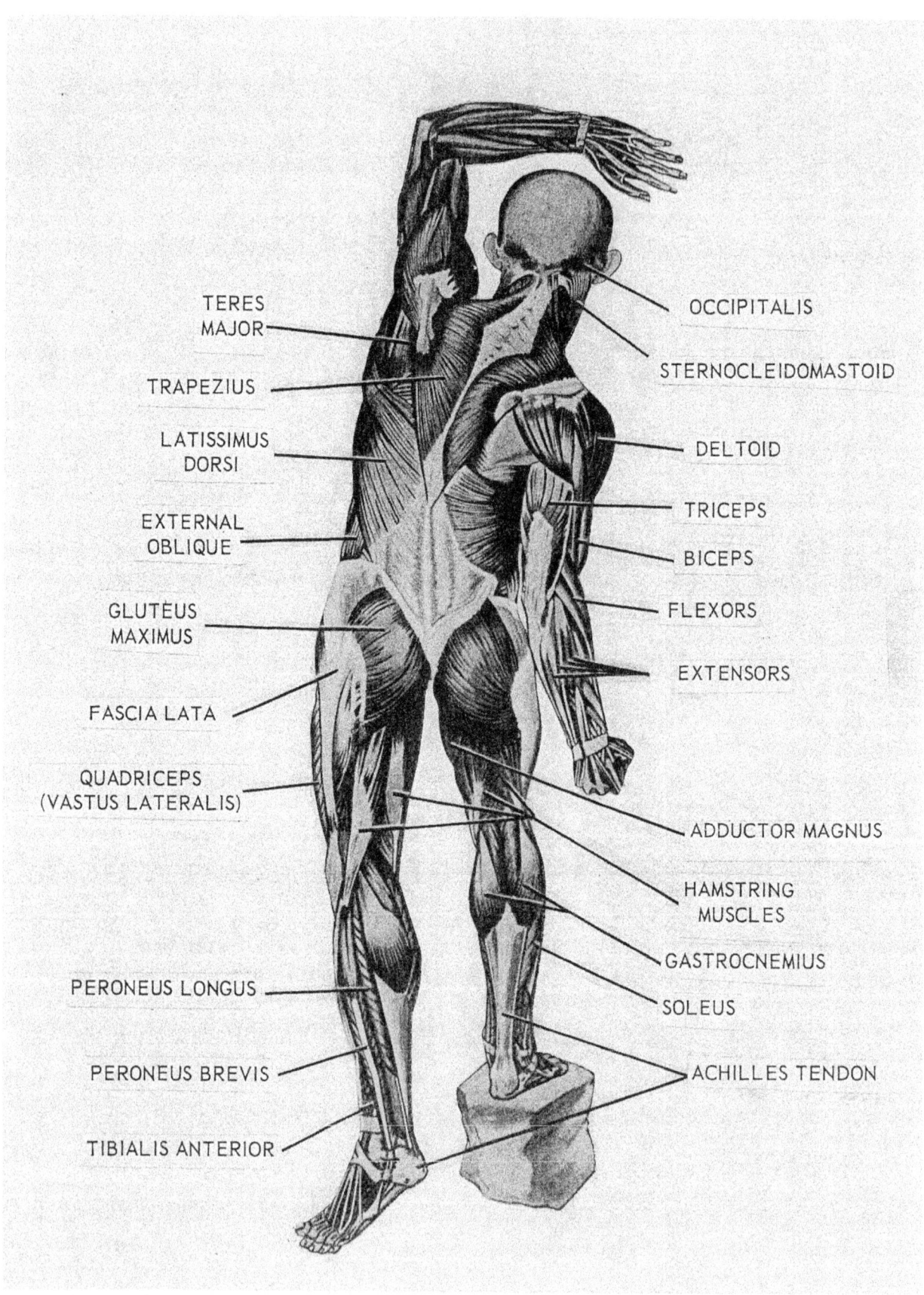

Figure 2-15—Continued.

(2) The biceps, a long, two-headed muscle located on the anterior arm, flexes the forearm at the elbow. It also helps to turn the arm palm up in supination.

(3) The triceps, a large three-headed muscle located on the posterior arm, extends the forearm at the elbow.

*e. Back.* The muscles of the back are large, and some are broad. Attached to vertebrae, the back muscles keep the trunk in an erect posture and aid it in bending and rotating. In the thoracic region, these muscles assist in respiration and in movements of the neck, arm, and trunk. Although the muscles of the midback are very powerful, the thigh and buttock muscles should be used in lifting to avoid straining the bony and ligamentous structures of the back.

*f. Abdominal.* The abdominal muscles form broad, thin layers which support the internal abdominal organs, assist in respiration, and help in flexion and rotation of the spine. Their names indicate their line of pull—external oblique, rectus abdominis (straight up and down), and transverse. Abdominal muscles also assist in urination and in defecation.

*g. Perineal.* The muscles of the perineum form the floor of the pelvic cavity and aid in defecation and in urination.

*h. Buttocks.* The thick, strong muscles of the buttocks help to stabilize the hip, and with the muscles of the posterior thigh, distribute weight to the pelvis in lifting and relieve the strain on the back muscles. This gluteus group includes the gluteus maximus, gluteus medius, and gluteus minimus. These muscles extend and rotate the thigh.

*i. Thigh.* The muscles located on the anterior and posterior of the thigh cross two joints, the hip and the knee. When they contract, they extend one joint and flex the other. The anterior thigh muscles include the quadriceps femoris and the posterior ones include the biceps femoris.

(1) *Quadriceps femoris.* This four-headed group of muscles located on the anterior of the thigh extends the leg at the knee. Its four muscles are the vastus lateralis, rectus femoris, vastus intermedius, and vastus medialis.

(2) *Biceps femoris (hamstring group).* This muscle group on the posterior of the thigh flexes the knee and extends the thigh.

*j. Leg.* The anterior muscle group of the leg includes the anterior tibialis, which flexes the foot on the leg, turning the foot upward in dorsiflexion. The largest posterior muscle of the leg is the gastrocnemius, the calf muscle, which attaches to the heel through the Achilles tendon. Contraction of the gastrocnemius causes the foot to turn downward in plantar flexion, or foot drop.

## Section V. THE SKIN

### 27. Integumentary System and Its Functions

The skin is called the integumentary or covering body system and serves the body in many important ways. The most obvious feature of skin is its outward appearance; indeed, the appearance and feel of the skin are important indications of general health and hygiene. Four functions of skin are protection, as a mechanical barrier to the entrance of bacteria; regulation of body temperature, through control of heat loss; sensory perception, through nerve endings that transmit sensations of touch, heat, cold, and pain; and excretion of body wastes, through sweat. Although this is not one of its normal functions, the skin can absorb water and other substances. This property of the skin is used to advantage in prescribing local application of certain drugs. It can be harmful, too, as when toxic agents such as "G" gas, lead salts in gasoline, and insecticides are absorbed and permitted to enter the body through the skin.

### 28. Structure

The skin has two principal layers, the epidermis, or outer layer, and the dermis, the inner layer or true skin. The epidermis and dermis (fig. 2–16) are supported by a subcutaneous (under-the-skin) layer which connects the skin to underlying muscles.

*a.* There are no blood vessels or nerve endings in the epidermis, which has two layers, outer and inner. The outer layer has flat, scaly, lifeless cells that are constantly being worn off by surface contacts. As this is happening, rapidly growing inner epidermis cells push up and replace the top layers. Skin pigment, found in the deepest parts of these inner epidermis cells, varies in individuals. It determines the darkness or lightness of skin color. However, the color of the skin is also due to the quantity and state of the blood circulating in the dermis, the inner skin layer. Pinkness, blueness (cyanosis), or pallor (paleness) of the skin surface is due to circulating blood.

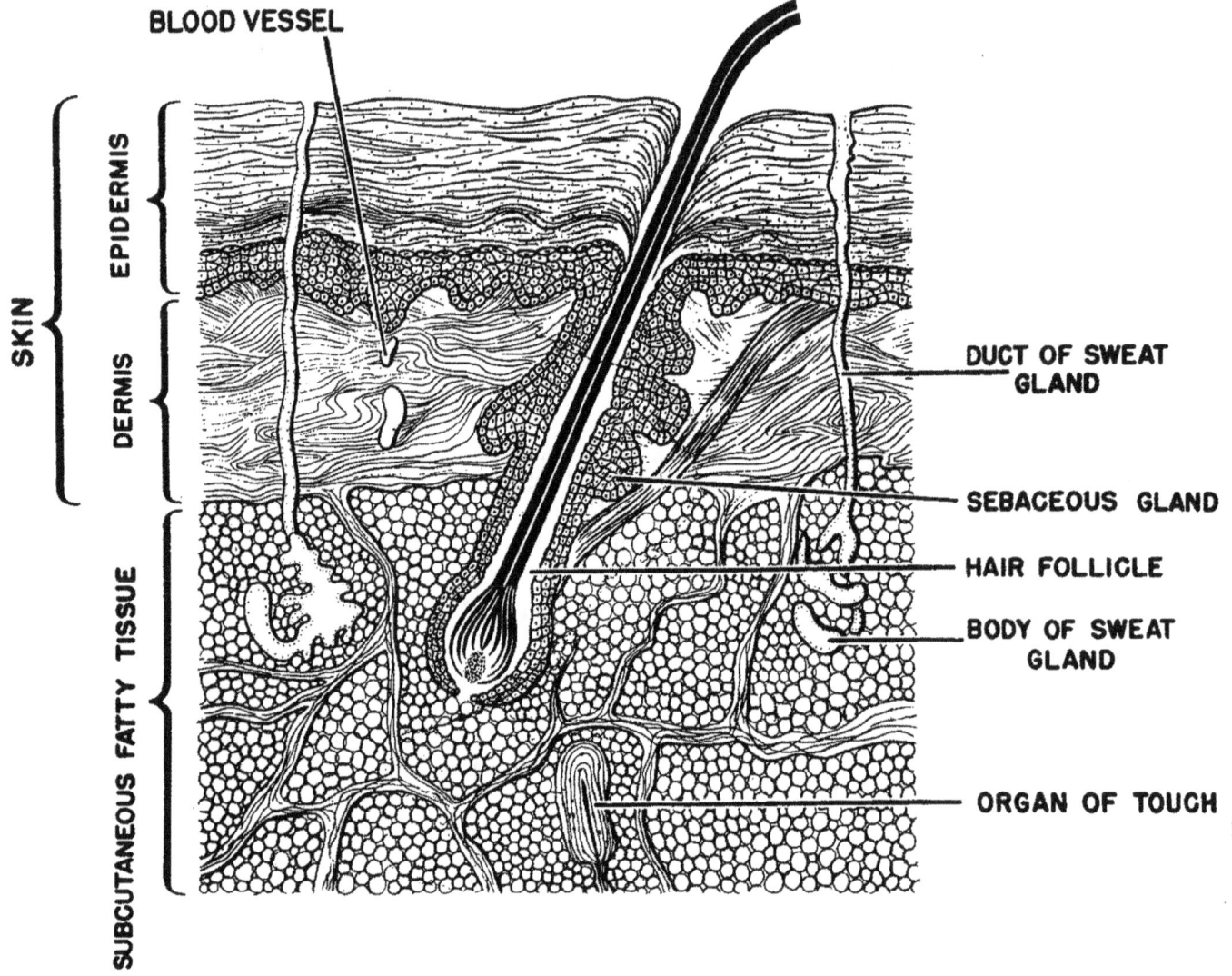

*Figure 2-16. Structure of the skin.*

b. The dermis is the deep, true skin layer. Nerves, blood vessels, glands, hair roots, and nail roots are in the dermis, supported by a connective tissue meshwork of elastic fibers. Tiny involuntary muscle fibers in the dermis contract and account for the reactions described as "hair standing on end" and "goose pimples."

c. The subcutaneous layer of tissue beneath the dermis is not skin. It is superficial fascia, a connective tissue. Fat and other connective tissues in the subcutaneous layer round out body surfaces and cushion bony parts. When a hypodermic injection is given, it is given into the subcutaneous tissue, below the skin layers.

## 29. Skin Accessory Organs

Hair, nails, sebaceous (oil) glands, and sweat glands are skin accessory organs. Each hair grows from a root embedded in the dermis, or below the dermis. A little tube, the hair follicle, incloses the root. Fingernails and toenails grow from nail beds buried at the proximal ends of the nails. The sebaceous glands secrete an oil called sebum, which lubricates the hair and the skin surface. This oily secretion keeps the skin pliable and helps keep it waterproof. When the openings of the sebaceous glands become plugged with dirt, they form blackheads. Sweat glands manufacture sweat, or perspiration, from fluid drawn from the blood. Sweat contains salts and organic wastes and is about 99 percent water. It is discharged through skin openings called the pores. As sweat evaporates, the body is cooled. Sweat formation and excretion is an important mechanism for losing body heat.

## 30. Skin as a Temperature Regulator

Skin helps regulate the temperature of the body

by controlling heat loss in two different ways. Blood vessels in the dermis can change size. *For example*, when blood vessels are dilated, warm blood is closer to the skin surface, and heat is lost more rapidly. When blood vessels constrict, the amount of blood at the skin surface is decreased, and heat is conserved. Because the surface of the skin is so large, heat loss by radiation is considerable. Added to this heat loss by radiation is the heat loss by evaporation of sweat. In very humid weather, evaporation of sweat from the skin and from saturated clothing decreases.

## Section VI. THE CIRCULATORY SYSTEM

### 31. Introduction

The circulatory system has two major fluid transportation systems, the cardiovascular and the lymphatic.

*a. Cardiovascular System.* This system, which contains the heart and blood vessels, is a closed system, transporting blood to all parts of the body. Blood flowing through the circuit formed by the heart and blood vessels (fig. 2-17) brings oxygen, food, and other chemical elements to tissue cells and removes carbon dioxide and other waste products resulting from cell activity.

*b. Lymphatic System.* This system, which provides drainage for tissue fluid, is an auxiliary part of the circulatory system, returning an important amount of tissue fluid to the blood stream through its own system of lymphatic vessels.

### 32. The Heart

The heart, designed to be a highly efficient pump, is a four-chambered muscular organ, lying within the chest, with about 2/3 of its mass to the left of the midline (fig. 2-18). It lies in the pericardial space in the thoracic cavity between the two lungs. In size and shape, it resembles a man's closed fist. Its lower point, the apex, lies just above the left diaphragm.

*a. Heart Covering.* The pericardium is a double-walled sac inclosing the heart. The outer fibrous surface gives support, and the inner lining prevents friction as the heart moves within its protecting jacket. The lining surfaces of the pericardial sac produce a small amount of pericardial fluid needed for lubrication to facilitate the normal movements of the heart.

*b. Heart Wall.* This muscular wall is made up of cardiac muscle called myocardium.

*c. Heart Chambers.* There are four chambers in the heart. These chambers are essentially the same size. The upper chambers, called the atria, are seemingly smaller than the lower chambers, the ventricles. The apparent difference in total size is due to the thickness of the myocardial layer. The right atrium communicates with the right ventricle; the left atrium communicates with the left ventricle. The septum (partition), dividing the interior of the heart into right and left sides, prevents direct communication of blood flow from right to left chambers or left to right chambers. This is important, because the right side of the heart receives deoxygenated blood returning from the systemic (body) circulation. The left side of the heart receives oxygenated blood returning from the pulmonary (lung) circulation. The special structure of the heart keeps the blood flowing in its proper direction to and from the heart chambers.

*d. Heart Valves.* The four chambers of the heart are lined with endocardium. At each opening from the chambers this lining folds on itself and extends into the opening to form valves. These valves allow the blood to pass from a chamber but prevent its return. The atrioventricular valves, between the upper and lower chambers, are within the heart itself. The semilunar valves are within arteries arising from the right and left ventricles.

(1) *Atrioventricular valves.* The tricuspid valve is located between the right atrium and right ventricle. It has three flaps or cusps. The bicuspid valve or mitral valve is located between the left atrium and left ventricle. It has two flaps or cusps.

(2) *Semilunar valves.* The pulmonary semilunar (half-moon shaped) valve is located at the opening into the pulmonary artery that arises from the right ventricle. The aortic semilunar valve is located at the opening into the aorta that arises from the left ventricle.

### 33. Flow of Blood Through the Heart

It is helpful to follow the flow of blood through the heart in order to understand the relationship

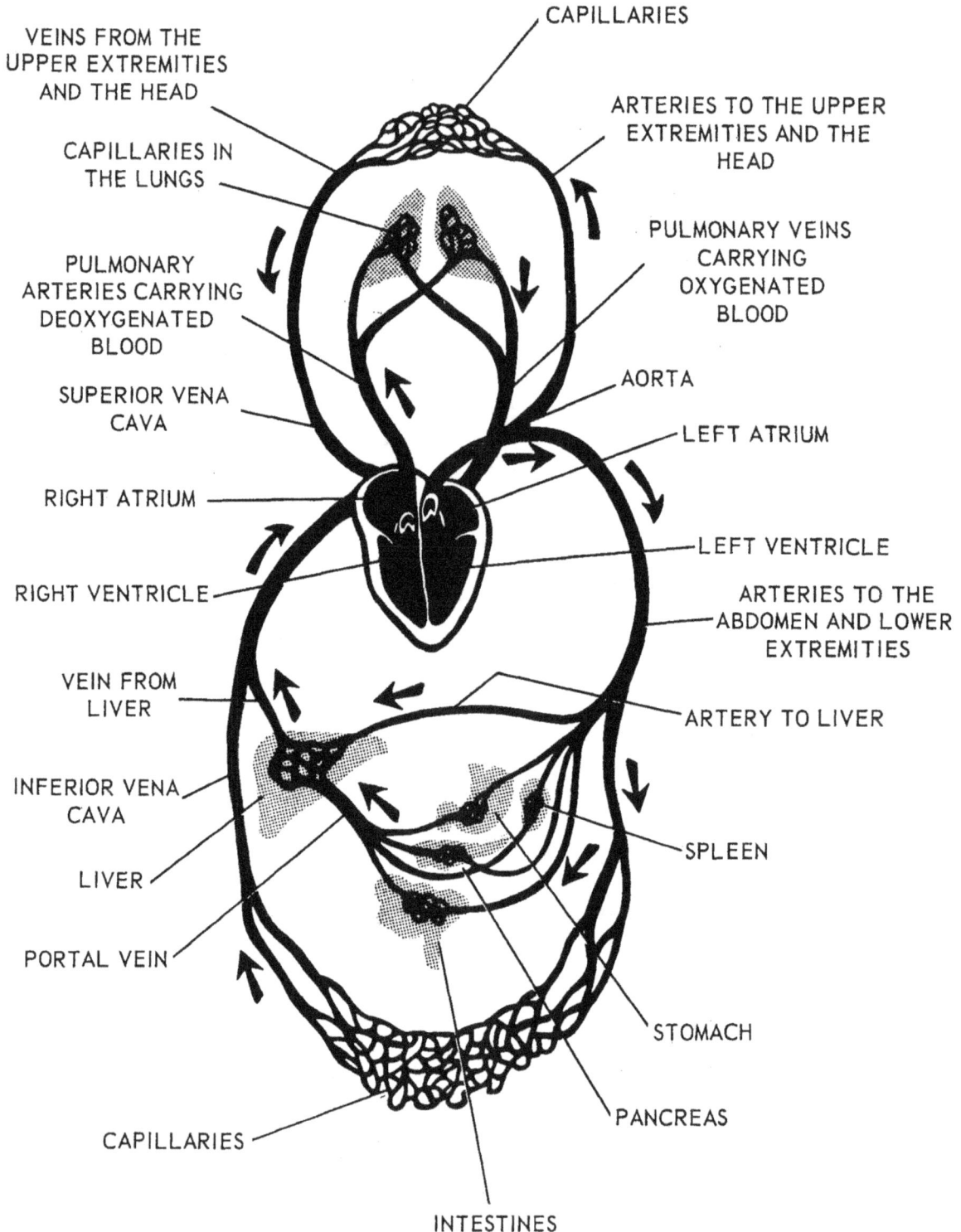

*Figure 2-17. Circulation of the blood (diagrammatic).*

of the heart structures. Remember, the heart is the pump and is also the connection between the systemic circulation and pulmonary circulation. All the blood returning from the systemic circulation must flow through the pulmonary circulation for exchange of carbon dioxide for oxygen. Blood from the upper part of the body enters the heart through a large vein, the superior vena cava, and from the lower part of the body by the inferior vena cava (fig. 2-19).

*a.* Blood from the superior vena cava and inferior vena cava enters the heart at the right

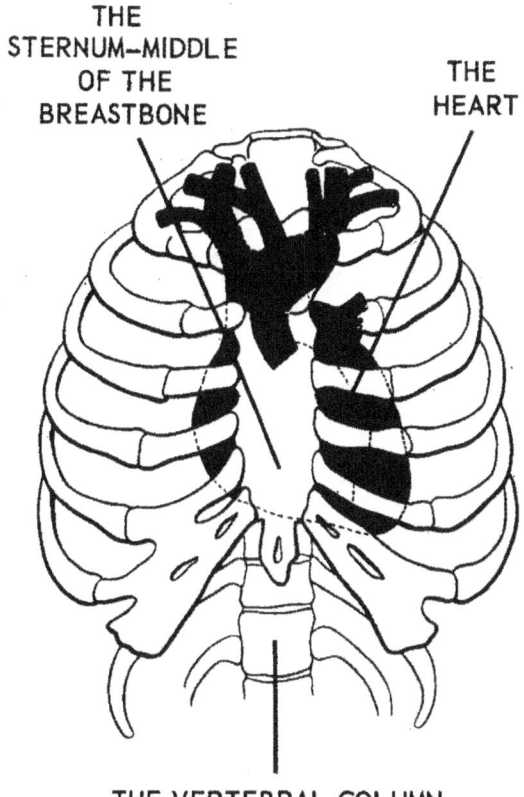

*Figure 2-18. Heart and thoracic cage.*

atrium. The right atrium contracts, and blood is forced through the open tricuspid valve into the relaxed right ventricle.

b. As the right ventricle contracts, the tricuspid valve is closed, preventing back flow into the atrium. The pulmonary semilunar valve opens as a result of the force and movement of the blood, and the right ventricle pumps the blood into the pulmonary artery.

c. The blood is carried through the lung tissues, exchanging its carbon dioxide for oxygen in the alveoli. This oxygenated blood is collected from the main pulmonary veins and delivered back to the left side of the heart to the left atrium.

d. As the left atrium contracts, the oxygenated blood flows through the open bicuspid (mitral) valve into the left ventricle.

e. As the left ventricle contracts, the bicuspid valve is closed. The aortic semilunar valve opens as a result of the force and movement of the blood, and the left ventricle pumps oxygenated blood through the aortic semilunar valve into the aorta, the main artery of the body. Oxygenated blood now starts its flow to all of the body cells and tissues. The systemic circulation starts from the left ventricle, the pulmonary circulation from the right ventricle.

### 34. Blood and Nerve Supply of the Heart

*a. Coronary Arteries.* The heart gets its blood supply from the right and left coronary arteries. These arteries branch off the aorta just above the heart, then subdivide into many smaller branches within the heart muscle. If any part of the heart muscle is deprived of its blood supply through interruption of blood flow through the coronary arteries and their branches, the muscle tissue deprived of blood cannot function and will die. This is called myocardial infarction. Blood from the heart tissue is returned by coronary veins to the right atrium.

*b. Nerve Supply.* The nerve supply to the heart is from two sets of nerves originating in the medulla of the brain. The nerves are part of the involuntary (autonomic) nervous system. One set, the branches from the vagus nerve, keeps the heart beating at a slow, regular rate. The other set, the cardiac accelerator nerves, speeds up the heart. Heart muscle has a special ability; it contracts automatically, but the nerve supply is needed to provide an effective contraction for blood circulation. Within the heart muscle itself, there are special groups of nerve fibers that conduct impulses for contraction. These groups make up the conduction system of the heart. When the conduction system does not operate properly, the heart muscle contractions are uncoordinated and ineffective. The impulses within the heart muscle are minute electric currents, which can be picked up and recorded by the electrocardiogram, the ECG.

### 35. The Heartbeat and Heart Sounds

*a. Heartbeat.* This is a complete cycle of heart action—contraction, or systole, and relaxation, or diastole. During systole, blood is forced from the chambers. During diastole, blood refills the chambers. The term cardiac cycle means the complete heart beat. The cardiac cycle, repeated continuously at a regular rhythm, occurs 70–80 times per minute. Each complete cycle takes less than one second—in this brief time, all of the heart action needed to move blood must take place, and the heart must be ready to repeat its cycle.

*b. Heart Sounds.* When heard through a stethoscope, heart sounds are described as "lubb-dup." The first sound, "lubb," is interpreted as the sound, or vibration, of the ventricles contracting

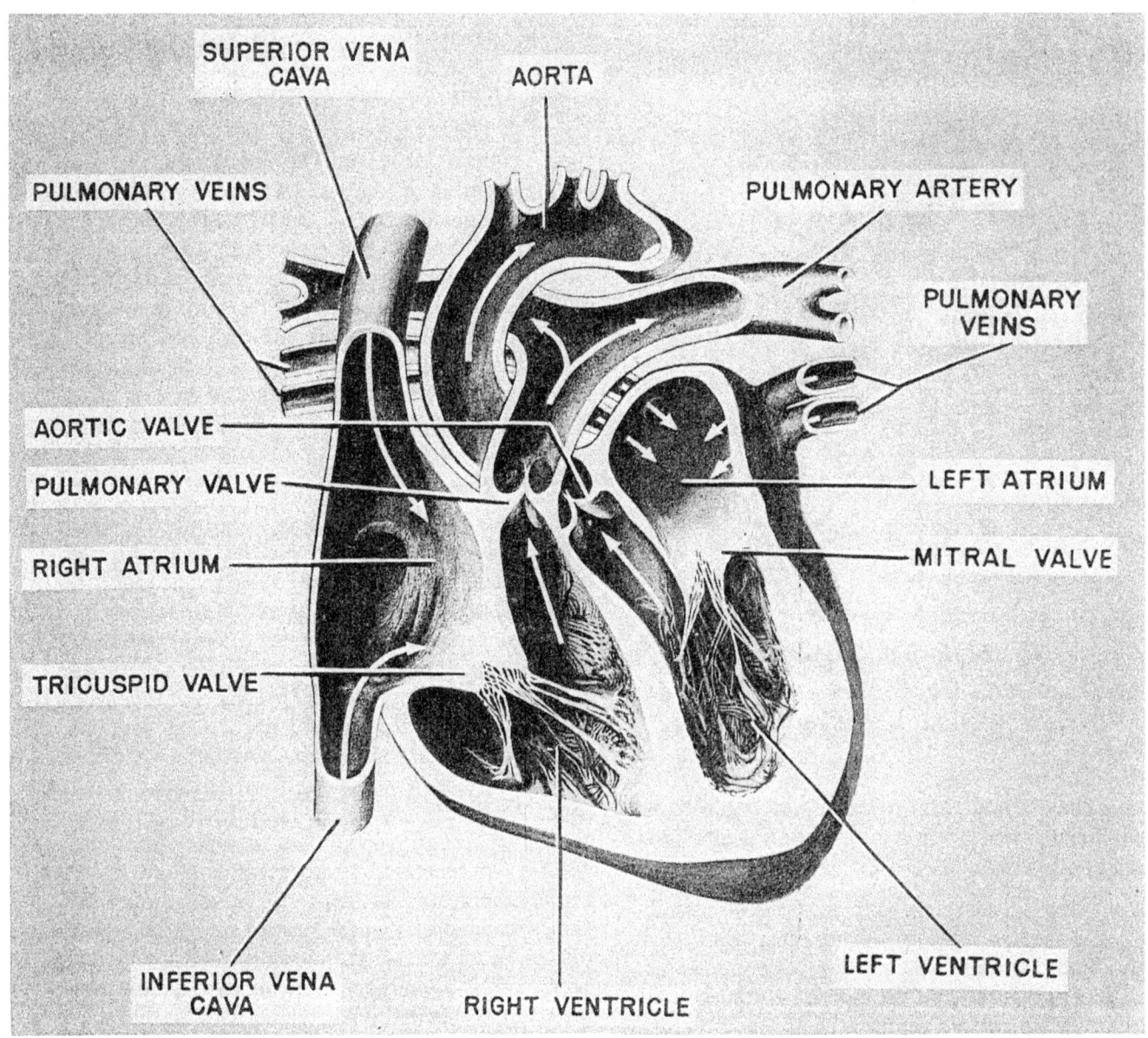

*Figure 2–19. The heart, chambers, and flow of blood.*

and atrioventricular valves closing. The second, higher-pitched sound, "dup," is interpreted as the sound of the semilunar valves closing. The doctor listening to the heart sounds can detect alterations of normal sounds; the interpretation of these heart sounds is part of the diagnosis of heart disease.

### 36. Blood Vessels

The blood vessels are the closed system of tubes through which the blood flows. The arteries and arterioles are distributors. The capillaries are the vessels through which all exchange of fluid, oxygen, and carbon dioxide take place between the blood and tissue cells. The venules and veins are collectors, carrying blood back to the heart. The capillaries are the smallest of these vessels but are of greatest importance functionally in the circulatory system.

*a. The Arteries and Arterioles.* The system of arteries (fig. 2–20) and arterioles is like a tree, with the large trunk, the aorta, giving off branches which repeatedly divide and subdivide. Arterioles are very small arteries, about the diameter of a hair. By way of comparison, the aorta is more than 1 inch in diameter.) An artery wall has a layer of elastic, muscular tissue which allows it to expand and recoil. When an artery is cut, this wall does not collapse, and bright red blood escapes from the artery in spurts. Arterial bleeding

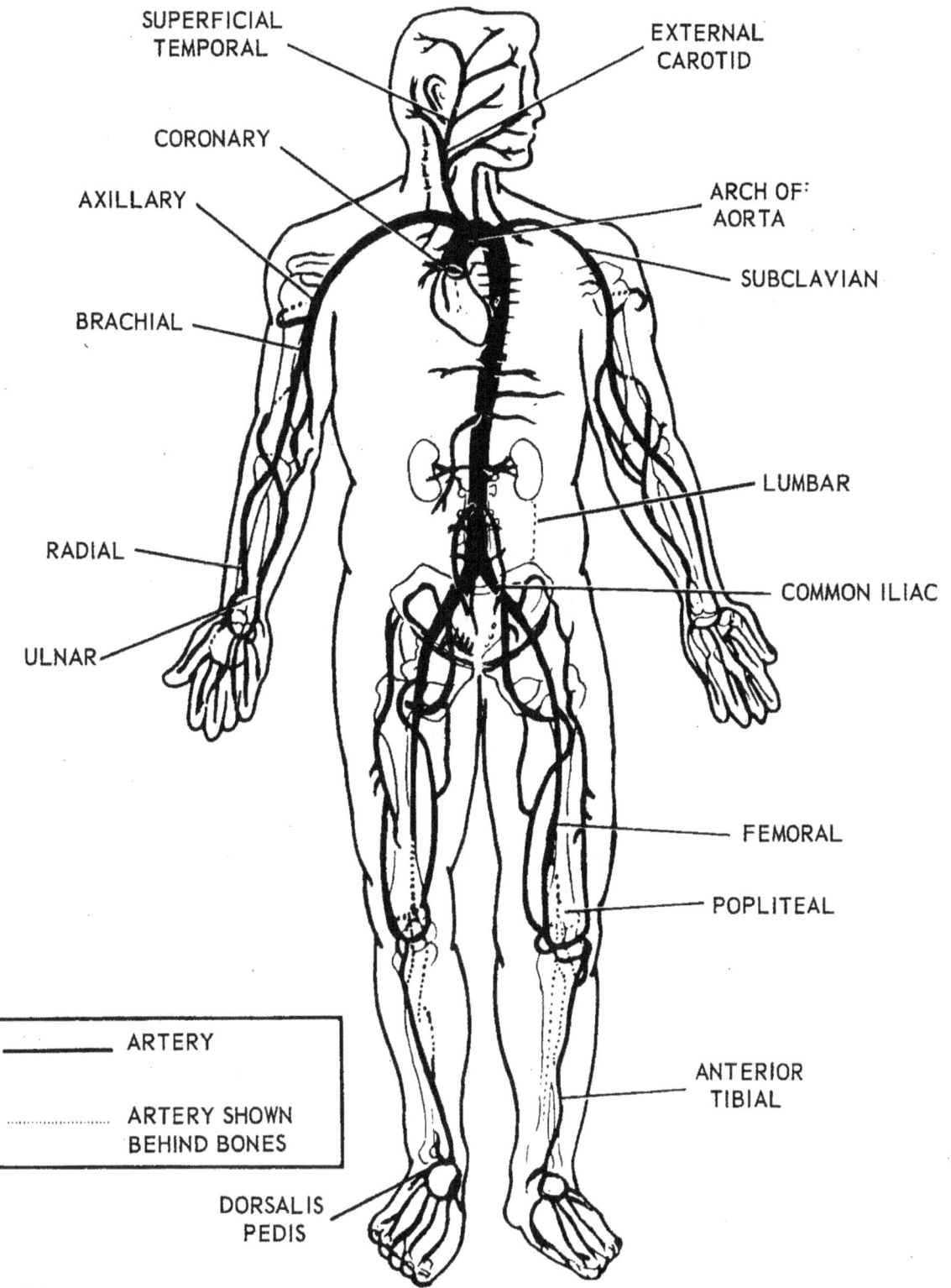

*Figure 2-20. Arterial system (diagrammatic).*

must often be controlled by clamping and tying off (ligating) the vessel. Some of the principal arteries and the area they supply with blood are—

(1) Carotid arteries, external and internal, supply the neck, head, and brain through their branches.

(2) Subclavian arteries supply the upper extremities.

(3) Femoral arteries supply the lower extremities.

*b. Capillaries.* Microscopic in size, capillaries

are so numerous that there is at least one or more near every living cell. A single layer of endothelial cells forms the walls of a capillary. Capillaries are the essential link between arterial and venous circulation. The vital exchange of substances from the blood in the capillary with tissue cells takes place through the capillary wall. Blood starts its route back to the heart as it leaves the capillaries.

*c. Veins.* Veins have thin walls and valves. Formed from the inner vein lining, these valves prevent blood from flowing back toward the capillaries. Venules, the smallest veins, unite into veins of larger and larger size as the blood is collected to return to the heart. The superior vena cava, collecting blood from all regions above the diaphragm, and the inferior vena cava, collecting blood from all regions below the diaphragm, return the venous blood to the right atrium of the heart. Superficial veins lie close to the surface of the body and can be seen through the skin.

(1) The median basilic vein (fig. 2-21) (at the antecubital fossa in the bend of the elbow) is commonly used for venipuncture to obtain blood specimens or to inject solutions of drugs or parenteral fluid intravenously.

(2) The great saphenous vein is the longest

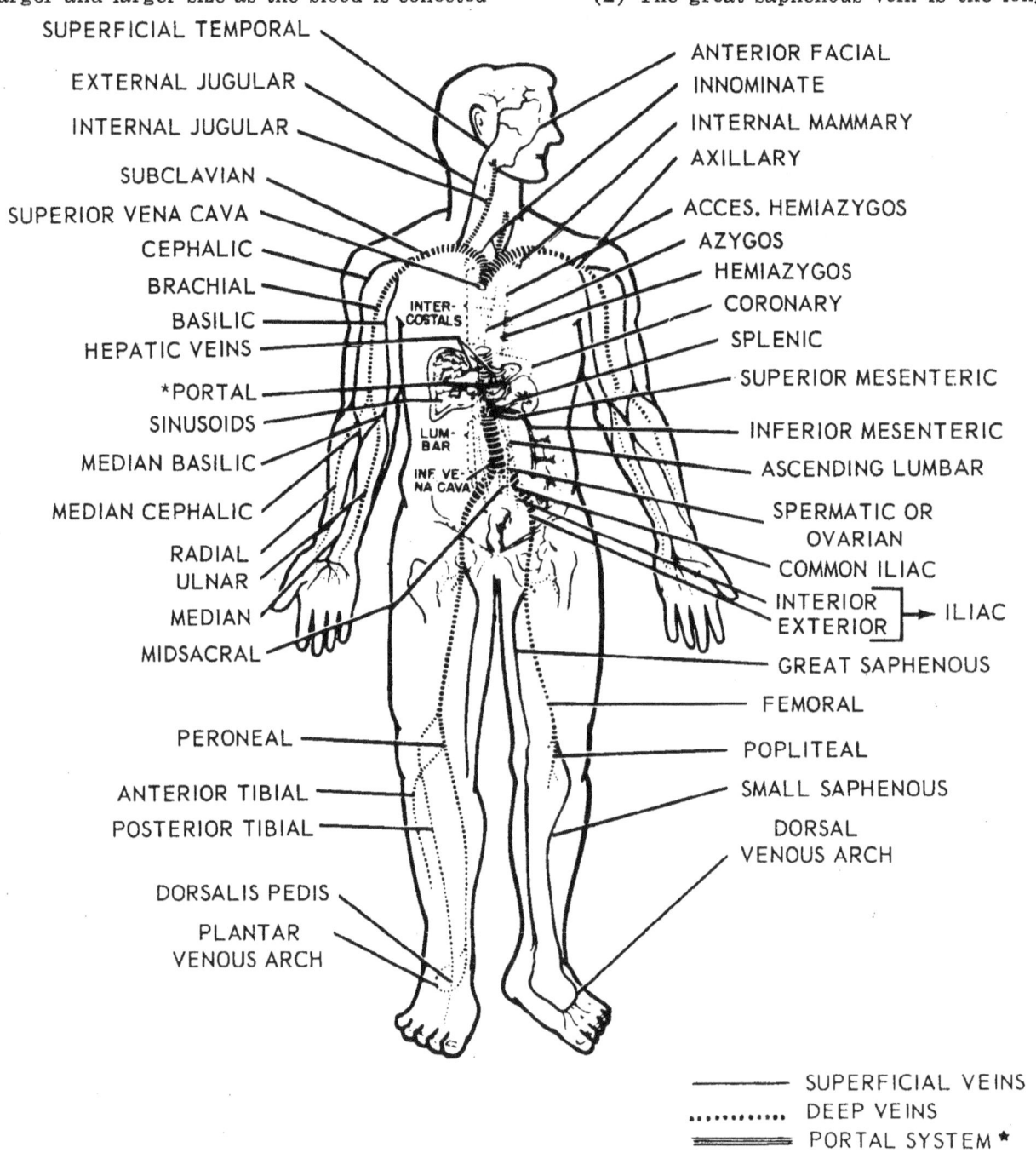

*Figure 2-21. Venous system (diagrammatic).*

vein in the body, extending from the foot to the groin. The saphenous vein has a long distance to lift blood against the force of gravity when an individual is in standing position. It is therefore susceptible to becoming dilated and stretched and the valves no longer function properly. When this occurs the vein is said to be varicosed.

### 37. Pulse and Blood Pressure

*a. Pulse.* This is a characteristic associated with the heartbeat and the subsequent wave of expansion and recoil set up in the wall of an artery. Pulse is defined as the alternate expansion and recoil of an artery. With each heartbeat, blood is forced into the arteries causing them to dilate (expand). Then the arteries contract (recoil) as the blood moves further along in the circulatory system. The pulse can be felt at certain points in the body where an artery lies close to the surface. The most common location for feeling the pulse is at the wrist, proximal to the thumb (radial artery) on the palm side of the hand. Alternate locations are in front of the ear (temporal artery), at the side of the neck (carotid artery), and on the top (dorsum) of the foot (dorsalis pedis).

*b. Blood Pressure.* The force that blood exerts on the walls of vessels through which it flows is called blood pressure. All parts of the blood vascular system are under pressure, but the term blood pressure usually refers to arterial pressure. Pressure in the arteries is highest when the ventricles contract during systole. Pressure is lowest when the ventricles relax during diastole. The brachial artery, in the upper arm, is the artery usually used for blood pressure measurement.

### 38. Lymphatic System

The lymphatic system consists of lymph, lymph vessels, and lymph nodes. The spleen belongs, in part, to the lymphatic system. Unlike the cardiovascular system, the lymphatic system has no pump to move the fluid which it collects, but muscle contractions and breathing movements aid in the movement of lymph through its channels and its return to the blood stream.

*a. Lymph and Tissue Fluid.* Lymph, fluid found in the lymph vessels, is clear and watery and is similar to tissue fluid, which is the colorless fluid that fills the spaces between tissues, between the cells of organs, and between cells and connective tissues. Tissue fluid serves as the "middleman" for the exchange between blood and body cells. Formed from plasma, it seeps out of capillary walls. The lymphatic system collects tissue fluid, and as lymph, the collected fluid is started on its way for return to the circulating blood.

*b. Lymph Vessels.* Starting as small blind ducts within the tissues, the lymphatic vessels enlarge to form lymphatic capillaries. These capillaries unite to form larger lymphatic vessels, which resemble veins in structure and arrangement. Valves in lymph vessels prevent backflow. Superficial lymph vessels collect lymph from the skin and subcutaneous tissue; deep vessels collect lymph from all other parts of the body. The two largest collecting vessels are the thoracic duct and the right lymphatic duct. The thoracic duct (fig. 2-22) receives lymph from all parts of the body except the upper right side. The lymph from the thoracic duct drains into the left subclavian vein, at the root of the neck on the left side. The right lymphatic duct drains into a corresponding vein on the right side.

*c. Lymph Nodes.* Occurring in groups up to a dozen or more, lymph nodes lie along the course of lymph vessels. Although variable in size, they are usually small oval bodies which are composed of lymphoid tissue. Lymph nodes act as filters for removal of infective organisms from the lymph stream. Important groups of these nodes are located in the axilla, the cervical region, the submaxillary region, the inguinal (groin) region, and the mesentric (abdominal) region.

*d. Infection and the Lymphatic System.* Lymph vessels and lymph nodes often become inflamed as the result of infection. An infection in the hand may cause inflammation of the lymph vessels as high as the axilla (armpit). Sore throat may cause inflammation and swelling of lymph nodes in the neck (submandibular nodes below the jaw and cervical nodes posteriorly).

*e. Spleen.* The largest collection of lymphoid tissue in the body, the spleen is located high in the abdominal cavity on the left side (LUQ), below the diaphragm and behind the stomach. It is somewhat long and ovoid (egg-shaped). Although it can be removed (splenectomy) without noticeable harmful effects, the spleen has useful functions, such as serving as a reservoir for blood and red blood cells.

### 39. The Blood

Blood is the red body fluid flowing through the arteries, capillaries, and veins. It varies in color

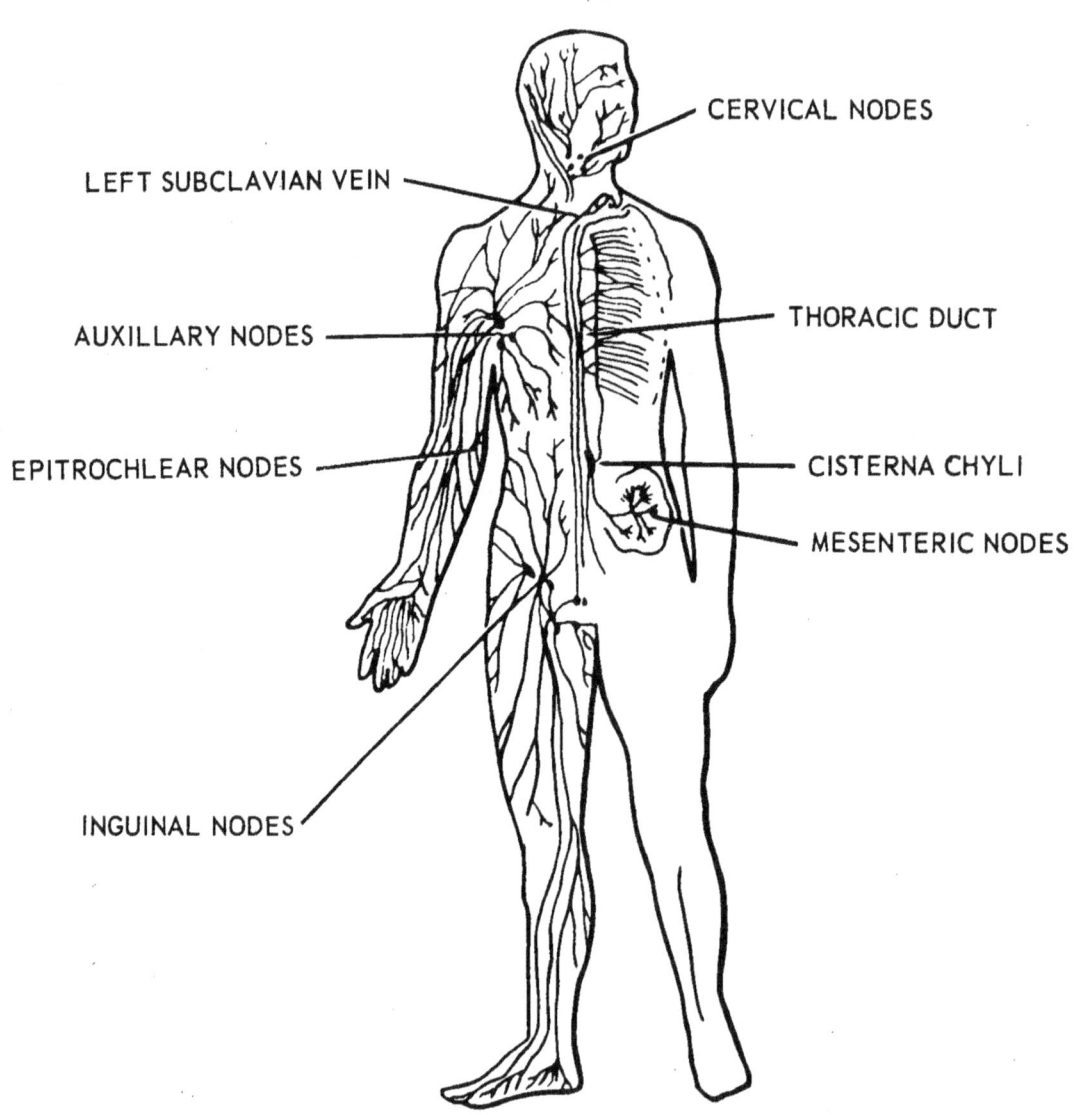

*Figure 2-22. Lymphatic system.*

from bright red (oxygenated blood) when it flows from arteries, to dark red (deoxygenated blood) when it flows from veins. The average man has about 6000 ml. of blood.

a. *Functions of Blood.* The six major functions of blood are all carried out when blood circulates normally through the blood vessels. These functions are—

(1) To carry oxygen from the lungs to tissue cells and carbon dioxide from the cells to the lungs.

(2) To carry food materials absorbed from the digestive tract to the tissue cells and to remove waste products for elimination by excretory organs—the kidneys, intestines, and skin.

(3) To carry hormones, which help regulate body functions, from ductless (endocrine) glands to the tissues of the body.

(4) To help regulate and equalize body temperature. Body cells generate large amounts of heat, and the circulating blood absorbs this heat.

(5) To protect the body against infection.

(6) To maintain the fluid balance in the body.

b. *Composition of Blood.* Blood is made up of a liquid portion, plasma, and formed elements, blood cells, suspended in the plasma.

(1) *Plasma.* Making up more than one-half of the total volume of blood, plasma is the carrier for blood cells and carbon dioxide and other dissolved wastes. It brings hormones and antibodies (protective substances) to the tissues. Other components of plasma are water, oxygen, nitrogen, fat, carbohydrates, and proteins. Fibrinogen, one of the plasma proteins, helps blood clotting. When blood clots, the liquid portion that remains is serum. Blood serum contains no blood cells.

(2) *Blood cells.* The cellular elements in the blood are red cells (erythrocytes, or rbc), white cells (leucocytes, or wbc) and blood platelets (thrombocytes).

### 40. Red Blood Cells (Erythrocytes)

There are about 5,000,000 red blood cells in 1 cubic millimeter (cmm.) of blood. (One cmm. is a very small amount, about 1/25 of a drop). When viewed under a microscope, an individual red blood cell is disc-shaped. An rbc is the only mature body cell that has no nucleus; this fact is important in the diagnosis of some blood disease, because immature red blood cells which do have a nucleus under normal circumstances do not appear in the blood. When nucleated rbc are found, there is a special significance since this may indicate a type of anemia. Red cells are formed in the adult by the red bone marrow in special protected bone areas. Millions of red cells are thought to be destroyed daily, either in the liver, the spleen, the lymph nodes, or in the vascular system itself. In a healthy person, the rate of destruction is equaled by the rate of production, so that a red count of about 5,000,000 per cubic millimeter remains constant. Red blood cells have an average life span of about 90 to 120 days before becoming worn out in service.

*a. Hemoglobin.* A pigment, hemoglobin, gives red cells their color. Hemoglobin (Hgb) has the power to combine with oxygen, carrying it from the lungs to the tissue cells. Hgb assists in transporting carbon dioxide from the cells to the lungs. This transportation of gases (oxygen and carbon dioxide) is the principal function of red cells. The oxygen content gives arterial blood its bright red color. In order to carry oxygen, hemoglobin needs the mineral, iron, which is ordinarily available in a nutritionally adequate diet.

*b. Anemia.* The condition known as anemia is due to a reduction in number of red cells or a reduction in the hemoglobin content of red cells.

### 41. White Cells (Leucocytes)

White cells vary in size and shape, and are larger and much fewer in number than red cells. The average number in an adult is 5,000 to 10,000 in 1 cmm. of blood. Their function is primarily one of protection. They can ingest and destroy foreign particles, such as bacteria, in the blood and tissues. This function is called phagocytosis, and the white cells performing it are phagocytes. White cells are capable of ameboid movement and thus can pass through the walls of capillaries into surrounding tissues. This ability to enter tissue makes them very useful in fighting infection—an area of infection is characterized by a great increase of white cells which gather about the site to destroy bacteria. An example of this is seen in an ordinary boil (furuncle). The pus contained in the boil is made up largely of white cells, plus bacteria and dissolved tissue. Many of the white cells are killed in their struggle with invading bacteria.

*a. Kinds of White Cells.* There are several kinds of white cells. The most numerous, neutrophils, make up about 65 percent of all white cells and are called polymorphonuclear granulocytes. Certain very potent drugs interfere with the formation of these valuable cells, and the condition agranulocytosis (absence of granulocytes) develops. When drugs with this known toxic effect must be used in treatment of a disease, the doctor orders frequent white cell blood counts as an important part of the treatment. Neutrophils are produced by the red bone marrow.

*b. Leucocytosis.* In various diseases, the number of white cells in the blood stream may increase considerably, especially in acute infections. This increase is leucocytosis, and it is an important body defense response. A common condition where there is a leucocytosis is acute appendicitis. (A subnormal white count is known as leucopenia.)

*c. Lymphocytes.* Lymphocytes are white cells produced in lymphoid tissue. One type of lymphocyte is a monocyte, the largest white cells.

### 42. Blood Platelets (Thrombocytes)

Blood platelets, which are smaller than red blood cells, are thought to be fragments of cells formed in the bone marrow. Platelets number about 300,000 per cmm. of blood. Their main function is to aid in the coagulation of blood at the site of a wound. Platelets when injured release a substance to hasten formation of a blood clot.

### 43. Coagulation of Blood

*a.* Blood coagulation, or clotting, is the body's major method of preventing excessive loss of blood when the walls of a blood vessel are broken or cut open. When undisturbed, blood circulates in its vascular system without showing a tendency to clot. However, when blood leaves its natural environment, certain physical and chemical factors are changed and it begins to clot almost at once. At first the clot is soft and jellylike, but it soon becomes firm and acts as a plug, preventing the further escape of blood.

*b.* It takes 3 to 5 minutes for blood to clot, but sometimes it is necessary to hold back the clotting process. This is done with drugs called anticoagulants.

### 44. Hemorrhage

Hemorrhage is bleeding, particularly excessive bleeding, from blood vessels due to a break in their walls. It may be caused by a wound or by disease. Whatever its cause, it can be a serious threat to life and calls for prompt control. Hemorrhage can occur either externally or internally. External hemorrhage is bleeding that can be seen, such as bleeding from a wound. In external hemorrhage, blood escapes to the outside and spills onto the surface of some part of the body. Internal hemorrhage happens inside the body, spilling blood into tissues, a body cavity, or an organ. It can occur without any blood being seen outside the body. Bleeding in some internal areas is evident, however, when blood accumulates in tissues (forming a hematoma), or is vomited, coughed up, or excreted in urine or feces.

*a. Effects of Hemorrhage.* The effects of hemorrhage depend on the amount of blood lost, the rate of loss, and the area into which internal bleeding occurs. Generally, blood pressure drops and breathing and pulse rates become rapid. When blood is lost rapidly, as in bleeding from an artery, blood pressure may drop suddenly. If only small vessels are injured and bleeding is slow, a large amount of blood may be lost without an immediate drop in blood pressure.

*b. Natural Measures to Control Hemorrhage.* When a blood vessel is opened, the body reacts with measures to check bleeding. Two natural body responses to bleeding are clotting of blood and retraction and constriction of blood vessels. The muscle in an injured artery contracts, and if the artery is severed, the contraction pulls the damaged vessel back into the tissues, thus tending to close the leak. As a rule, these natural responses must be helped by artificial means for controlling hemorrhage and for restoring the blood. Artificial means for controlling external hemorrhage include two important first aid measures—elevation of bleeding extremities and applying pressure dressings.

### 45. Blood Types

All human blood may be divided into four main types or groups—O, A, B, AB. This system of typing is used to prevent incompatible blood transfusion, which causes serious reactions and sometimes death. Certain types of blood are incompatible or not suited to each other if combined. Two bloods are said to be incompatible when the plasma or serum of one blood causes clumping of the cells of the other. Two bloods are said to be compatible and safe for transfusion if the cells of each can be suspended in the plasma or serum of the other without clumping. Blood typing and cross-matching are done by highly trained laboratory technicians. Table 2-2 shows blood compatibilities and incompatibilities.

*a. Importance of Blood Types.* From table 2-2, it is evident that if the donor's blood is type "O" it is compatible with all types of recipient blood; or, in other words, type "O" is the universal donor. If the recipient's blood is type "AB", it is compatible with all types of donor blood, or, in other words, type "AB" is the universal recipient. When a blood transfusion is given, the blood type of both donor and recipient should be identical, and their compatibility must be proved by a cross-matching test. However, when blood of the same type is not available and death may result if transfusion is delayed, a type "O" donor (universal donor) may be used if the cross-matching is satisfactory.

*Table 2-2. Blood Types*

| Donor | Recipient | | | |
|---|---|---|---|---|
| | O | A | B | AB |
| O | Compatible | Compatible | Compatible | Compatible |
| A | Incompatible | Compatible | Incompatible | Compatible |
| B | Incompatible | Incompatible | Compatible | Compatible |
| AB | Incompatible | Incompatible | Incompatible | Compatible |

*b. Rh Factor.* In addition to blood grouping and cross-matching for compatibility, the Rh factor must be considered. The Rh factor is carried in red cells, and about 85 percent of all individuals have this factor and are, therefore, Rh positive. Individuals who do not have the Rh factor are Rh negative. As a general rule, Rh negative blood can be given to anyone, provided it is compatible in the ABO typing system, but Rh positive blood should not be given to an Rh negative individual.

## Section VII. THE RESPIRATORY SYSTEM

### 46. Introduction

*a.* The cells of the body require a constant supply of oxygen to carry on the chemical processes necessary to life. As a result of these processes, a waste product, carbon dioxide, is formed that must be removed from the body. Oxygen and carbon dioxide are continually being exchanged, both between the body and the atmosphere and within the body, by the process known as respiration. The system which performs this exchange of gases is the respiratory system.

*b.* The respiratory system consists of the lungs and a series of air passages that connect the lungs to the outside atmosphere. The organs serving as air passages are the nose, the pharynx, the larynx, the trachea, and the bronchi. They carry air into the depths of the lungs and end there in thin-walled sacs, the alveoli, where carbon dioxide is exchanged for oxygen.

### 47. Structure and Function of the Respiratory System

*a. Nose.* The nose consists of two portions, one external and the other internal (nasal cavity). The external nose is a triangular framework of bone and cartilage covered by skin. On its under surface are the nostrils, the two external openings of the nasal cavity. The nasal cavity is divided in two by the nasal septum, and is separated from the mouth by the palate. Inhaled air is warmed, moistened, and filtered by the nasal cavity. The filtering is done by cilia of the mucous membrane lining the nasal passages. Cilia are numerous, long, microscopic processes which beat or wave together and cause movement of materials across the surface and out of the body. Ciliary movement is important in draining the sinuses.

*b. Air Sinuses.* Air spaces in several bones of the face and head open into the nasal cavity. They serve as resonance chambers in the production of voice and decrease the weight of the skull. These air sinuses (fig. 2–23) take the name of the bone in which they are found. They are lined with mucous membrane continuous with that lining the nasal cavity.

*c. Pharynx.* The pharynx, or throat, connects the nose and mouth with the lower air passages and esophagus. It is divided into three parts: the nasopharynx, the oropharynx, and the laryngopharynx. It is continued as the esophagus. Both air and food pass through the pharynx. It carries air from the nose to the larynx, food from the mouth to the esophagus. The walls of the pharynx contain masses of lymphoid tissues called the adenoids and tonsils.

*d. Larynx.* The larynx, or voice box, connects the pharynx with the trachea (fig. 2–23). It is located in the upper and anterior part of the neck. The larynx is shaped like a triangular box. It is made of 9 cartilages joined by ligaments and controlled by skeletal muscles. The thyroid cartilage is the largest. It forms the landmark in the neck called the "Adam's apple." Another of the cartilages is the epiglottis. During swallowing, the epiglottis closes the larynx, the soft palate closes the nasal cavity, and the lips close the mouth. Thus food is forced into the only remaining opening, the esophagus. Except during swallowing or when the throat is voluntarily closed, the air passages are wide open and air is free to pass from the mouth and nose into the lungs. Two membranous bands in the wall of the larynx are called vocal cords. Vibration of the vocal cords produce sounds. The cricoid cartilage, located just below the prominent thyroid cartilage, is joined to the thyroid cartilage by a membrane. The emergency procedure of cricothyroidotomy to produce an airway is performed by puncturing this connecting membrane.

*e. Trachea.* The trachea, or windpipe, is a tube held open by cartilaginous rings. It carries air from the larynx to the bronchi (fig. 2–24). The trachea is lined with cilia and mucous glands whose secretions provide a sticky film to keep dust and dirt out of the lungs.

*f. Bronchi.* The trachea divides to form the two bronchi. One bronchus enters each lung and there divides into many small air passages, called bronchioles or bronchial tubes which lead air into the final air spaces within the lungs.

*g. The Lungs.*

(1) The lungs (fig. 2–24) are the soft, air-filled, essential organs of respiration. They are elastic structures, almost filling the left and right

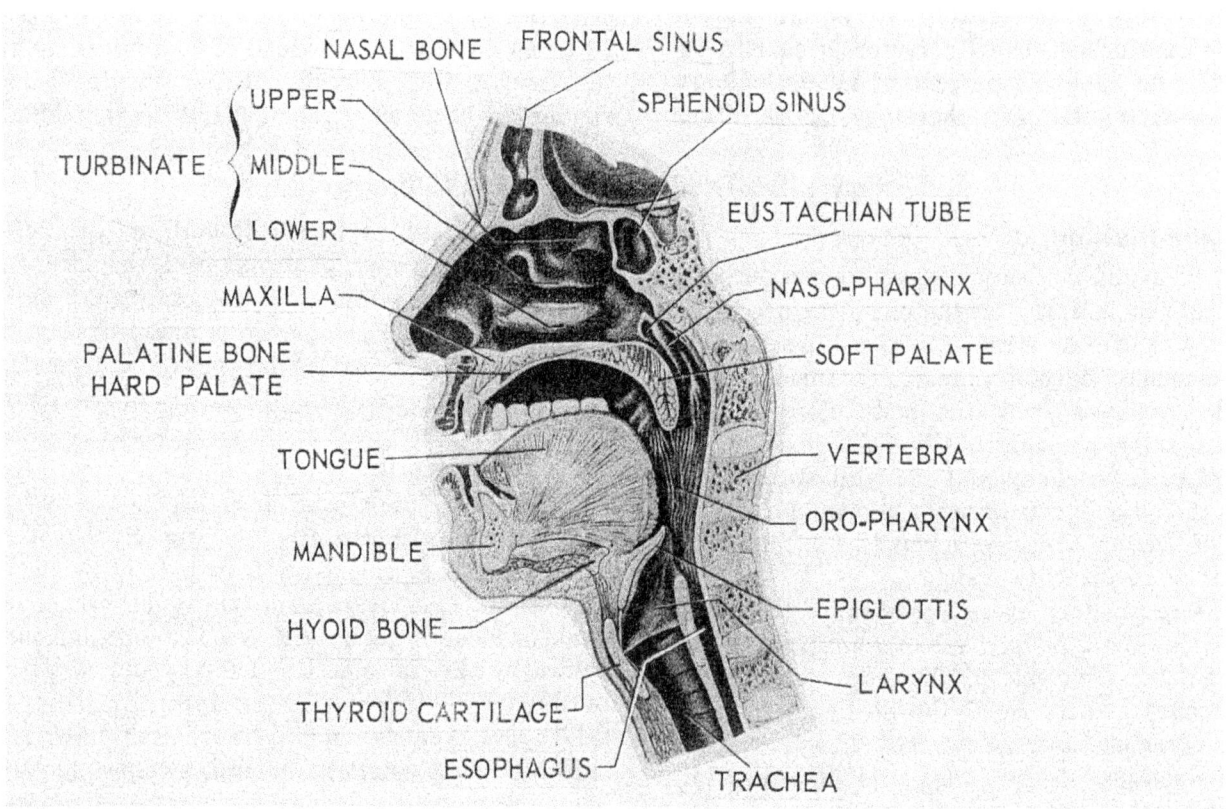

*Figure 2-23. Upper respiratory tract.*

sections of the thoracic cavity. The upper, pointed margin of each lung, the apex, extends above the clavicle. The lower border, the base, fits upon the dome-shaped surface of the diaphragm. Between the two lungs is the mediastinum (fig. 2–25), the central thoracic cavity containing the heart, great blood vessels, esophagus, and lower trachea. The right lung has three lobes; the left lung has two. Within each lobe are separate branches of the main bronchus, and the lobes themselves are divided into segments. The last subdivisions of the air passages to the lungs are alveoli, which are surrounded by networks of capillaries. The alveoli are air chambers.

(2) Each lung is inclosed by a membranous sac formed of two layers of serous membranes called the pleurae (or singly, pleura). One layer covers the lungs (visceral pleura); the other lines the chest cavity (parietal pleura). If air enters the pleural sac, it expands to form a large cavity and the lung collapses (fig. 2–25). This condition of air in the chest outside the lungs is called pneumothorax. If air can move through a hole into the chest, it is called open pneumothorax, a life-endangering condition. An open pneumothorax can result from a bullet wound, stab wound, or other injury that makes a hole in the chest.

### 48. Physiological Process of Respiration

The walls of the alveoli are very thin and it is here that oxygen passes into the bloodstream and carbon dioxide is taken from it. This exchange of oxygen and carbon dioxide in the lungs is called external respiration. The oxygen which enters the blood is carried by the red blood cells in chemical combination with hemoglobin. The blood, oxygenated in the lungs, returns to the heart, then is pumped through the arteries to the capillaries. Here oxygen from the blood passes to the tissue cells and carbon dioxide from the cells passes into the blood to be carried back by the veins to the heart. The exchange of gases between the capillary blood and the tissue cells is called internal respiration.

### 49. Mechanical Process of Respiration

The act of breathing, the cycle of inspiration and expiration, is repeated about 16 to 20 times per minute in an adult at rest. Breathing is regulated primarily by a respiratory center in the brain. The respiratory center is sensitive to changes in blood composition, temperature, and pressure, and adjusts breathing according to the body's needs.

*a. Inspiration.* This is an active movement. The diaphragm, the large, dome-shaped muscle form-

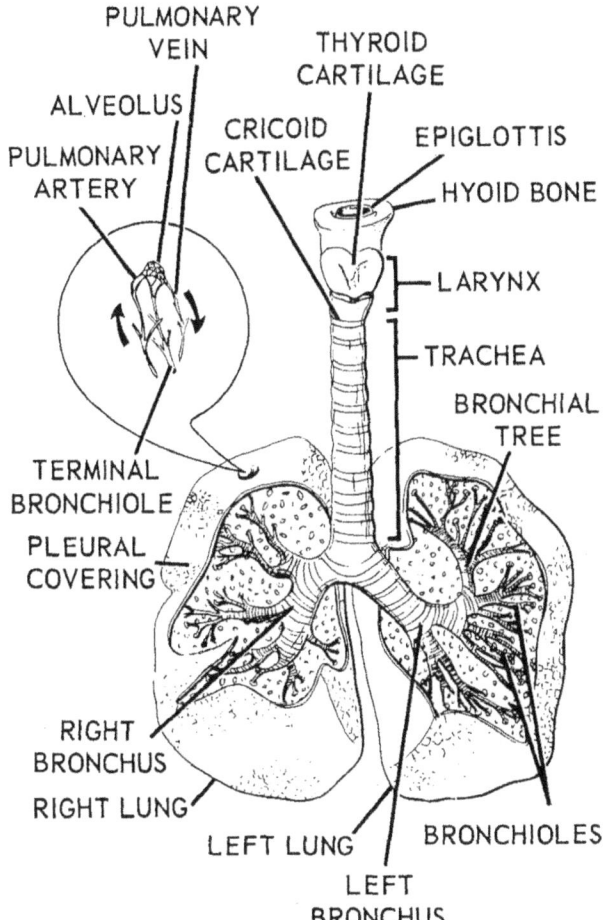

*Figure 2-24. Lungs and air passages.*

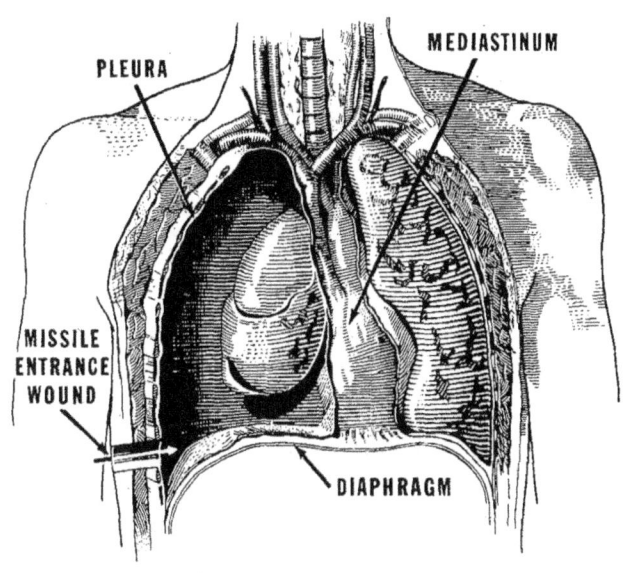

*Figure 2-25. Collapse of lungs by a sucking chest wound.*

ing the floor of the thoracic cavity, contracts, flattening its domed upper surface and increasing the size of the cavity. At about the same time, muscles attached to the ribs (intercostals) contract to elevate and spread the ribs. This further increases the size of the cavity. Air rushes into the lungs and they expand, filling the enlarged cavity.

  b. *Expiration.* At rest, during quiet breathing, expiration is a passive movement. The diaphragm, as it relaxes, is forced upward by intra-abdominal pressure. Muscles attached to the ribs relax, permitting the chest to flatten. These actions reduce the size of the thoracic cavity, allowing the elastic recoil of the stretched lungs to drive out the air. More air can be expelled from the lungs by forced expiration. This is done by contraction of the abdominal muscles, forcing the diaphragm upward, and of the muscles attached to the ribs, flattening the chest to compress the lungs and drive out the air. When breathing becomes forced, as with exercise, expiration also becomes active.

  c. *Volume.* About 500 milliliters (1 pint) of air are inhaled during normal respiration. By deep inspiration it is possible to inhale an additional 1,500 milliliters.

  d. *Sounds.* Sounds caused by air moving in the lungs change with some diseases. These changes, heard with a stethoscope, assist in diagnosis of diseases of the lungs such as pneumonia or tuberculosis.

## Section VIII. THE DIGESTIVE SYSTEM

### 50. Description

  a. The digestive system is made up of the alimentary tract (food passage) and the accessory organs of digestion. Its main functions are to ingest and carry food so that digestion and absorption can occur, and to eliminate unused waste material. The products of the accessory organs help to prepare food for its absorption and use (metabolism) by the tissues of the body.

  b. Digestion consists of two processes, one mechanical and the other chemical. The mechanical part of digestion includes chewing, swallowing, peristalsis, and defecation. The chemical part of digestion consists of breaking foodstuffs into simple components which can be absorbed and used by the body. In this process, foodstuffs are broken down by enzymes, or digestive juices, formed by digestive glands. Carbohydrates are broken into simple sugar (glucose). Fats are changed into fatty acids. Proteins are converted to amino acids.

## 51. Structure of Digestive System
(fig. 2-26)

a. The alimentary canal is about 28 feet long, extending from the lips to the anus, and is divided as follows:

Mouth cavity:
 Teeth
 Tongue
Pharynx
Esophagus
Stomach
Small intestine
Large intestine (colon)
Rectum
Anus

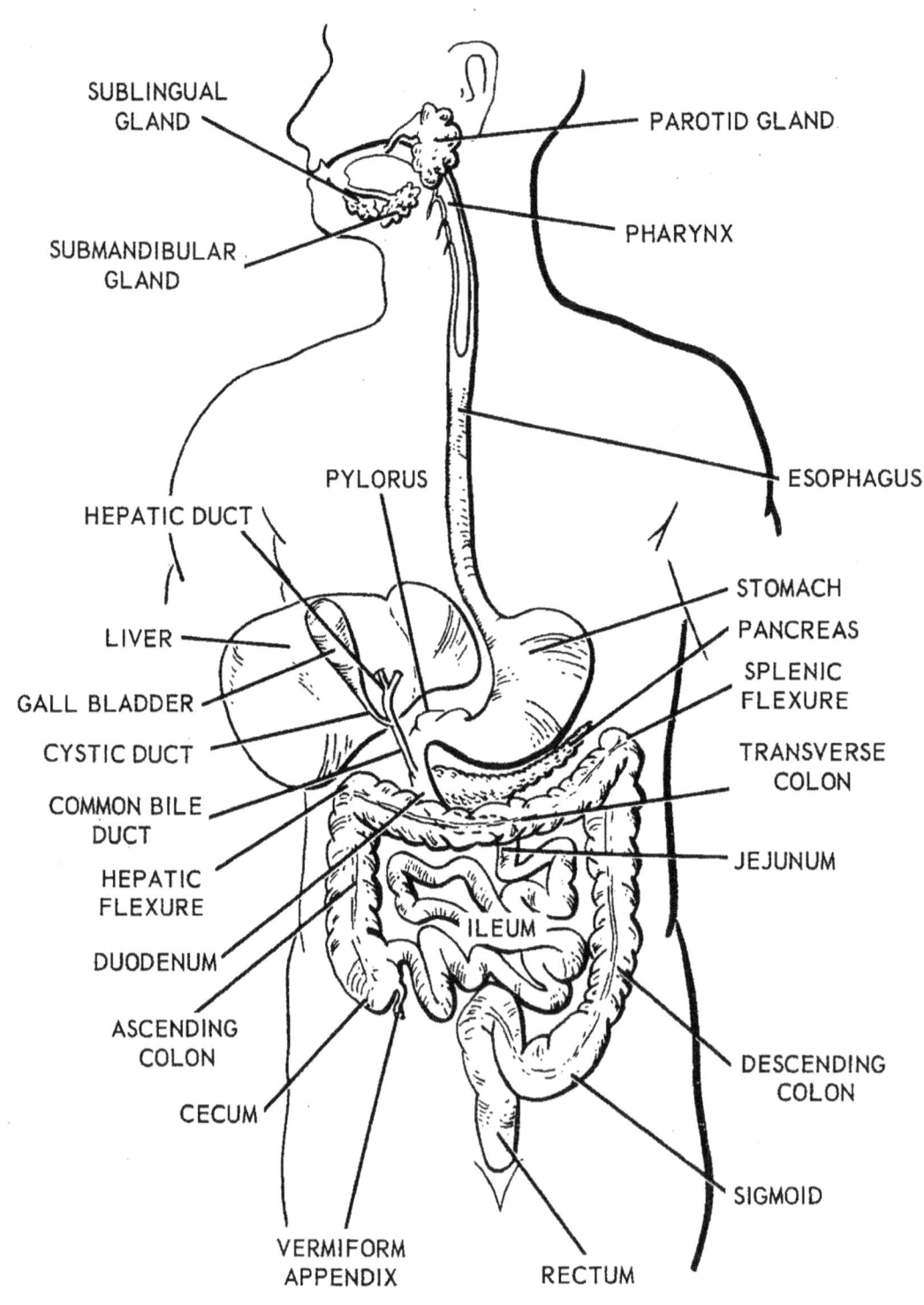

Figure 2-26. Digestive system.

b. The accessory organs that aid the process of digestion are: the salivary glands, pancreas, liver, gall bladder, and intestinal glands.

## 52. The Mouth

The mouth, or oral cavity, is the beginning of the digestive tract. Here food taken into the body is broken into small particles and mixed with saliva so that it can be swallowed.

*a. Teeth.*

(1) A person develops two sets of teeth during his life, a deciduous (or temporary) set and a permanent set. There are 20 deciduous teeth and these erupt during the first 3 years of life. They are replaced during the period between the 6th and 14th years by permanent teeth. There are 32 permanent teeth in the normal mouth; 4 incisors, 2 cuspids, 4 bicuspids, and 6 molars in each jaw. Each tooth is divided into two main parts: the crown, that part which is visible above the gums; and the root, that part which is not visible and which is embedded in the bony structure of the jaw. The crown of the tooth is protected by enamel. Tooth decay is from the outside in; once the protective enamel is broken, microorganisms attack the less resistant parts of the tooth.

(2) The primary function of the teeth is to chew or masticate food. Secondarily, the teeth help to modify sound as produced by the larynx and as used in forming words.

*b. Salivary Glands.* These glands are the first accessory organs of digestion. There are three pairs of salivary glands. They secrete saliva into the mouth through small ducts. One pair, the parotid glands, is located at the side of the face below and in front of the ears. The second pair, the submandibular glands, lies on either side of the mandible. The third pair, the sublingual glands, lies just below the mucous membrane in the floor of the mouth. The flow of saliva is begun in several ways. Placing food in the mouth affects the nerve endings there. These nerve endings stimulate cells of the glands to excrete a small amount of thick fluid. The sight, thought, or smell of food also activates the brain and induces a large flow of saliva. About 1,500 ml. of saliva are secreted daily. The saliva moistens the food, which makes chewing easier. It lubricates the food mass to aid in the act of swallowing. Saliva contains two enzymes, chemical ferments which change foods into simpler elements. The enzymes act upon starches and break them down into sugars.

*c. Tongue.* The tongue is a muscular organ attached at the back of the mouth and projecting upward into the oral cavity. It is concerned in taste, speech, mastication, salivation, and swallowing. After food has been masticated, the tongue propels it from the mouth into the pharynx. This is the first stage of swallowing. Mucus secreted by glands in the tongue lubricates the food and makes swallowing easier. Taste buds situated in the tongue make it the principal organ of the sense of taste. Stimulation of the taste buds causes secretion of gastric juices needed for the breaking down of food in the stomach.

## 53. Pharynx

The pharynx is a muscular canal which leads from the nose and mouth to the esophagus. The passage of food from the pharynx into the esophagus is the second stage of swallowing. When food is being swallowed, the larynx is closed off from the pharynx to keep food from getting into the respiratory tract.

## 54. The Esophagus

The esophagus is a muscular tube about 10 inches long, lined with a mucous membrane. It leads from the pharynx through the chest to the upper end of the stomach (fig. 2–26). Its function is to complete the act of swallowing. The involuntary movement of material down the esophagus is carried out by the process known as peristalsis, which is the wavelike action produced by contraction of the muscular wall. This is the method by which food is moved throughout the alimentary canal.

## 55. The Stomach

The stomach is an elongated pouchlike structure (fig. 2–26) lying just below the diaphragm, with most of it to the left of the midline. It has three divisions: the fundus, the enlarged portion to the left and above the entrance of the esophagus; the body, the central portion; and the pylorus, the lower portion. Circular sphincter muscles which act as valves guard the opening of the stomach. (The cardiac sphincter is at the esophageal opening, and the pyloric sphincter is at the junction of the stomach and the duodenum, the first portion of the small intestine.) The cardiac sphincter prevents stomach contents from re-entering the esophagus except when vomiting occurs. In the digestive process (fig. 2–27), two of the important functions of the stomach are—

*a.* It acts as a storehouse for food, receiving fairly large amounts, churning it, and breaking it down further for mixing with digestive juices. Semiliquid food is released in small amounts by the pyloric valve into the duodenum, the first part of the small intestine.

*b.* The glands in the stomach lining produce gastric juices (which contain enzymes) and hyrochloric acid. The enzymes in the gastric juice start the digestion of protein foods, milk, and fats. Hydrochloric acid aids enzyme action. The mucous membrane lining the stomach protects the stomach itself from being digested by the strong acid and powerful enzymes.

### 56. Small Intestine

The small intestine is a tube about 22 feet long. The intestine is attached to the margin of a thin band of tissue called the mesentery, which is a portion of the peritoneum, the serous membrane lining the abdominal cavity. The mesentery supports the intestine, and the vessels which carry blood to and from the intestine lie within this membrane. The other edge of the mesentery is drawn together like a fan; the gathered margin is attached to the posterior wall of the abdomen. This arrangement permits folding and coiling of the intestine so that this long organ can be packed into a small space. The intestine is divided into three continuous parts: duodenum, jejunum, and ileum. It receives digestive juices from three accessory organs of digestion: the pancreas, liver, and gall bladder (fig. 2–26).

*a. Pancreas.* The pancreas is a long, tapering organ lying behind the stomach. The head of the gland lies in the curve of the small intestine near the pyloric valve. The body of the pancreas extends to the left toward the spleen. The pancreas secretes a juice which acts on all types of food. Two enzymes in pancreatic juice act on proteins. Other enzymes change starches into sugars. Another enzyme changes fats into their simplest forms. The pancreas has another important function, the production of insulin (para 2–83).

*b. Liver.* The liver is the largest organ in the body. It is located in the upper part of the abdomen with its larger (right) lobe to the right of the midline. It is just under the diaphragm and above the lower end of the stomach. The liver has several important functions. One is the secretion of bile, which is stored in the gall bladder and discharged into the small intestine when digestion is in process. The bile contains no enzymes but it breaks up the fat particles so that enzymes can act faster. The liver performs other important functions. It is a storehouse for the sugar of the body (glycogen) and for iron and vitamin B. It plays a part in the destruction of bacteria and wornout red blood cells. Many chemicals such as poisons or medicines are detoxified by the liver; others are excreted by the liver through bile ducts. The liver manufactures part of the proteins of blood plasma. The blood flow in the liver is of special importance. All the blood returning from the spleen, stomach, intestines, and pancreas is detoured through the liver by the portal vein in the portal circulation (fig. 2–17). Blood drains from the liver by hepatic veins which join the inferior vena cava.

*c. Gall Bladder.* The gall bladder is a dark green sac, shaped like a blackjack and lodged in a hollow on the underside of the liver. Its ducts join with the duct of the liver to conduct bile to the upper end of the small intestine. The main function of the gall bladder is the storage and concentration of the bile when it is not needed for digestion.

*d. Ileum.* Most of the absorption of food takes place in the ileum. The walls of the ileum are covered with extremely small, finger-like structures called villi which provide a large surface for absorption. After food has been digested, it is absorbed into the capillaries of the villi. Then it is carried to all parts of the body by the blood and lymph.

### 57. Large Intestine (Colon)

*a.* The large intestine is about 5 feet long. The cecum (fig. 2–26), located on the lower right side of the abdomen, is the first portion of the large intestine into which food is emptied from the small intestine. The appendix extends from the lower portion of the cecum and is a blind sac. Although the appendix usually is found lying just below the cecum, by virtue of its free end it can extend in several different directions, depending upon its mobility.

*b.* The colon extends along the right side of the abdomen from the cecum up to the region of the liver (ascending colon). There the colon bends (hepatic flexure) and is continued across the upper portion of the abdomen (transverse colon) to the spleen. The colon bends again (splenic flexure) and goes down the left side of the abdomen

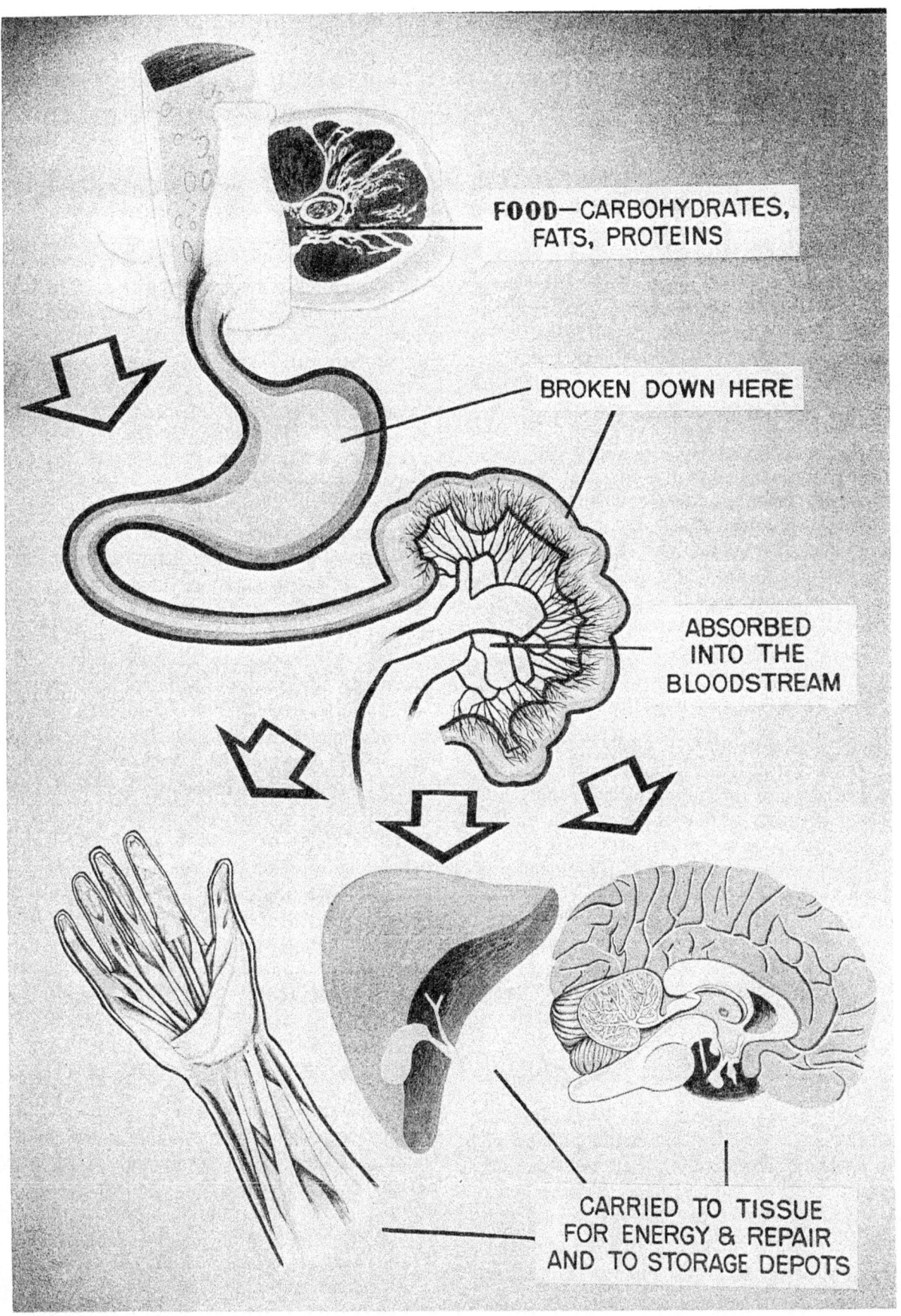

*Figure 2-27. Assimilation of food.*

(descending colon). The last portion makes an S curve (sigmoid) toward the center and posterior of the abdomen and ends in the rectum.

*c.* The main function of the large intestine is the recovery of water from the mass of undigested food it receives from the small intestine. As this mass passes through the colon, water is absorbed and returned to the tissues. Waste materials, or feces, become more solid as they are pushed along by peristaltic movements. Constipation is caused by delay in movement of intestinal contents and removal of too much water from them. Diarrhea results when movement of the intestinal contents is so rapid that not enough water is removed.

### 58. The Rectum and Anus

The rectum is about 5 inches long and follows the curve of the sacrum and coccyx until it bends back into the short anal canal. The anus is the external opening at the lower end of the digestive system. It is kept closed by a strong sphincter muscle. The rectum receives feces and periodically expels this material through the anus. This elimination of refuse is called defecation.

### 59. Time Required for Digestion

Within a few minutes after a meal reaches the stomach, it begins to pass through the lower valve of the stomach. After the first hour the stomach is half empty, and at the end of the sixth hour none of the meal is present in the stomach. The meal goes through the small intestine, and the first part of it reaches the cecum in 20 minutes to 2 hours. At the end of the sixth hour most of it should have passed into the colon; in 12 hours all should be in the colon. Twenty-four hours from the time when food is eaten, the meal should reach the rectum. However, part of a meal may be defecated at one time and the rest at another.

### 60. Absorption of Digested Food
(fig. 2-27)

There is very little absorption in the stomach. Most absorption takes place in the small intestine. The final products of digestion pass through the mucous membrane lining of the gastrointestinal tract and are carried to the liver and from there to the rest of the body. There is marked absorption of water in the large intestine. The residue is concentrated and expelled as feces.

### 61. Defecation

The passage of feces is called defecation. It is begun voluntarily by contraction of the abdominal muscles. At the same time, the sphincter muscles of the anus relax and there is a peristaltic contraction wave of the colon and rectum. Feces are expelled as a result of all these actions. Feces consist of undigested food residue, secretions from the digestive glands, bile, mucus, and millions of bacteria. Mucus is derived from the many mucous glands which pour secretions into the intestine. Bacteria are especially numerous in the large intestine. They act upon food material, causing putrefaction of proteins and fermentation of carbohydrates. Although the bacteria normally in the large intestine serve a useful purpose internally, they are contaminants outside the intestine.

## Section IX. THE URINARY SYSTEM

### 62. Description

The urinary system (fig. 2-28), which filters and excretes waste materials from the blood, consists of two kidneys, two ureters, one urinary bladder, and one urethra. The urinary system helps the body maintain its delicate balance of water and various chemicals in the proportions needed for health and survival. During the process of urine formation, waste products are removed from circulating blood for elimination, and useful products are returned to the blood.

### 63. Kidney

*a.* The kidneys are bean-shaped organs (fig. 2-28), about 4½ inches long, 2 inches wide, and 1 inch thick. They lie on each side of the spinal column, against the posterior wall of the abdominal cavity, near the level of the last thoracic vertebra and the first lumbar vertebra. The right kidney is usually slightly lower than the left. Near the center of the medial side of each kidney is the central notch or hilum, where blood vessels and nerves enter and leave and from which the ureter leaves.

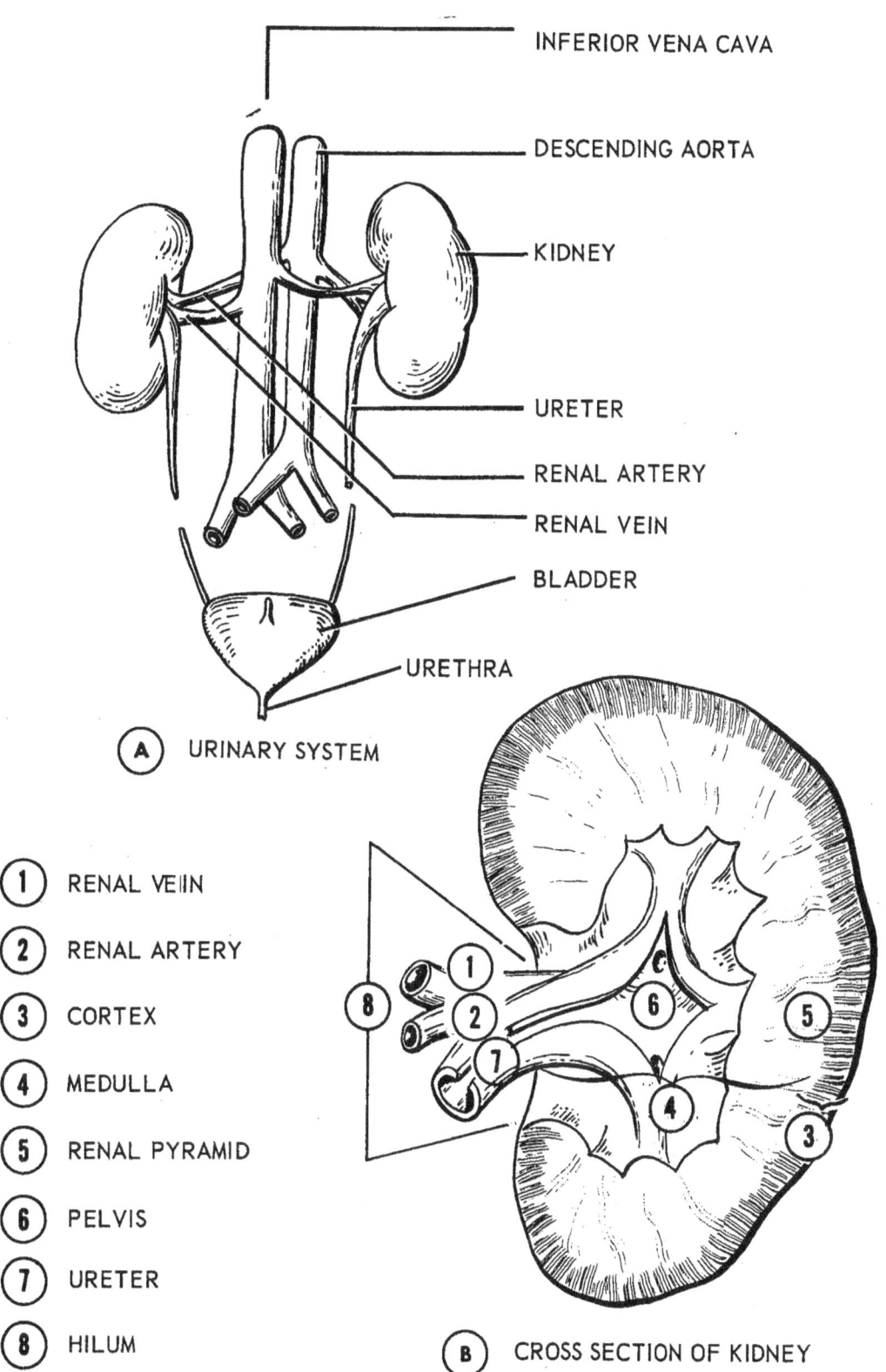

Figure 2-28. *Urinary system and cross section of kidney.*

b. The kidney is composed of an outer shell or cortex, and an inner layer, the medulla. The cortex is made of firm, reddish-brown tissue containing millions of microscopic filtration plants, called nephrons. Each nephron is a urine-forming unit. The nephron units receive and filter all the body's blood about once every 12 minutes. During this period, they draw off and filter the liquid portion of blood, remove liquid wastes (urine), and return the usable portion to the circulation to maintain the body's fluid balance.

(1) Nephrons are very complicated struc-

tures. Each nephron has a capsule containing a cluster of capillaries called glomerulus. Leading from the capsule is a continuous looped tubule. The glomerulus filters the blood; the water, salts, waste products, and usable products pass from the capsule to the tubule; usable products and water are reabsorbed; and the final waste product, urine, drains from the last loop of the tubule. The glomerulus, the capsule, and the loops of tubule together form a nephron. Each part is essential for the coordinated filtration, reabsorption, and excretion process.

(2) Channels called collecting tubules form larger tubes and deliver the urine to the pelvis of the kidney.

### 64. Ureters

The pelvis of each kidney is drained by a ureter, a muscular tube extending from the hilus to the posterior portion of the urinary bladder. Ureters are smooth muscle structures, and urine is passed through each ureter by peristalsis. Drop by drop, urine passes into the bladder. Ureters are about 15 to 18 inches in length and about $\frac{1}{5}$ inch in diameter.

### 65. Urinary Bladder

The urinary bladder, a muscular sac located in the lowest part of the abdominal cavity, stores urine. Normally it holds 300 to 500 ml. The bladder is emptied by contraction of muscles in its walls which force urine out through the urethra.

### 66. Urethra

The urethra is the tube that carries urine from the urinary bladder to the external opening, the urinary meatus. In the male, the urethra will vary in length. Including the portion within the body, it is approximately 6 to $7\frac{1}{2}$ inches in length. It is divided into three areas: the prostatic which passes through the prostate gland; the membranous area, beneath the prostate; and the penile area (anterior), which passes through the penis (para 2–85). The female urethra, about $1\frac{1}{2}$ inch long, extends from the bladder to the meatus, which is located above the vaginal opening.

### 67. Urine

Normal urine is an aromatic, transparent (clear) fluid. The color of normal urine varies from amber or pale yellow to a brownish hue. Freshly voided urine has a characteristic aromatic odor, while stale urine has strong ammonia odor. The average quantity of urine excreted by a normal adult in 24 hours ranges from 1,500 to 2,000 ml., depending upon the fluid intake, amount of perspiration, and other factors. Urine contains protein wastes (urea), salts in solution, hormones, and pigments. (Normal urine should not contain blood, albumin, sugar, or pus cells.)

### 68. Urination

Urination is the discharge or voiding of urine. It is done by a contraction of the bladder and relaxation of the sphincters. In the adult, the act of voiding, although dependent on involuntary reflexes, is partly under voluntary control. Voluntary contraction of abdominal muscles usually accompanies and aids urination.

## Section X. THE NERVOUS SYSTEM

### 69. General

*a.* The nervous system has two major functions, communication and control. It enables the individual to be aware of and to react to his environment. It coordinates the body's responses to stimuli and keeps body systems working together. (Stimuli are changes in environment that require adjustment of body activities.)

*b.* The nervous system consists of nerve centers and of nerves that branch off from them and lead to tissues and organs. Most nerve centers are in the brain and spinal cord. Nerves carry impulses from tissues and organs to nerve centers, and from these centers to tissues and organs. The neurons that carry impulses from the skin and other sense organs to the central nervous system are sensory neurons. They make the body aware of its environment. The neurons that carry impulses from the central nervous system to muscles and glands are motor neurons. They cause the body to react to its environment.

*c.* For study, parts of the nervous system may be considered separately as: the central nervous system, which consists of the brain and spinal cord; the peripheral nervous system, where the nerves are located outside the brain and spinal cord; and the autonomic nervous system, which influences the activities of involuntary muscle and gland tissue.

## 70. The Neuron and Nerves

*a.* The basic unit of the nervous system is the neuron, a cell specialized to respond to stimuli by transmitting impulses. Neurons differ in shape and function from all other body cells. Each neuron has three parts: a cell body and two kinds of processes extending from it (fig. 2–2 ⒟). Many branched processes, the dendrites, conduct impulses toward the cell body. A single process, the axon, conducts impulses away from the cell body. Impulses are the messages carried by the processes. All communication between nerve cells is carried out through these dendrites and axons at the region of contact (synapse) between processes of 2 adjacent neurons.

*b.* The neuron processes, whether dendrite or axon, are called fibers. These nerve fibers are wrapped in an insulating material, the myelin sheath. In addition to the myelin sheath, nerve fibers that extend outside the brain and spinal cord (peripheral nerves) have an outside wrapping called neurilemma. The neurilemma and the nerve cell body are essential for nerve regeneration following injury. In time, if the nerve cell body has not been destroyed, a peripheral nerve fiber can regenerate.

*c.* Nerve cells and nerve processes are bound together and supported by special connective tissue cells called neuroglia. Neuroglia literally means nerve glue. Several different kinds of neuroglia cells help form nerve tissue.

*d.* Nerves, which appear as whitish cords, are bundles of nerve fibers bound together by a connective tissue sheath.

## 71. The Central Nervous System

The central nervous system (CNS) consists of the brain and spinal cord. These are delicate structures that are protected by two coverings, bones and special membranes. The brain is encased by the bones of the skull that form the cranium; the spinal cord by the vertebrae. The membranes enclosing both brain and spinal cord are the meninges.

*a. The Meninges.* Three layers of protective membranes, the meninges, surround the brain and spinal cord. The outer layer of strong fibrous tissue is called the dura mater. The middle layer of delicate cobwebby tissue is the arachnoid. The innermost layer, adherent to the outer surface of the brain and spinal cord, is the pia mater. Between the dura mater and arachnoid is the subdural space; between the arachnoid and pia mater is the subarachnoid space.

*b. Cerebrospinal Fluid.* In addition to protective bones and membranes, nature provides a cushion of fluid around and within the subarachnoid space, in the spaces within the brain called the ventricles, and in the central canal of the spinal cord. Cerebrospinal fluid, which is similar to lymph, filters out from networks of capillaries in the ventricles. It is formed constantly, circulated constantly, and part of it is reabsorbed constantly into the venous blood of the brain. At any one time, an adult has about 135 ml. of this fluid circulating, although over 500 ml. is produced daily. If anything interferes with its circulation or its reabsorption, the fluid accumulates. An abnormal accumulation of cerebrospinal fluid is hydrocephalus (water on the brain).

*c. The Brain.* The brain (fig. 2–29), a mass of nervous tissue, is the highest level of the nervous system. It coordinates activities of the entire body; carries on the learning, thinking, and reasoning processes; and directs voluntary movements of the body. The brain may be divided into three parts: the cerebrum, cerebellum, and the brain-stem, the last consisting of the forebrain, midbrain, pons, and medulla. The midbrain serves as a connecting pathway between the right and left halves of the cerebrum and also between the cerebellum and the rest of the brain.

(1) *Cerebrum.* The cerebrum is described as resembling many small sausages bound together. It is the largest part of the brain, divided, not quite completely, into two hemispheres. Each hemisphere has five lobes. The outer surface, or cortex, of the brain is made up of gray matter, which is composed of nerve cells. The white matter within the brain is made up of nerve fibers, which lead to and from the cell bodies in the gray matter. Certain areas of the cerebrum are localized for certain functions, but it is believed that no one area functions independently. In the frontal lobe is the motor area, which controls voluntary movements, the speech center, and the writing center. In the parietal lobe is the general sensory area which perceives sensations of heat, cold, touch, pressure, pain, and position. In the temporal lobe are the centers for hearing and smelling. In the occipital lobe is the visual center.

(2) *Cerebellum.* The cerebellum lies below the posterior part of the cerebrum. It coordinates muscular activity at an unconscious level. It also

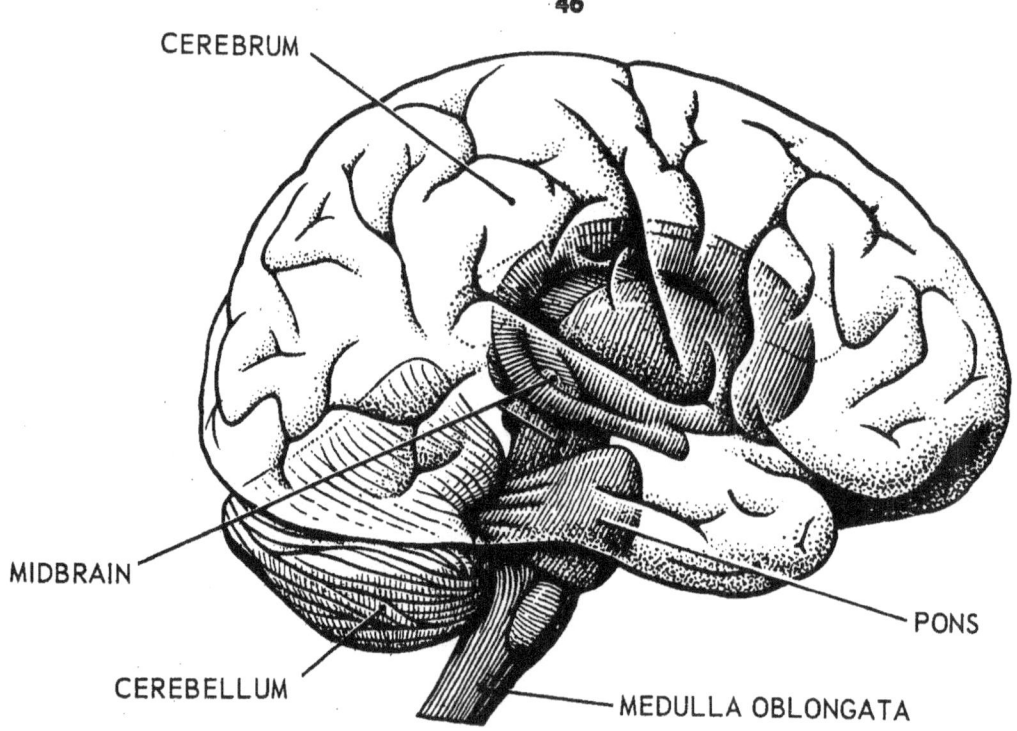

*Figure 2-29. The brain, sagittal section.*

coordinates with the cerebrum to produce skilled movements. The cerebellum helps control posture and controls skeletal muscles to maintain equilibrium. If the cerebellum is injured, movements will be jerky and trembly.

(3) *The pons.* The pons is a bridgelike structure, forming the part of the brain stem above the medulla. Nerve pathways between the spinal cord and other parts of the brain go through the pons.

(4) *The medulla.* The medulla oblongata, a bulblike structure attaching the brain to the spinal cord, is a part of the brain stem. It contains vital centers controlling heart action, blood vessel diameter, and respirations. Mechanisms controlling nonvital functions such as sneezing, hiccoughing, and vomiting are also functions of the medulla. Nerve fibers cross from one side to the other in the medulla, a fact that explains why one side of the brain is said to control the opposite side of the body.

*d. The Spinal Cord.* The spinal cord, protected by meninges and vertebrae, is about 18 inches in length. The cord is continuous with the medulla of the brain and terminates at a level between the first and second lumbar vertebrae (fig. 2-9).

(1) The meninges inclosing the cord continue down below the termination of the cord and are anchored at the sacrum and coccyx. This anatomical feature makes it possible for a physician to withdraw samples of cerebrospinal fluid without danger of injuring the cord. When a patient is placed on his side and his back is arched by drawing his knees and chest together, the space between the fourth and fifth lumbar vertebrae is enlarged. A lumbar puncture needle can be inserted through the intervertebral space into the subarachnoid space to obtain spinal fluid for diagnostic tests. This feature also makes it possible to administer spinal anesthesia.

(2) The spinal cord has two major functions —conduction and connection. Many nerves enter and leave the spinal cord at different levels. These nerves all connect with nerve centers located within the spinal cord or with nerve centers in the brain. Nerve centers within the cord form the gray matter of the cord's inner core. Surrounding the gray matter are columns of nerve fibers, forming the white matter. The nerve fiber columns in the spinal cord are called tracts; these tracts connect the different levels of the nervous system. Tracts which transmit upward, the ascending tracts, are all sensory nerve fibers. Tracts which transmit impulses downward, the descending tracts, are all motor nerve fibers, controlling both voluntary and involuntary muscles. When the spinal cord is damaged, the extent of disability depends upon which nerve centers and which tracts are damaged.

(3) The soft spinal cord can be compressed by vertebrae fractures or by dislocation and displacement of vertebrae or vertebrae discs. If the

pressure can be relieved by surgical procedures or by traction, permanent damage may be avoided. Careful and knowledgeable moving and transporting of all patients suspected of having a spinal injury is essential to minimize injury to the spinal cord. If the cord is severed, or if all cord tracts have been damaged, patients lose feeling because sensory impulses cannot reach the brain; they are paralyzed, because motor impulses from the brain can no longer reach muscles located below the injury. Damage to the cord in the cervical area is particularly disabling because all of the cord tracts below the injury are involved. Disease, injury, or chemicals (drugs) can cause loss of function by interrupting the conduction and connection pathways.

(4) All sensory impulses coming into the cord do not have to travel all the way to the brain to get a motor impulse reaction. The gray matter in the spinal cord contains reflex centers, the places where incoming sensory impulses become outgoing motor impulses. There are reflex centers in both the brain and the spinal cord. The knee jerk is an example of a spinal cord reflex. When the doctor taps the patellar tendon, the sensation is transmitted to a segment of the spinal cord at the lumbar level, and a motor impulse causes extension of the lower leg. This kind of reflex is an involuntary response. If lumbar segments of the cord are damaged, the knee jerk is absent. The doctor tests for these different reflexes during a neurological examination because in certain diseases they deviate from normal.

## 72. The Peripheral Nervous System

The peripheral nervous system is composed of the nerves located outside the brain and spinal cord. Cranial nerves and their branches stem from the brain; spinal nerves and their branches stem from the spinal cord.

*a. The Cranial Nerves.* The 12 pairs of cranial nerves arise from the undersurface of the brain and pass through openings in the skull to their destinations (table 2-3). The nerves are numbered and have names that describe their distribution or their function; *for example,* the vagus nerve (fig. 2-30), the cranial nerve, is an important nerve in the autonomic nervous system, with both sensory and motor fibers distributed to organs in the thorax and abdomen. The cranial nerves supply organs of special sense, such as the eye, nose, ears, tongue, and their associated muscles, and also control muscles of the face, neck, thorax, and abdomen.

### NOTE
Cranial nerves are usually indicated by Roman numerals.

*b. The Spinal Nerves.* The 31 pairs of spinal nerves arise from the spinal cord and pass through lateral openings between the vertebrae. Spinal nerves are numbered according to the level of the spinal column at which they emerge. The lumbar, sacral, and coccygeal nerves descend from the terminal end of the spinal cord and emerge in sequence from their respective vertebrae. These lower spinal nerves form the cauda equina (horse's tail) within the spinal cavity. Spinal nerves branch and subdivide into many lesser nerves after emerging from the spinal cavity.

(1) *Nerve plexuses.* A nerve plexus is a network of spinal nerve subdivisions that appear as tangled masses in areas outside the spinal cord. The brachial plexus (fig. 2-30) is in the shoulder region. Nerves emerging from this tangle go to the skin, the arm, and the hand. Pressure and/or

*Table 2-3. The 12 Cranial Nerves*

| Number and name | Origin | Associated with— |
|---|---|---|
| I. Olfactory (sensory) | Nasal chamber | Sense of smell |
| II. Optic (sensory) | Retina | Sense of sight |
| III. Oculomotor (motor) | Midbrain | Eyeball muscles |
| IV. Trochlear (motor) | Midbrain | Eyeball muscles |
| V. Trigeminal (sensory and mixed). | Pons | (Three branches) eye, upper portion of face, ear, lower lip, teeth, gums. |
| VI. Abducens (motor) | Pons | Eyeball muscles |
| VII. Facial (mixed) | Pons | Facial muscles, middle ear, taste |
| VIII. Auditory (sensory) | Pons | Sense of hearing and balance |
| XI. Glossopharyngeal (mixed) | Medulla | Taste, swallowing |
| X. Vagus (mixed) | Medulla | Swallowing, hunger, speech muscles, breathing, heart rate, peristalsis, control of glands in stomach and pancreas. |
| XI. Spinal accessory (motor) | Medulla | Muscles of neck and upper back. |
| XII. Hypoglossal (motor) | Medulla | Muscles of tongue |

stretching of the brachial plexus can cause paralysis of the arm and hand. If an unconscious patient's arm is allowed to dangle off a litter or bed, the plexus can be overstretched. Pressure from a plaster cast can also damage this area. The sacral plexus in the pelvic cavity supplies nerves to the lower extremity. The largest nerve in the body, the sciatic nerve, emerges from the sacral plexus. From the buttocks, the sciatic nerve runs down the back of the thigh; its branches supply posterior thigh muscles, leg, and foot. The sciatic nerve must be avoided when intramuscular injections are given into the buttocks.

(2) *Nerve fibers.* All spinal nerves carry both sensory and motor fibers. Some of the fibers supply skeletal muscle and others supply visceral (smooth) muscle. The spinal nerves are two-way conductors, and if anything happens to them, there can be both anesthesia, loss of sensation, and paralysis, loss of motion.

### 73. The Autonomic Nervous System

The autonomic nervous system is part of the nervous system that sends nerve fibers from nerve centers to smooth muscle, cardiac muscle, and gland tissue. Autonomic nerve fibers supply nerve impulses to body structures that are thought of as operating outside conscious control. Organs supplied are the heart, blood vessels, iris and ciliary muscles of the eye, bronchial tubes, parts of the esophagus, and abdominal organs. The autonomic nervous system is a part of the central and peripheral nervous system. It is not separate and independent. It has two divisions, sympathetic and parasympathetic. These divisions receive impulses from the CNS by way of the ganglia.

*a.* Ganglia are the relay stations of the autonomic nervous system. Neurons originating in the cord, or in the brain, conduct impulses to an autonomic ganglion. Other neurons conduct impulses from the ganglion to the tissue or organ. Ganglia of the sympathetic division are in a chain formation, like a string of beads, one on each side of the spinal column. Ganglia of the parasympathetic division are located in or near the organs to which they send impulses (table 2–4).

*b.* The sympathetic division regulates activities to prepare the body for maximum effort as a response to hazardous conditions. Sympathetic stimulation and response to stress go together.

*c.* The parasympathetic division regulates activities to conserve energy and to promote digestion and elimination.

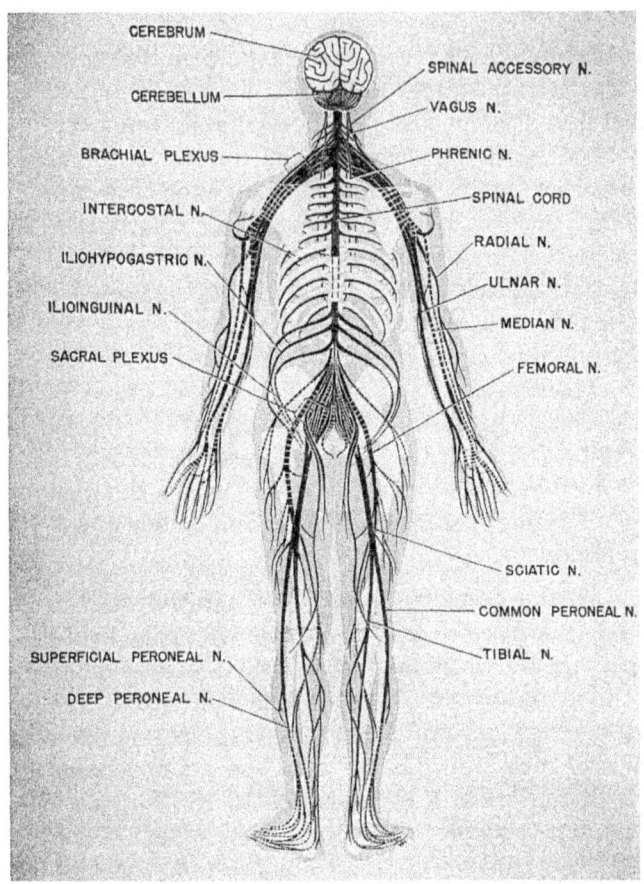

*Figure 2–30. Principal nerve trunks.*

### 74. Special Senses

Sensations of smell, taste, sight, hearing, and equilibrium are usually referred to as special senses because these sensations are received through specialized sense organs or receptors which are sensitive to specific types of stimuli. Other very important sensations such as touch, pressure, pain, heat, and cold are received through receptors widely distributed in the skin and underlying tissue and in viscera. Impulses from receptors for both special and other senses are carried by sensory nerve pathways to the cerebrum. There the impulses are converted into sensation and perception (awareness or consciousness of sensation). The parts of the sensory mechanism are (1) the sense organ or receptor, (2) the pathway by which the impulse is conducted into the central nervous system, and (3) the sensory center in the cerebrum. The sensory mechanisms of the special senses are summarized as follows:

*a. Smell.* Cells located in the olfactory membrane of the nose are stimulated by odors. The olfactory membrane is located in the uppermost part of the nose, in the area above the upper turbinates. Impulses from receptors for odors are

*Table 2-4. Functions of the Autonomic Nervous System*

| Increased sympathetic tone results in— | Increased parasympathetic tone results in— |
|---|---|
| 1. Dilation of pupils. | 1. Contraction of pupils. |
| 2. Decreased tones of ciliary muscles, so that the eyes are accommodated to see distant objects. | 2. Contraction of ciliary muscles, so that the eyes are accommodated to see objects near at hand. |
| 3. Dilation of bronchial tubes. | 3. Contraction of bronchial tubes. |
| 4. Quickened and strengthened heart action. | 4. Slowed heart action. |
| 5. Contraction of blood vessels of the skin and viscera so that more blood goes to the muscles where it is needed for "fight or flight." | 5. Dilation of blood vessels. |
| 6. Relaxation of gastrointestinal tract and bladder. | 6. Increased contractions of gastrointestinal tract and muscle tone of bladder. |
| 7. Decreased secretions of glands (except sweat glands which secrete more). | 7. Increased secretions of glands (except sweat glands). |
| 8. Contraction of sphincters which prevents emptying of bowels and bladder. | 8. Relaxation of sphincters which allows emptying of bowels or bladder. |

transmitted by the olfactory nerve to the temporal lobe of the brain. Although olfactory receptor cells are quite sensitive, they can also become fatigued, and odors that at first may be very noticeable may be less so upon continued exposure. Smell is considered a primitive sense and the detection of odors is more highly developed in animals than in man.

*b. Taste.* Sense organs for taste are taste buds located in the surface of the tongue. The primary taste sensations are sweet, sour, salty and bitter. The actual sensation of taste, particularly for distinctive flavors, is influenced by the sense of smell. Taste sensation is usually dulled when nasal membranes are congested or when the nostrils are pinched shut while eating foods. Impulses from taste receptors are transmitted by nerve fibers from two cranial nerves, facial and glossopharyngeal, to the temporal lobe.

*c. Sight.* Cells in the retina of the eye (fig. 2-3 Ⓐ) are stimulated by light rays entering the eye. These stimuli create impulses that are carried by the optic nerve to the visual center of the occipital lobe of the brain.

*d. Hearing.* Cells in the cochlea of the inner ear (fig. 2-32 Ⓑ) are stimulated by vibration of sound waves. These stimuli create impulses that are carried by the cochlear branch of the acoustic (auditory) nerve to the auditory center of the temporal lobe.

*e. Equilibrium.* In addition to receptors for hearing, the internal ear contains three semicircular canals which regulate the sense of equilibrium. Change in position of the head causes movement of fluid within the canals. The fluid movement stimulates nerve endings in the walls of the canals which send impulses to the brain by the vestibular branch of the auditory nerve.

## 75. The Eye

The eye is specialized for the reception of light. Each eye is located in a bony socket or cavity called the orbit, which is formed by several bones in the skull. The orbit provides protection, support, and attachment for the eye and its muscles, nerves, and blood vessels.

*a. The Eyeball.* The interior of the eye (fig. 2-31 Ⓐ) is divided into an anterior cavity (anterior to the lens) and a posterior cavity (posterior to the lens). A clear watery solution, the aqueous fluid, is formed and circulated in the anterior cavity. A transparent, semifluid material, the vitreous fluid, is contained in the posterior cavity. The globular form and firmness of the eyeball is maintained by its fluid contents, which also function in the transmission of light.

(1) *Eye tissue coats.* The eyeball has an outer coat, a middle coat, and an inner coat.

(a) *Outer coat.* The outer coat consists of a normally invisible, transparent anterior portion, the cornea, and a fibrous, white, nontransparent portion, the sclera, which is directly continuous with the cornea. The transparent cornea focuses and transmits light to the interior of the eye. The surface of the cornea must be moist at all times to maintain its transparency. The sclera helps to maintain the shape of the eyeball and protects the delicate structures within.

(b) *Middle coat.* The middle coat consists of the choroid, the iris, and the ciliary body. These three structures are referred to as the uveal tract. The choroid, the vascular middle layer of the eyeball, lies beneath the sclera and lines the posterior portion of the eye from the ciliary body to the optic nerve. The iris is a circular, colored, muscular membrane which is suspended between

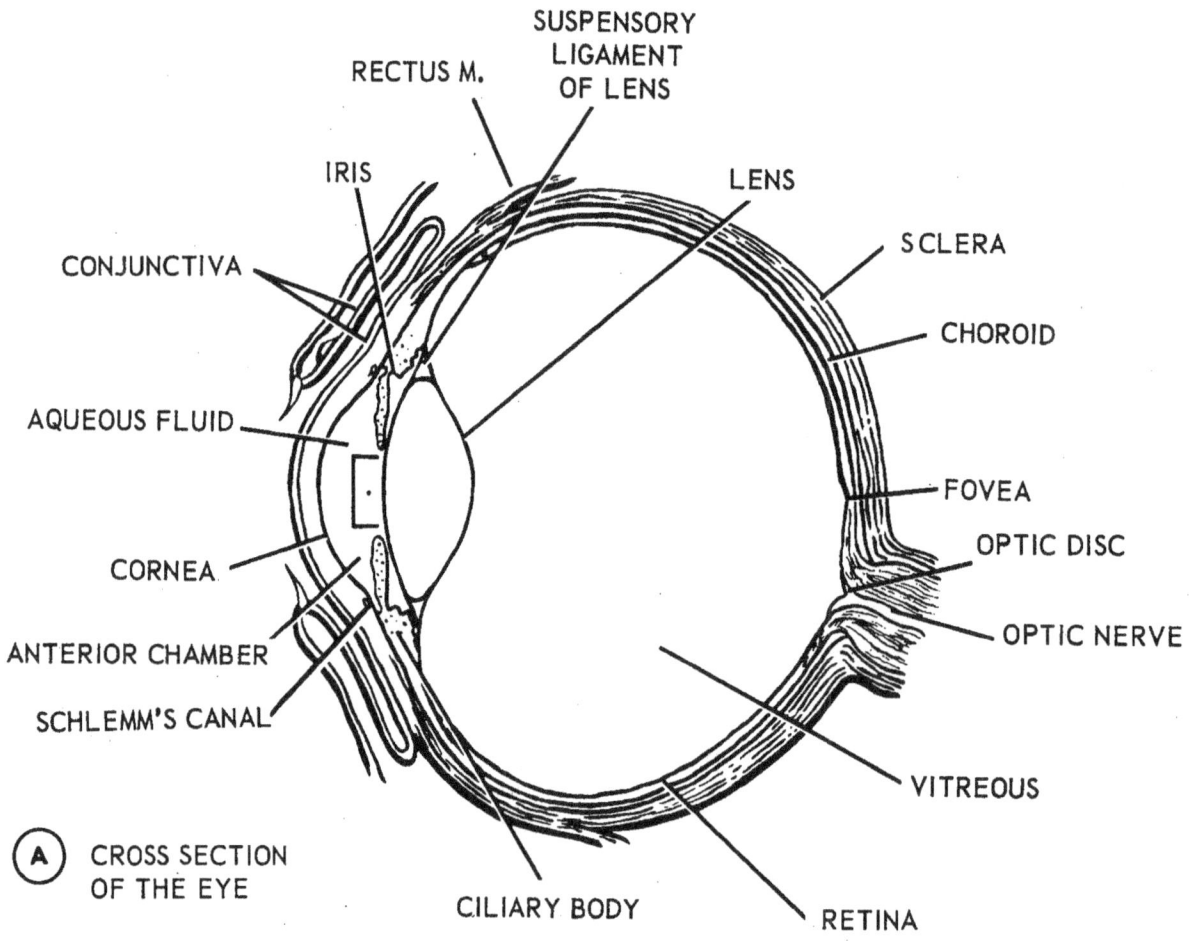

*Figure 2-31. The eye.*

the cornea and the lens. The pigment material in the iris gives the eye its characteristic color. The round opening in its center is the pupil. The muscle structure of the iris adjusts the size of the pupil to adapt the eye to existing brightness of light. The ciliary body lies between the iris and choroid; it has a muscular function, changing the focus of the lens, and a secretory function, producing aqueous fluid.

(c) *Inner coat.* The inner coat is the retina, which lines the interior of the eye except toward its anterior inner surface. The visual nerve cells (rods and cones) are arranged closest together at the central portion of the retina, the macula lutea. A slight depression in the macula lutea, the fovea centralis, is in a direct line back from the center of the cornea and lens and is the area of the retina most sensitive to light. Medial to the fovea centralis is the area called the optic disc, the site of exit of the optic nerve and entry of the retinal artery. Here there is a natural defect in the retina; there are no visual cells at the exit of the optic nerve and in every eye there is, therefore, a physiological "blind spot." When the doctor examines the interior of the eye with an ophthalmoscope, he can see the posterior surface of the retina and examine the appearance of the optic disc. The inner surface of the retina is in contact with the vitreous and the outer surface with the choroid. The condition known as "detached retina" means that some portion of the retina has become separated from the supporting choroid.

(2) *The lens.* The lens is a small, disc-shaped, transparent structure about ⅓ inch in diameter. It is situated immediately behind the iris and in front of the vitreous cavity. The lens is suspended in a capsule within the globe of the eye by a circular ligament, the suspensory ligament of the lens. This ligament is attached to the ciliary body. Muscular movements of the ciliary body affect the suspensory ligament and the consequent focus of the lens. The condition of "cataract" means that some portion of the lens has lost its transparency and has become cloudy or opaque.

(3) *Aqueous fluid.* The aqueous fluid is formed by a portion of the ciliary body and fills the two divisions of the anterior cavity of the eye, called the anterior and the posterior chamber.

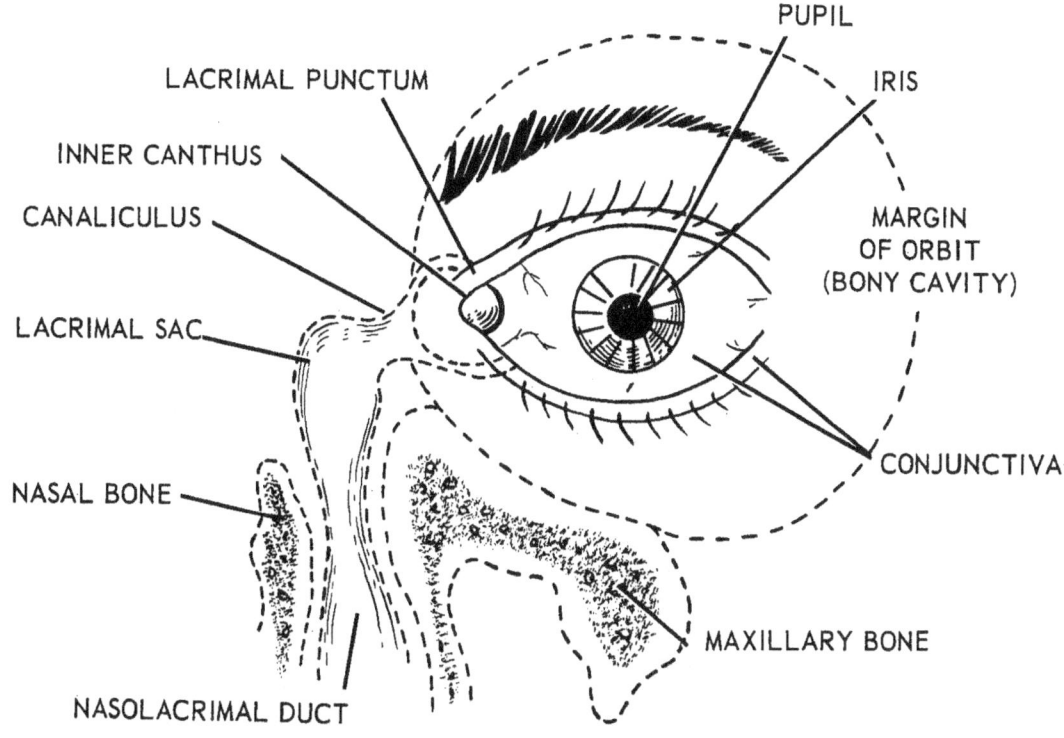

B) THE EYE (FRONTAL, EXTERIOR VIEW) AND LACRIMAL APPARATUS.

*Figure 2-31—Continued.*

Aqueous fluid is normally crystal clear for transmission of light rays and its formation and flow helps maintain the normal intraocular pressure. The aqueous fluid flows from the posterior chamber to the anterior chamber and drains by means of a series of channels into the venous blood. The largest of these drainage channels is the canal of Schlemm. Interference with the normal formation and flow of aqueous fluid can lead to development of excessively high intraocular pressure, a condition called glaucoma. Glaucoma will cause blindness. Fortunately, glaucoma can be detected by a tonometry examination, the measurement of internal eye pressure by means of a measuring instrument, a tonometer. With early detection, glaucoma can be treated successfully and blindness can be prevented.

*b. The External Eye and Accessory Structures.* Viewed from the surface of the body, the anterior surface of the eye and some of its accessory structures such as eyebrows, lids, lashes, and conjunctiva are readily visible. An additional essential accessory structure, the lacrimal (tear) apparatus, is indicated in figure 2-31 ⓑ.

(1) *Eyebrows and eyelashes.* The eyebrow and lashes are usually considered to have a cosmetic (decorative) function, but the eyelashes also help protect against the entrance of foreign objects into the eyes. An eyelash becomes a foreign body itself if it becomes detached and falls on the eye surface. On the margin of the eyelids near the attachment of the eyelashes are the openings of a number of glands. Infection in these glands is commonly called a sty.

(2) *Eyelids.* The eyelids are thin, moveable, protective coverings for the eyes. The junctions of the upper and lower eyelids of each eye are canthi; the inner canthus (fig. 2-31 ⓑ) is at the nasal junction and the outer canthus is at the temporal junction. A sheet of connective tissue called the tarsal plate maintains the shape of the eyelids. The tarsal plate and the orbicularis oculi muscle hold the eyelids in proper position against the eye; a levator (lifting) muscle opens the upper lid by pulling the lid upward into the orbit. The circular orbicularis oculi muscle closes the eyelids.

(3) *Conjunctiva.* The conjunctiva (fig. 2-31 ⓑ) is a delicate mucous membrane which lines the inside of the eyelids and covers the front surface of the eyeball, continuing over the cornea as the corneal epithelium. The edge or margin where the conjunctiva overlaps the cornea is called the limbus; it is sometimes visible at the periphery of

the iris. The semitransparent conjunctiva appears while on the front surface of the eyeball where it covers the sclera and pink where it overlies lid tissue. Should the conjunctiva itself become inflamed or infected it appears red and swollen; one type of acute bacterial infection of the conjunctiva is commonly called "pinkeye."

(4) *The lacrimal apparatus.* The lacrimal apparatus consists of the lacrimal gland, lacrimal ducts (canaliculi), lacrimal sac, and the nasolacrimal duct (fig. 2-31 ⑧). Its function is the secretion and drainage of tears. The lacrimal gland (not illustrated) is about the shape and size of a small almond and is located in a small depression on the lateral side of the frontal bone of the orbit. Many small ducts drain tears secreted by the gland to the conjunctival surface; the tears drain downward and toward the inner angle of the eye. The normal regular blinking of the eyelids helps to spread the tears evenly to provide a lubricating, protective, moist film over the exposed surface of the cornea. The tears drain into openings near the nasal portion of each eyelid (lacrimal puncti) and then into the tear ducts, the sac, and finally into the nose through the nasolacrimal duct. This normal formation and drainage of tears is the natural way in which the eye surface is kept clean and moist.

(5) *Extraocular muscles.* In addition to the levator muscles of the eyelids and the orbicularis oculi, there are six sets of muscles located outside the eyeball. These muscles raise, lower, or rotate the eyeball within its socket. The muscles of the two eyes normally function in a coordinated manner so that both eyes move simultaneously and are aimed in the same direction. Divergence or crossing of the eyes is called strabismus.

### 76. The Ear

The ear, the organ of hearing, consists of three parts; the external ear, the middle ear (tympanic cavity), and the internal ear (the labyrinth). These divisions are commonly referred to as the outer ear, the middle ear, and the inner ear. They provide the reception and conduction of sound and contain one of the principal mechanisms for the maintenance of equilibrium. The structures of the ear, except the part protruding from the head, are situated within portions of the temporal bone of the skull.

*a.* The external ear (fig. 2-32 Ⓐ) consists of the shell-shaped portion of the ear, called the auricle or pinna, which projects from the side of the head and of the external acoustic meatus, which is the external auditory canal leading inward toward the middle ear. The principal function of the external ear is the collection and conduction of sound waves to the middle and the inner ear. The auricle or pinna is composed of cartilage covered with membrane (called the perichondrium) and the skin.

(1) The prominent folded rim of the ear is the helix.

(2) A deep cavity, the concha, leads into the external auditory canal.

(3) In front of the concha and projecting backward over the entrance to the external auditory canal is a small, triangular eminence of cartilage called the tragus. The tragus protects, but does not touch, the entrance to the external auditory canal. The undersurface of the tragus is usually covered with soft hairs which help to prevent insects and other foreign bodies from entering the ear.

(4) The lobule, or lobe, is located inferior to the tragus and to the lowest point of the helix. The lobule contains no cartilage, is composed of adipose (fatty) tissue and of connective tissue, and lacks the firmness of the rest of the auricle.

*b.* The external auditory canal extends about 1¼ inches from its entrance at the bottom of the concha to the tympanic membrane, or eardrum, which closes its inner end. The canal is formed of two parts, its outer, or cartilaginous, part which is formed of cartilage and membrane; and its inner, or bony portion, formed by a passage in the temporal bone. The cartilage of the auricle is continuous with that forming the outer portion of the canal.

(1) Two or more deep fissures are present in

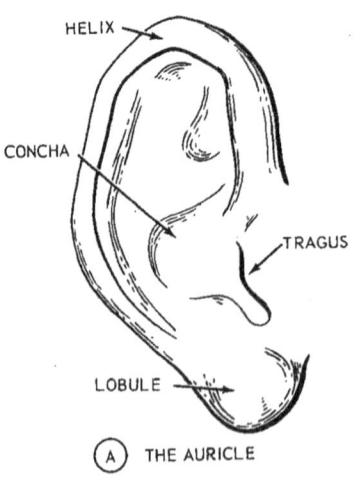

*Figure 2-32. The ear.*

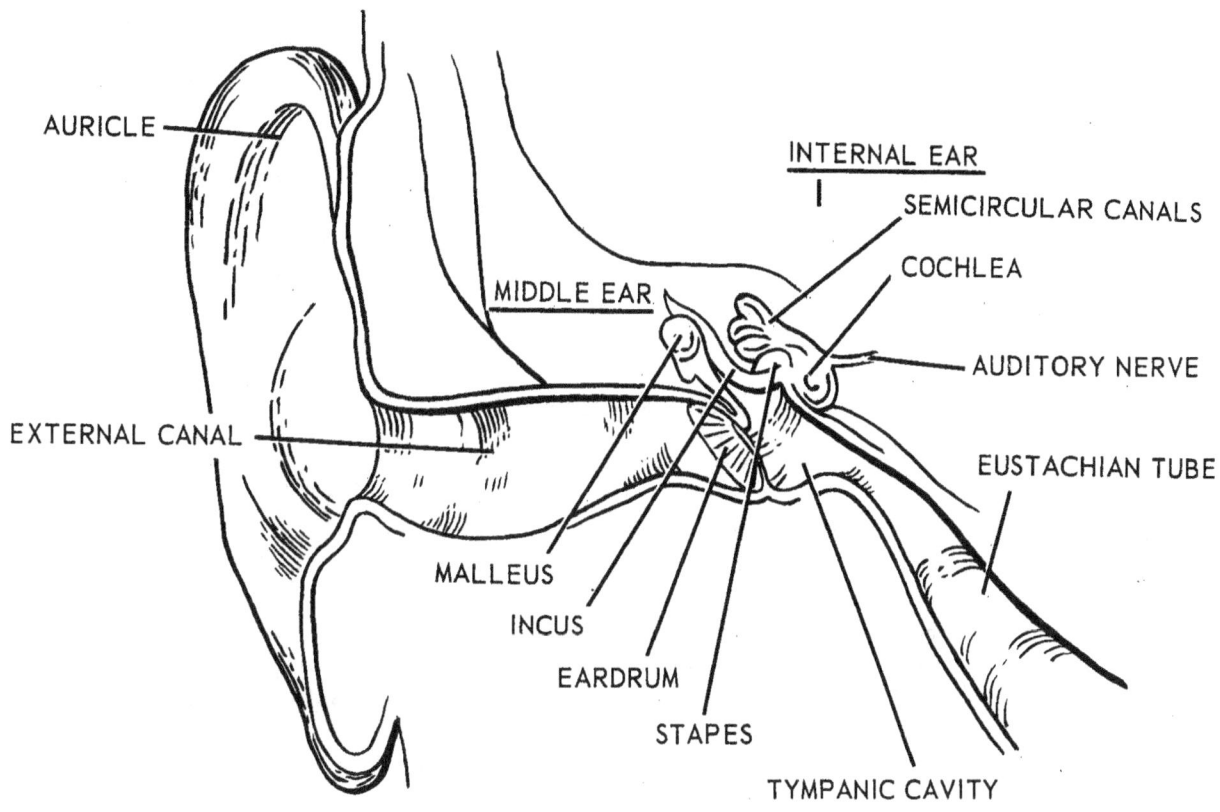

B  THE EXTERNAL, MIDDLE, AND INTERNAL EAR, FRONTAL VIEW

*Figure 2-32*—Continued

the anterior wall of the cartilaginous portion of the canal and are filled with fibrous membrane which allows for the flexibility of the canal. If the auricle (helix area) is pulled up and back, this portion of the canal straightens and may be examined or treated more easily. The entire passage is lined with skin. Near the entrance of the canal, the skin contains wax-producing glands and hair follicles. This wax, called cerumen, also helps to prevent the entry of foreign objects into the ear.

(2) The tympanic membrane, or eardrum, separates the inner end of the canal from the middle ear. The medical officer examines the external canal and the eardrum by means of a lighted instrument, an otoscope. The normal eardrum is translucent (partly transparent) and shiny gray (pearl-like). When inflamed, it appears pink or dull red.

c. The middle ear (tympanic cavity) is an irregular space in the temporal bone filled with air and containing the three ossicles of the ear: malleus (hammer), incus (anvil), and stapes (stirrup).

These bones conduct vibrations from the eardrum to the internal ear.

(1) The eustachian tube which connects the middle ear with the nasopharynx is about 1½ inches long. The trumpet-shaped opening of the eustachian tube into the pharynx remains closed except during the act of yawning or of swallowing, when it opens to admit air into the middle ear, thus performing its principal function of keeping the air pressure equal on either side of the eardrum. This is also an avenue of infection by which disease spreads from the throat to the middle ear.

(2) The roof or superior wall of the middle ear is composed of a very thin plate of bone which separates it from the dura. This bony plate is quite susceptible to fracture in head trauma and to spread of infection from the middle ear (otitis media), either of which can result in intracranial disease.

d. Internal ear (labyrinth). The internal ear contains receptors for hearing and equilibrium.

The receptor for hearing, the organ of Corti, lies within a structure called the cochlea which is coiled and resembles the shell of a snail.

(1) Sound waves, which pass through the external auditory canal, vibrate the eardrum and ossicles and are finally transmitted through the fluid of the inner ear. Nerve impulses travel through the acoustic (auditory) nerve from the organ of Corti to the auditory center of the cerebral cortex. The acoustic nerve is the final link in the chain of mechanisms which convey the sensation of sound to the brain for perception.

(2) The internal ear also contains three semicircular canals which control equilibrium. Change in the position of the head causes movement of the fluid within the canals and this fluid movement stimulates nerve endings in the wall of the canal. These nerve endings serve as receptors and transmit impulses along the acoustic nerve to the cerebellum.

## Section XI. THE ENDOCRINE SYSTEM

### 77. Components

The endocrine system is made up of glands classified as glands of internal secretion (ductless glands). These glands are located in different parts of the body (fig. 2-33). Secretions produced by endocrine glands are hormones, which are secreted directly into the circulating blood, reach every part of the body, and influence the activities of specific organs and tissues, as well as the activities of the body as a whole. Small in quantity but powerful in action, hormones are part of the body's chemical coordinating and regulating system. There are six recognized endocrine glands—the thyroid, parathyroid, adrenals, pituitary (hypophysis), the testes or ovaries (male or female gonads, the glands of sex), and the pancreas.

### 78. The Thyroid

The thyroid gland, located in front of the neck, has two lobes, one on either side of the larynx. The hormone produced by the thyroid is thyroxin. This hormone is associated with metabolism, regulating heat and energy production in body cells. Thyroid gland cells need a mineral, iodine, to manufacture thyroxin. Iodine is ordinarily obtained from foods included in normal diet; however, certain geographical areas have an iodine deficiency. In these areas, iodized table salt can be used to insure an adequate amount of iodine for normal thyroid function. (This use of iodized salt is an example of a preventive health measure.) Disorders of thyroid function include hyperthyroidism, which, when severe, causes a dangerous increase in the metabolic rate; and hypothyroidism, an opposite condition, which causes physical and mental sluggishness. An enlargement of the thyroid gland is called a goiter. When the enlargement is a nodular tumor, it is called an adenoma. During a physical examination, the doctor may

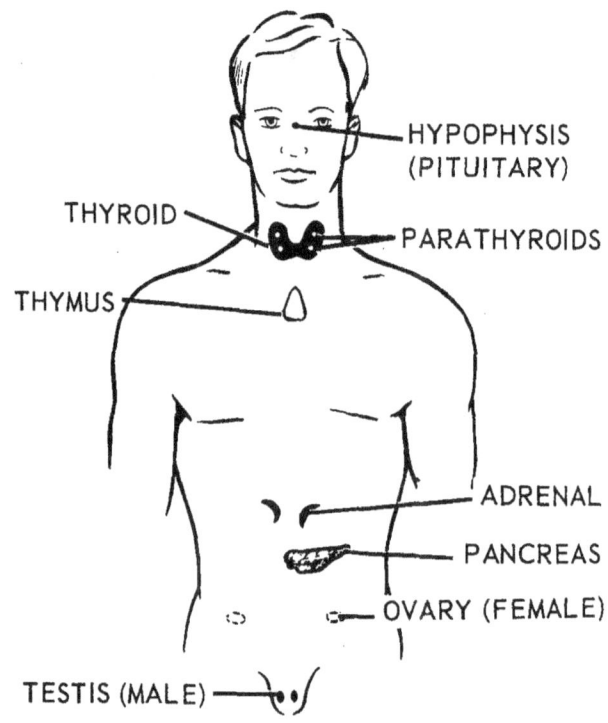

*Figure 2-33. Endocrine system.*

palpate the neck tissues to determine the size and consistency of thyroid tissue.

### 79. The Parathyroids

The parathyroid glands, usually four in number, are located on the posterior surfaces of the lobes of the thyroid gland. These glands produce the hormone, parathormone, which helps to regulate the amount of calcium in the blood. Calcium, normally stored in the bones, is released into the blood as required for normal nerve and muscle tissue function. When there is too little calcium in the blood, a type of muscle twitching called tetany develops. Because of the location of the parathyroid glands in relation to the thyroid, special observation for tetany may be required in the immediate postoperative period following thyroid surgery. Calcium is given by intravenous infusion to relieve the symptoms of tetany.

## 80. The Adrenal Glands

The two adrenal glands are located one above each kidney (suprarenal glands). Each adrenal gland actually functions as two separate glands, producing different hormones from its two parts, the medulla and the cortex. The medulla is the inner part of the adrenal gland. It produces epinephrine, the "fight or flight" hormone. The medulla is stimulated to produce epinephrine by the sympathetic branch of the autonomic nervous system in order to give the body the extra push it needs in responding to emergencies. The cortex, the outer part of the adrenal glands, produces a series of adrenocortical hormones, which include hydrocortisone. The adrenocortical hormones influence the salt and water balance of the body, the metabolism of foods, and the ability of the body to handle stress. The cortex of the adrenal glands requires stimulation by a hormone produced by the pituitary gland.

## 81. The Pituitary Gland

The pituitary gland, located deep within the skull, is also called the hypophysis. This small gland has two lobes, each producing distinctive hormones. The anterior lobe hormones stimulate other endocrine glands to produce their distinctive secretions; for this reason, the pituitary gland is called the master gland of the endocrine system. The four hormones produced by the anterior lobe of the pituitary have names with the suffix "trophic," meaning nourishing. Somatotrophic hormone (STH) means body nourishing. This hormone influences skeletal and soft tissue growth. Adrenocorticotrophic hormone (ACTH) stimulates the cortex of the adrenal gland to produce its cortisone-type hormones. Gonadotrophic hormone stimulates the normal development of the gonads, the testes or ovaries, and controls the development of the male and female reproductive systems. Thyrotrophic hormone stimulates the thyroid gland to produce its hormone. The posterior lobe of the pituitary gland produces a hormone that stimulates the contraction of the smooth muscle of the uterus, so it is important in childbirth. Another posterior lobe hormone which helps prevent excessive water excretion from the kidneys is called the antidiuretic hormone.

## 82. The Testes and Ovaries (the Gonads)

The male testes are located in the scrotum; the female ovaries, in the lower abdominal cavity. Hormones produced by these glands stimulate the development of sexual characteristics that normally appear at the development period called puberty (sexual maturity). They are responsible for the appearance of the secondary sexual characteristics: the pubic and axillary hair, the beard and the changing of the voice, and mammary (breast) development in the female. These hormones also help maintain the reproductive system organs in their adult state.

## 83. The Pancreas

Part of the pancreas functions as an accessory organ of the digestive system and part functions as an endocrine gland. Its endocrine gland function is carried out by groups of pancreas cells called the islands of Langerhans, which produce the hormone insulin. This hormone is necessary for the normal use of sugar by body cells. If insulin is not produced in sufficient amounts, the sugar normally present in the blood cannot be properly used by body cells, and the disease, diabetes mellitus, develops. A patient with diabetes mellitus requires continuous medical treatment—a combination of diet modification, education in modified living habits, and special medication as needed. As a medication, insulin must be given by hypodermic injection, because it is destroyed by digestive juices when taken by mouth. However, some patients requiring medication for diabetes mellitus can be treated with oral medications which are NOT insulin but which apparently stimulate underfunctioning pancreatic cells to produce insulin. An example of such a medication is tolbutamide (orinase). Other types of oral medication (such as phenformin) for diabetes promote the utilization of glucose by muscle tissue instead of stimulating underfunctioning pancreatic cells.

## Section XII. THE REPRODUCTIVE SYSTEM

### 84. General

The male and female reproductive systems have their own specialized internal and external organs, passageways, and supportive structures. The parts and functions of these systems are designed to make the process of fertilization possible. The female cell, the ovum, must be fertilized by the male cell, the spermatozoa. The normal result of fertilization is reproduction. (Pregnancy and childbirth will be discussed in chapter 7.)

### 85. The Male Reproductive System

The major parts of the male reproductive system (fig. 2–34) are the scrotum, testis, epididymis, ductus deferens (also referred to as vas deferens or seminal duct), seminal vesicles, ejaculatory ducts, prostate gland, urethra, and penis. The penis, testes, and scrotum are referred to as external genitalia.

*a. The Scrotum, the Testes, and the Epididymis.* There are two testes, one on each side of the septum of the scrotum. A testis is an oval-shaped gland, about 1½ to 2 inches in length, which produces the male germ cells, spermatozoa (or sperm), and the male hormone, testosterone. Sperm are produced in great numbers, starting at the age of puberty. Although microscopic in size, each sperm has a head, which contains the cell nucleus, and an elongated tail for movement.

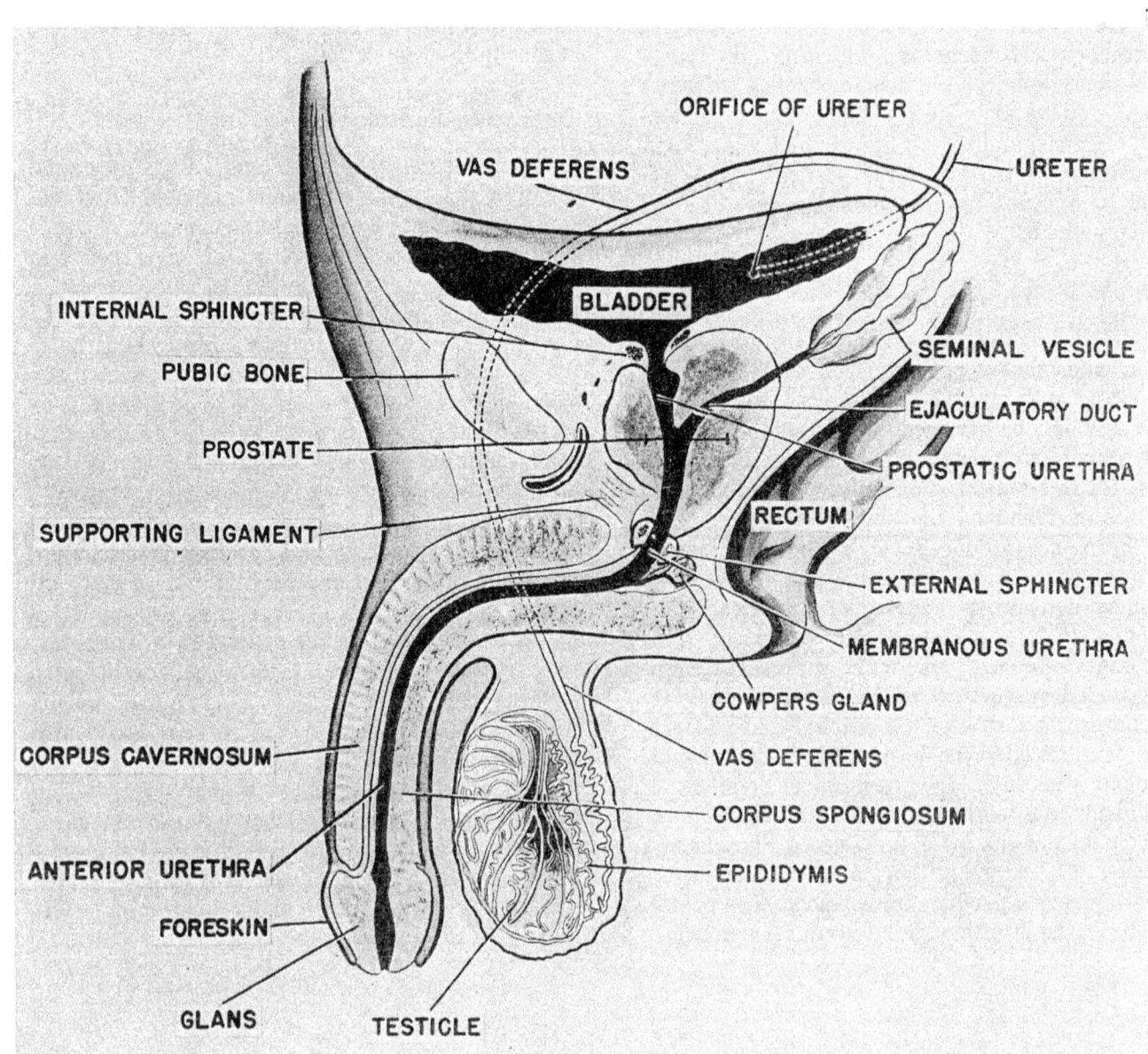

*Figure 2–34. Male urogenital system.*

Sperm travels from the testis to the tightly coiled tube, the epididymis. A continuation of the epididymis is the ductus deferens (or vas deferens) (fig. 2-35).

b. *The Ductus Deferens.* This duct carries sperm from the scrotum to the pelvic cavity. As the duct leaves the scrotum, it passes through the inguinal canal into the pelvic cavity as part of the spermatic cord. Spermatic cords, one in each groin, are supporting structures. Each ductus deferens curves around the bladder and delivers the sperm to one of two storage pouches, called the seminal vesicles.

c. *The Seminal Vesicles and Ejaculatory Ducts.* The seminal vesicles are located behind the bladder. During the storage of sperm in these vesicles, secretions are added to them to keep them alive and motile. The secretions and the sperm form the seminal fluid, or semen. Ejaculatory ducts carry the seminal fluid from the seminal vesicles, through the prostate gland, to the urethra.

d. *The Prostate Gland.* This gland is located around the urethra at the neck of the bladder (fig. 2-35). Prostatic secretions are added to the seminal fluid to protect it from urethral secretions and female vaginal secretions. When the prostate gland becomes enlarged (hypertrophied), it can seriously constrict the urethra. The size and consistency of the prostate gland is determined by the doctor by means of a rectal examination.

e. *The Urethra and the Penis.* The urethra, a passageway for seminal fluid and for urine, has its longest segment in the penis. Several glands add secretions to the urethra, the largest being two bulbo-urethral (or Cowper's) glands (fig. 2-35). The terminal opening of the urethra is in the glans penis, which is surrounded by a retractable fold of skin called the foreskin, or prepuce. Surgical removal of the foreskin is circumcision, which is performed to reduce the possibility of an abnormal constriction of the glans, called phimosis, or to reduce the possibility of irritation from secretions that accumulate under the foreskin. The penis has spongy tissues which become distended from a greatly increased blood supply during penile erection.

## 86. The Female Reproductive System

The major parts of the female reproductive system (fig. 2-36) are the ovaries; fallopian tubes; uterus; vagina; and the external genitalia, the vulva. The supportive structures for the internal reproductive organs are a complicated arrangement of pelvic ligaments, which are formed in part, from folds of peritoneum that line the abdomino-pelvic cavity.

a. *The Ovaries.* These are described as two almond-shaped glands (fig. 2-37), one on either side of the abdomino-pelvic cavity. They produce female germ cells, ova, and female hormones, estrogen and progesterone. These hormones maintain

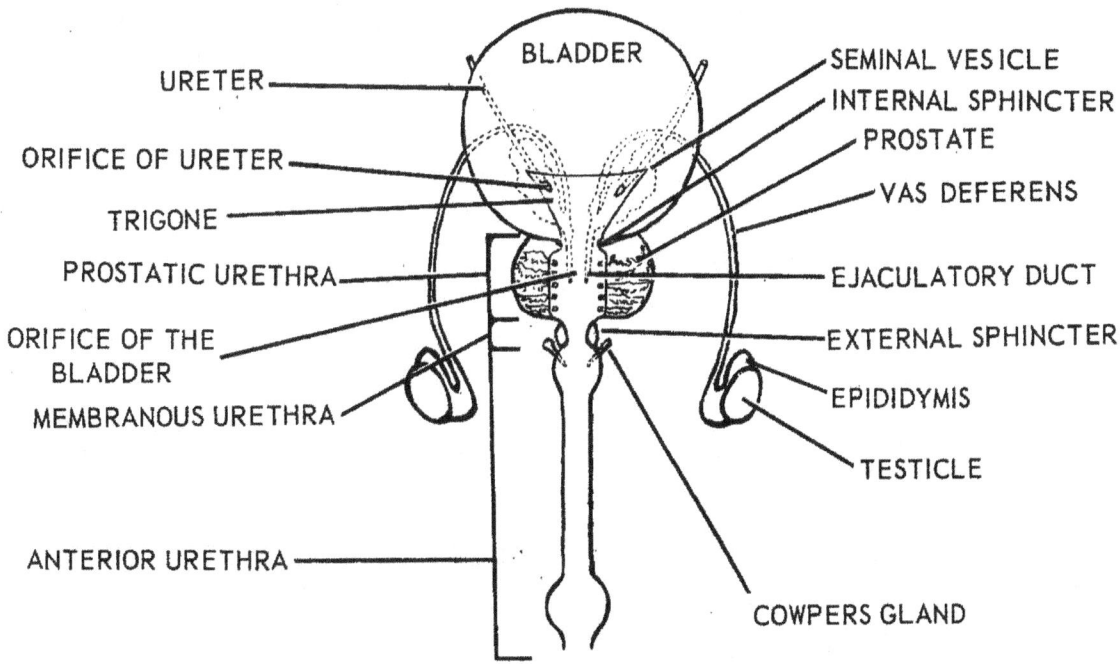

*Figure 2-35. Diagram of male reproductive system.*

the normal menstrual cycle An ovum is expelled from the surface of an ovary in a process called ovulation, which occurs about halfway between each menstrual period. An expelled ovum is picked up by the free end of a fallopian tube for transportation to the uterus.

  b. *Fallopian Tubes.* There are two fallopian tubes (oviducts) each curving outward from the upper part of the uterus. About four inches in length, each tube has a free end which curves around, but is not attached to, an ovary. The fringed surface of the free end of the fallopian tube carries an expelled ovum into the tube, and the ovum moves slowly on its way to the uterus. If fertilization takes place, it normally occurs as the ovum moves through a tube. The male germ cell, the sperm, must therefore travel up the female reproductive tract in order to unite with the female germ cell, the ovum. Of the millions of sperm produced, only one must unite with one ovum for fertilization to occur.

  c. *The Uterus.* The uterus, shaped somewhat like a pear, is suspended in the pelvic cavity, supported between the bladder and the rectum by its system of eight ligaments. The normal position of the body of the uterus is anteflexion (bent for-

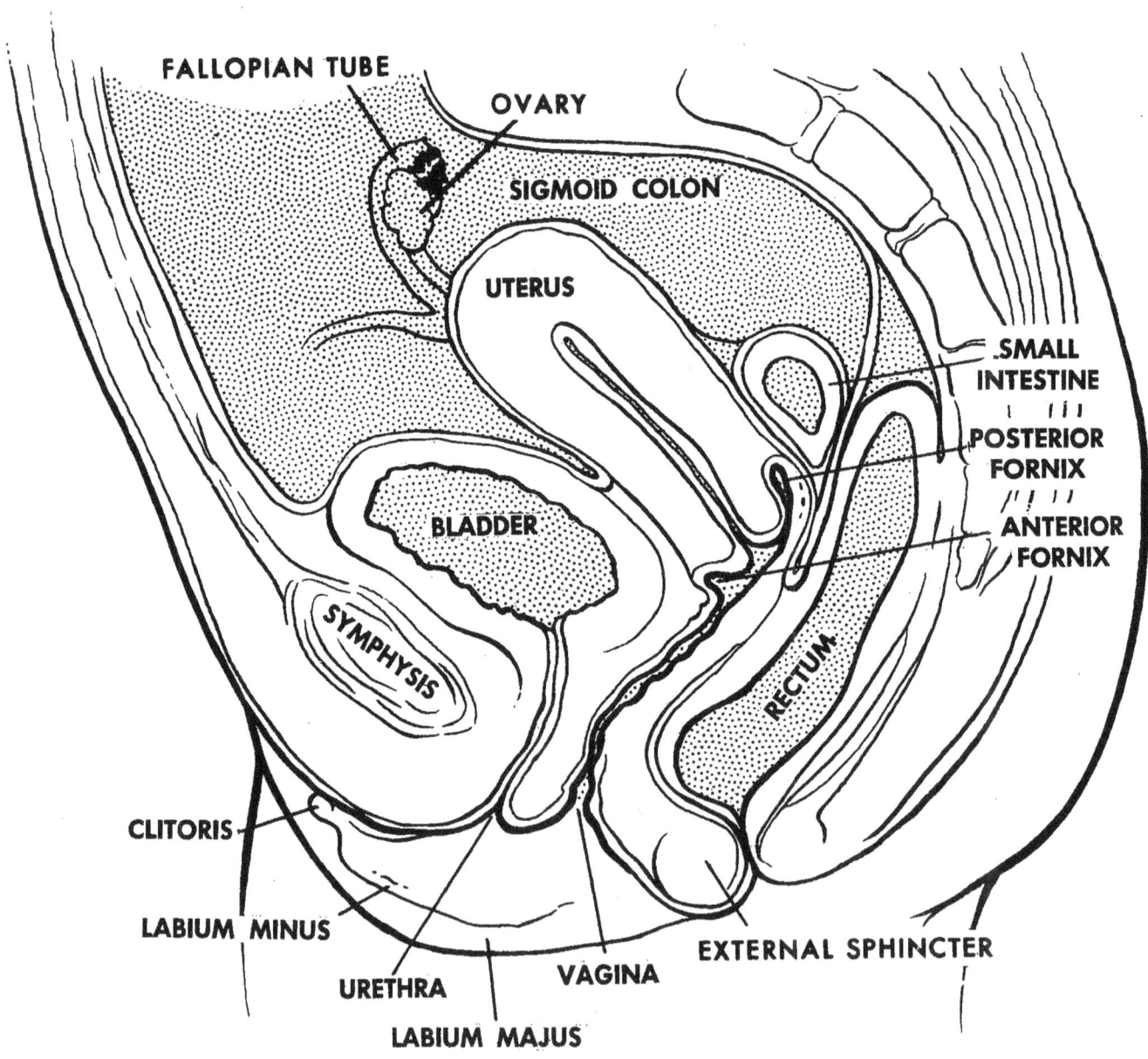

Figure 2-36. *Female urogenital system.*

ward over the bladder) (fig. 2-36). The uterus is about three inches long and three inches thick at its widest part. It has a thick wall of smooth muscle and a relatively small inner cavity. During pregnancy, it can increase about 20 times in size. The upper dome-shaped portion of the uterus is the fundus, the main part is the body, and the lower neck portion is the cervix (fig. 2-37). The cervix is a canal opening into the vagina. The inner lining of the uterus, the endometrium, undergoes periodic changes during the regular menstrual cycle, to make the uterus ready to receive a fertilized ovum. If the ovum is not fertilized, the endometrium gets a message from hormone influences and sheds its surface cells and built-up secretions. Some of the extra blood supply, the surface cells, and uterine secretions are eliminated as menstrual flow.

*d. The Vagina.* This muscular canal extends from the cervix of the uterus to the vaginal opening in the vestibule of the vulva. The vaginal canal is capable of stretching widely and serves as the birth canal. Part of the cervix protrudes into the uppermost portion of the vagina. An important part of a female pelvic examination is the physical examination of the visible surface of the cervix and vagina, plus a laboratory examination of cervical and vaginal secretions. A Pap (Papanicolaou) smear is made by obtaining these secretions for laboratory examination.

*e. The Vulva.* The several structures that make up the female external genitalia form the vulva. These are the mons pubis, the labia, the clitoris, and the vestibule. The labia, two parallel sets of liplike tissues, are the labia majora, the larger outer folds of tissue, and the labia minora, the smaller inner folds. The clitoris is located at the upper meeting point of the labia majora and the labia minora. Between the labia minora is the vestibule, a shallow depression into which the urethra and the vagina open. The urethral opening is above the vaginal opening. A series of glands, which can become infected, open into the vestibule, the largest being the Bartholin glands at the vaginal opening.

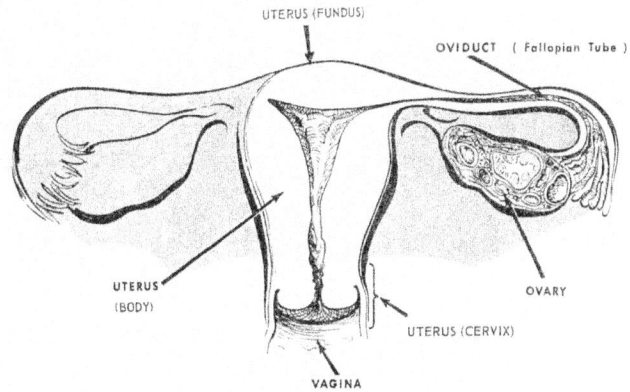

**Internal Organs - Female Reproductive System**

*Figure 2-37. Female reproductive organs (frontal section).*

### 87. Menstruation

In preparing to receive the ovum, the mucous lining (mucosa) of the uterus becomes soft and swollen and uterine blood vessels are dilated. If the ovum is not fertilized, the unneeded blood and mucosa are expelled from the uterus through the vagina. This process, called menstruation, begins at puberty and is repeated, except when interrupted by disease or pregnancy, about every 28 days until the age of 40 to 50 years.

# SKELETAL ANATOMY

# A TABLE OF THE BONES

## Contents

|  | Page |
|---|---|
| Head | 1 |
| Face | 1 |
| Ear | 2 |
| Neck | 2 |
| Vertebrae | 2 |
| Upper Extremities | 3 |
| Lower Extremities | 4 |

# SKELETAL ANATOMY

# A TABLE OF THE BONES

| NAME | PRINCIPAL FEATURES | ARTICULATION |
|---|---|---|
| **HEAD** | | |
| OCCIPITAL (1) | Back part and base of cranium. | Parietal (2): Temporal (2) Sphenoid: Atlas. |
| PARIETAL (2) | Form sides and roof of skull. | Opposite Parietal; Occipital; Frontal; Temporal; Sphenoid |
| FRONTAL (1) | The forehead bone; and enters into formation of the orbits and nasal cavity. | Parietal (2); Sphenoid; Ethnoid; Nasal (2); Maxillary (2); Lacrimal (2); Malar (2) |
| TEMPORAL (2) | Situated at side and base of skull | Occipital; Parietal; Sphenoid; Inferior maxillary; Malar |
| SPHENOID (1) | Anterior part of base of skull, and binds the other cranial bones together. | All the cranial bones; Malar (2); Palate (2); Vomer |
| ETHMOID (1) | Forms part of the orbits, nasal fossae, and base of cranium. | Sphenoid; Frontal; Nasal (2); Maxillary (2); Lacrimal (2); Vomer; Palate (2) |
| **FACE** | | |
| NASAL (2) | Form the bridge of the nose | Frontal; Ethmoid; opposite Nasal; Maxillary. |
| MALAR (2) | The cheek bones; form the prominence of the cheek; and part of the outer wall and floor of the orbit. | Frontal; Sphenoid; Temporal; Maxillary. |
| MAXILLA (2) | The upper jaw bones; assist in forming part of the floor of the orbit; the floor and outer wall of the nasal fossae; and the greater part of the roof of the mouth. | Frontal; Ethmoid; Nasal; Malar; Lacrimal; Palate; Vomer; opposite Maxilla |
| MANDIBLE | The lower jaw bones; serves for the reception of the lower teeth. | Temporal |
| LACRIMAL (2) | Situated at the front part of the inner wall of the orbit. Contain part of the canal through which the tear duct runs. | Frontal; Ethmoid; Maxillary; Inferior Turbinated |

| | | |
|---|---|---|
| VOMER | Situated at the lower and back part of the nasal cavity; forms part of the central septum of the nose. | Sphenoid; Ethmoid; Maxillary (2); Palate (2); Septal Cartilage |
| PALATE (2) | Back part of nasal cavity; help to form floor and outer wall of nose, the roof of the mouth, and floor of the orbit. | Sphenoid, Ethmoid, Maxillary; Vomer; opposite Palate |
| INFERIOR TURBINATED | Situated in the nostril, on the outer wall of each side. | Ethmoid; Maxilla, Lacrimal; Palate |
| **EAR**<br>MALLEUS (2)<br>INCUS (2)<br>STAPES (2) | | |
| **NECK**<br>HYOID | An isolated U-shaped Bone lying in front of throat; supports the tongue. | None |
| **VERTEBRAE**<br>CERVICAL (7)<br><br>THORACIC or DORSAL (12)<br>LUMBAR (5)<br>SACRAL (5)<br>COCCYGEAL (4) | Each vertebra consists of two essential parts, — a ventral solid portion or body, and a dorsal portion or arch. Each arch has seven processes:- 4 articular (2 to connect with bone above, and 2 to connect with bone below); 2 transverse, one at each side; and one spinous process, projecting backwards | 1. The 1st cervical vertebra, the Atlas, articulates with the occiput, supports the head.<br>2. The 2nd cervical vertebra, the Axis, acts as a pivot for rotating the head.<br>3. The different vertebrae are connected by (a) the articular processes; (b) by discs of intervertebral fibrocartilage (containing nuclear material) placed between the vertebral bodies; and (c) by broad thin ligaments called the "ligamenta flava" which connect the transverse processes.<br>4. The dorsal vertebrae articulate with the ribs.<br>5. The sacral vertebrae articulate with the ilium of the pelvis. |

| | | |
|---|---|---|
| RIBS<br>(12 each side) | Situated 12 on each side of thoracic cavity. The first 7 pairs are "true" ribs. The 8th, 9th, and 10th pairs are attached in front to the costal cartilages of the next rib above. The 2 lowest pairs are unattached in front and are termed "floating" ribs. | All 12 pairs are attached in back to the dorsal vertebrae. The first 7 pairs (true ribs) are connected with the Sternum in front through the costal cartilages. |
| STERNUM | The breastbone, situated in the median line, in front of chest. The upper part is the "manubrium", the middle and largest section is the "gladiolus" and the lowest portion is the "uniform" or "xiphoid" process. | Clavicles (2) through clavicular notches of manubrium; first 7 pairs of ribs. |
| **UPPER EXTREMITIES**<br>CLAVICLE | Collar bone, situated horizontally above the thorax | Sternum; Scapula through clavicular facet; cartilage of 1st rib. |
| SCAPULA | Shoulder blade, situated between 2nd and 8th ribs on back part of thorax. | Clavicle, through acromial process of scapula; Humerus, through glenoid cavity. |
| HUMERUS | Upper-arm bone. Upper end consists of a rounded "head" joined to the shaft by a constricted "neck", and of two eminences, called the "greater" and "lesser Tuberosities". Lower end consists of a broad articular surface called the "trochlea" which is divided by a ridge into the internal and external condyles. | The "head" articulates with glenoid cavity of scapula.<br><br>The external and internal condyles and trochlea articulate with the radius and ulna. |
| ULNA | Occupies the inner (little finger) side of forearm. Upper end consists of two larger curved processes and two concave cavities. The larger process is the "olecranon process"; the smaller, the "coronoid process." Between these processes is the "greater sigmoid" cavity. On the outer side of the coronoid is the "lesser sigmoid" cavity. The lower end of the ulna ends in two prominences, — an outer, or "head" and an inner, "styloid process". | The greater sigmoid cavity articulates with the trochlea of the humerus. The lesser sigmoid cavity receives the head of the radius. The lower head of the ulna articulates with the lower end of the radius. The styloid process serves for the attachment of ligaments from the wrist. The ulna does not articulate with the wrist bones. |
| RADIUS | Occupies the outer (thumb) side of forearm. Upper end contains a disc-shaped "head" which is shallowly depressed for articulation with the humerus, and has a prominent ridge about it, like the head of a nail, by means | See under "Principal Features" for articulation. |

| | | |
|---|---|---|
| | of which it rotates within the lesser sigmoid cavity of the ulna. Lower end widens out on bottom to a styloid process and two smooth portions which articulate with the semilunar and scaphoid bones of the carpus. | |
| CARPUS (8 each hand) | The wrist bones. Are arranged in two rows; 1st row (proximal); scaphoid (or navicular), cuneiform, pisiform, semilunar; -2nd row (distal); trapizium, trapezoid, os magnum, unciform. | 1st row articulates with radius, through scaphoid and semilunar bones. 2nd row articulates with metacarpal bones. |
| METACARPUS (5 each side) | The bones of the palm, one in line with each finger. | At their bases with each other, and with the 2nd row of carpal bones. At their heads, with the first row of phalanges. |
| PHALANGES | The bones of the fingers, three for each finger, and two for the thumb. | The proximal row articulates with the metacarpals, and with the second row, etc. |
| **LOWER EXTREMITIES** | | |
| HIP BONE PELVIS | The two hip bones together form the sides and front wall of the pelvic cavity. Each bone has three separate parts, which unite in the adult. These parts are the "ilium", which forms the prominence of the hip, the "ischium" and the "pubis." Where these bones meet and finally unite is a deep socket, the "Acetabulum", into which the head of the femur fits. Both hip bones join at the inner margins of each pubis to form the "symphasis pubis." The sacrum articulates on either side with the inner margins of each ilium to form the "sacroiliac" joints. | Femur through glenoid cavity, Sacrum through sacroiliac joint. |
| FEMUR | The thigh bone. Upper end consists of a rounded head, joined to the shaft by a constricted neck, and of two eminences, the "greater" and "lesser trochanters." The lower end is divided into two large eminences, the "medial" and "external condyles", separated by an intervening notch. | "Head" articulates with the glenoid cavity of the hip bone; Patella; Tibia, through the medial and lateral semi-lunar cartilages. |
| PATELLA | The knee cap. | Articulates with the two condyles of the femur. |

| | | |
|---|---|---|
| TIBIA | The shin bone, situated at the front and medial side of the leg. Upper end is large and expanded into two eminences with concave surfaces, which receive the condyles of the femur. The lower end is prolonged downward into a process called the "medial malleolus". | Articulates with the condyles of the femur, and on the lower end with the fibula and the astragalus of the tarsus. |
| FIBULA | Situated at outer side of leg, running parallel to tibia. Upper end has a "head" which articulates with tibia. The lower end is prolonged downward into a pointed process, the "lateral" or "external malleolus". | Articulates with the tibia above and below, and with the astragalus of the tarsus. |
| TARSUS (7 each foot) | The ankle bones. Consists of the Calcaneum or Os Calcis (heel bone); Astragalus; Cuboid; Scaphoid; External Cuneiform; Internal Cuneiform; and middle Cuneiform. | Astragalus articulates with Tibia and fibula. Also articulates with metatarsal bones. |
| METATARSUS (5 each side) | The sole or instep bones, one in line with each toe. | With the tarsal bones on one end, and the first row of toe phalanges on the other. |
| PHALANGES | The bones of the toes; three for each toe, and two for the great toe. | The proximal row articulates with the metatarsals, and with the second row, etc. |

# GLOSSARY OF ANATOMIC SCIENCES

## CONTENTS

| | Page |
|---|---|
| Achilles Tendon ............... Concha | 1 |
| Costal...............................Iliacus | 2 |
| Iliocostal............................ Pubis | 3 |
| Radius.......................... Zygoma | 4 |

# GLOSSARY OF ANATOMIC SCIENCES

**ACHILLES TENDON**
The tendon which attaches to the heel and originates from the muscles in the calf (gastrocnemius and soleus muscles).
**ANCONEUS**
This muscle extends from humerus in upper forearm to ulna in forearm. Its function is to straighten the elbow joint.
**ARYEPIGLOTTIC**
From the arytenoid cartilage to the epiglottis (the structure which closes the windpipe when swallowing). Its function is to close entrance to larynx.
**ARYTENOID**
From one arytenoid cartilage to other, its function is to close the larynx.
**ASTRAGALUS**
Located just below tibia and fibula (leg bones) in ankle. It connects with the heel bone.
**ATLAS**
First vertebra lying just beneath the skull.
**AXIS**
Second vertebra in neck, just below Atlas.

### B

**BRACHIALIS**
Extends from upper and lower jaw bones too muscles about the mouth. Its function is to pull back angles of the mouth and tighten the cheeks.
**BULBO-CAVERNOSUS**
Extends from perineum (a point below the genitals) to penis. Its function is to compress urethra.

### C

**CALCANEUS**
Heel bone.
**CALVARIUM**
Bones which form top of skull.
**CAPITATE**
Largest bone in wrist, located toward center of wrist joint.
**CARPAL**
Eight small bones of wrist greater multangular, lesser multangular, lunate, capitate, hamate, navicular, triquetrum, and pisiform bones.
**CILIARY**
Extends from membrane around iris to ciliary process of iris in the eye. Its function is to open and close the pupil of the eye.
**CLAVICLE**
Collarbone extending from sternum (breastbone) to shoulder tip.
**COCCYX**
Tailbone, the last vertebrae at base of spine.
**CONCHA**
Shell-shaped small bone located along the outer side of the nasal cavity.

**COSTAL**
Ribs; 12 bones on each side, arising from the spinal column.
**COXAE**
Hipbone; joins with sacrum and other hipbone to form the bon pelvis. The Coxae is composed of 3 fused bones: ilium, ischium, and pubis.
**CRICOARYTENOID**
From cricoid cartilages to arytenoid cartilages in the neck. It function is to open and close the vocal chords.
**CUROID**
Cube-shaped small bone of foot.

## D

**DELTOID**
Extends from the collarbone and the scapula, over the shoulder, to the humerus in the upper arm. Its function is to lift the upper arm away from the body.

## E

**ETHMOID**
Small bone located in front of base of skull, forming part of orbit and nose. Within it are spaces, making up the ethmoid sinuses.
**EXTENSOR CARPI RADIALIS**
From humerus to bones of wrist. Its function is to straighten the wrist.

## F

**FEMUR**
The thighbone, extending from hip to knee.
**FIBULA**
Outer bone of leg, extending from knee to ankle
**FLEXOR CARPI RADIALIS**
Extends from humerus to bones in front of the wrist. Its function is to bend the wrist.
**FRONTAL**
Bones of forehead, parts of orbit and nose.

## G

**GASTROCNEMIUS**
Extends down leg from femur to heel bone. Its function is to bend ankle in downward direction and to help flex knee.

## H

**HAMSTRING**
Three large muscles extending down back of the thigh from ischium to tibia below the knee. Its function is to flex the knee joint.
**HUMERUS**
Arm bone, extending from shoulder to elbow.
**HYOID**
Thin U-shaped bone beneath the chin and above the larynx.

**ILIACUS**
Extends from pelvis bones to femur in the thigh. Its function is to flex hip joint.

**ILIOCOSTAL**
From ribs to vertebral column. Its function is to straighten spinal column and bend trunk sideways.
**ILLIUM**
Part of hipbone, into which the femur fits.
**INCUS**
The anvil. One of 3 small bones of middle ear, adjacent to eardrum.
**ISCHIUM**
Part of hipbone

## L

**LONGISSIMUS**
Extends up back near spine. Its function is to straighten spine. LONGUS CAPITIS
Extends from vertebrae in neck to base of the skull. Its function is to flex the head.

## M

**MALAR**
Cheekbone; the zygoma.
**MALLEUS**
The hammer. One of 3 small bones of middle ear; adjacent to eardrum.
**MANDIBLE**
Jawbone. Attached to the skull at the temperanandibular joint in front of the ear.
**MASSETER**
Extends from cheekbone to the lower jawbone. Its function is to close the mouth.
**MAXILLA**
Upper jawbone. Makes up part of the face, orbit, nose, etc.
**METACARPAL**
The 5 bones of the hand to which the finger bones are attached.
**METATARSAL**
The 5 bones of the foot to which the toe bones are attached.

## N

**NASALIS**
Maxillary bone of face to bridge. Alters expression of face.
**NAVICULAR**
Small bones of the hands and feet; shaped like a boat.

## O

**OBTURATOR**
Extends from bones of pubis to femur (thighbone). Rotates thigh outward.
**OCCIPITAL**
The back and part of base of the skull.

## P

**PALMARIS**
Extends down front of forearm to palm of the hand. Helps to flex the wrist and make "hollow of the hand."
**PARIETAL**
This bone makes up part of the side and top of the skull.
**PATELLA**
The kneecap.
**PELVIS**
The bony pelvis is made up of the hipbones, sacrum, and coccyx.
**PHALANGES**
The bones of the fingers and toes.
**PUBIS**
The bone in front of the pelvis.

## R

**RADIUS**
Long bone on outer side of the forearm, extending from elbow to wrist.

## S

**SACRUM**
Five fused vertebrae in lower back which make up the back part of the bony pelvis.

**SCALENE**
Extends from vertebra in the neck to the first and second ribs. Bends the head and neck sideways.

**SCAPULA**
The shoulder blade (wing bone).

**SPHENOID**
Irregularly shaped bone making up front portion of the base of the skull and parts of the orbit and nose.

**SPLENIUS**
Extends from the vertebrae in the chest and the neck to back of the head. Straightens the head and spine.

**STAPES**
The stirrup. One of 3 small bones of middle ear adjacent to the eardrum.

**STERNUM**
The breastbone.

## T

**TALUS**
The same as the astragalus.

**TARSAL**
The same as the foot bones.

**TEMPORAL**
The bone forming front portion of the side of the skull and part of the base. Extends from temple to lower jaw. Closes the mouth.

**TIBIA**
The large inner bone of the leg, extending from knee to the ankle (It is responsible for weight bearing.)

**TURBINATE**
Three bones located on the outer side of the nasal cavity.

## U

**ULNA**
The long bone on the inner side of the forearm, extending from the elbow to the wrist.

## V

**VASTUS**
It extends down the entire front of the thigh to the kneecap and tibia in the leg its function is to straighten the knee.

**VOMER**
This bone forms the back segment of the nasal septum which separates the two side of the nose

## Z

**ZYGOMA**
The cheekbone; the malar bone.

# Glossary of Dietary Terms

## CONTENTS

| | Page |
|---|---|
| Absorption ................................................................. Available | 1 |
| Avidin ............................................................................ Carbohydrate | 2 |
| Carob powder .............................................................. Denaturation | 3 |
| Dixtrin ........................................................................... Exchange list | 4 |
| Excipient ...................................................................... Hyperkalemia | 5 |
| Hyperlipoproteinemia ................................................. Lactose intolerance | 6 |
| Lecithin ........................................................................ Mineral oil | 7 |
| Monosaccharides ........................................................ Pasteurized | 8 |
| Pellagra ....................................................................... Saccharin | 9 |
| Salt .............................................................................. Urea | 10 |
| Uremia ......................................................................... Zinc | 11 |

# Glossary of Dietary Terms

**Absorption.** Assimilation or taking up of nutrients, fluids, gases, or other substances by the stomach or intestinal walls following digestion.

**Acetone (dimethyl ketone).** Product of incomplete oxidation of fats. May occur in diabetes mellitus, giving a fruity odor to the breath.

**Acid-forming foods.** Foods in which the acidic residue exceeds the alkaline residue.

**Acidosis.** An abnormal increase of acids in the blood caused by accumulation of an excess of acids in the body or by excessive loss of base; characterized by a fall in the pH of the blood or decrease in the alkali reserve in the body. Examples of acidosis include the ketosis (of diabetes mellitus), phosphoric, sulfuric, and hydrochloric acids (of renal insufficiency), lactic acid (or prolonged exercise), and carbonic acid (in respiratory disease).

**ADA.** Abbreviation for the American Dietetic Association, American Diabetes Association, and American Dental Association.

**Adipose.** Fat or fatty.

**Alcohol.** Ethanol. Ethyl alcohol. Distilled from the products of anaerobic fermentation of carbohydrate. An ingredient in a variety of beverages including beer, wine, liqueurs, cordials, and mixed or straight drinks. Pure alcohol itself yields about seven Calories per gram, of which more than 75 percent is available to the body.

**Alkaline-forming foods.** Foods in which the alkaline residue exceeds the acidic residue.

**Alkalosis.** An excess of base in the body, commonly resulting from persistent vomiting, excessive sodium bicarbonate intake, or hyperventilation. An abnormal condition of elevated blood pH caused by excessive loss of acids from the body without comparable loss of base or more supply of base than can be neutralized or eliminated.

**Allergen.** Any agent or substance (usually protein) capable of producing an allergic reaction.

**Amino acid (AA).** Chief components of proteins. Each amino acid molecule contains one or more amino group ($-NH_2$) and carboxyl group ($-COOH$). Amino acids may be acid, basic, or neutral.

**Anabolism.** Process of building simple substances into more complex substances.

**Anemia.** Deficiency in the circulating hemoglobin, red blood cells, or packed cell volume resulting in decreased capacity of the blood to carry oxygen. Macrocytic (large cell size) anemias may result from folacin and $B_{12}$ deficiencies. Microcytic (small cell size), hypochromic (low color index) anemia may result from iron deficiency. Iron, protein, folic acid, vitamin $B_{12}$, and vitamin C are the major nutrients essential in blood formation.

**Anorexia.** Lack or loss of appetite for food.

**Antibiotic.** A substance that destroys or inhibits the growth of bacteria and other micro-organisms.

**Antioxidant.** A substance which delays or prevents oxidation.

**Antivitamin.** A substance which may inactivate or destroy a vitamin.

**Anuria.** Suppression or absence of urinary excretion.

**Apatite.** Complex calcium phosphate salt giving strength to bones.

**Appetite.** Natural desire or craving for food.

**Arteriosclerosis.** Hardening, thickening, and loss of elasticity of the inner walls of arteries and capillaries.

**Artificial sweeteners.** See saccharin, sorbitol, mannitol, and cyclamate.

**Ascorbic acid.** Reduced form of vitamin C; water soluble vitamin; prevents scurvy.

**Ash.** Mineral residue remaining after burning or oxidizing all organic matter.

**As Purchased (AP).** The weight of food before removing or trimming inedible parts.

**Atherosclerosis.** A fatty degeneration of the blood vessels and connective tissue of arterial walls. A kind of arteriosclerosis. The fatty deposits, including cholesterol, phospholipids, triglycerides, and other substances, decrease the internal channel size of the blood vessel.

**Atony.** Lack of normal tone or strength.

**Atrophy.** A wasting away of the cell, tissue, or organ.

**Available.** A nutrient that is in a form readily

absorbed by the digestive tract and usable by the body.

**Avidin.** A protein in raw egg white which binds with the B vitamin, biotin, and prevents its absorption from the digestive tract. Cooking inactivates avidin.

**Avitaminosis.** A condition due to inadequate vitamin intake or absorption, increased body require. ment, or antivitamins.

**Azotemia uremia.** Retention of urea or other nitrogenous substances in the urine.

**Balance study.** Quantitative method of measuring amount of a nutrient ingested and excreted to determine retention (positive balance) or loss (negative balance).

**Basal metabolism.** Energy expended at complete physical and mental rest (12-to-16 hours after food ingestion and in thermally neutral temperature). Includes energy for respiration, circulation, gastrointestinal contractions, muscle tone, body temperature, and organ function. Basal metabolic rate (BMR) for an adult is approximately one Calorie per kilogram body weight per hour.

**Beikost.** Foods other than milk or formula.

**Beriberi.** Nutritional deficiency of thiamin (vitamin $B_1$) resulting in loss of appetite, general weakness, progressive edema, polyneuritis, and enlarged heart.

**Bile.** A fluid produced in the liver, stored, and concentrated in the gallbladder, and emptied into the duodenum to aid in digestion of fat.

**Biological value (BV).** The efficiency of food protein in supplying amino acids in the proper amounts for protein synthesis in the body. For example, meat has a high biological value (HBV) and beans have a low value. The Thomas-Mitchell equation for calculating BV follows:

$$\%BV = 100\% \times \frac{N\ intake - [(FN - MN) + (UN - EN)]}{N\ intake - (FN - MN)}$$

where N = nitrogen, FN = fecal nitrogen, MN = metabolic nitrogen, UN = urinary nitrogen, and EN = endogenous nitrogen.

**Biotin.** A member of the water-soluble vitamin B complex; aids in fixation of carbon dioxide in fatty acid synthesis. Widely distributed in foodstuffs and synthesized by intestinal bacteria. Deficiency may be induced by large amount of avidin, causing scaly dermatitis, muscle pains, general malaise, and depression.

**Bland.** Any food that is not irritating to the gastric mucosa.

**Blood lipids.** Primarily cholesterol, phospholipid, and triglyceride which are bound to protein and circulate in the plasma.

**Blood sugar level (BSL).** The level of glucose (blood sugar) per 100 ml blood.

**Bowel.** The intestines.

**Bran.** The outer layer of whole grain. It contains iron, phosphorus, B vitamins, and fiber. Fiber absorbs water, softens and increases the bulk of stools, and facilitates elimination.

**Brat diet.** Diet consisting of banana, rice, applesauce, and toast; prescribed for diarrhea, especially for infants and children.

**Bulk.** The indigestible portion of carbohydrates which cannot he hydrolyzed by gastrointestinal enzymes.

**Bulking agent.** A metabolically inert substance which increases food volume without increasing calories.

**BUN.** Blood urea nitrogen.

**Caffeine.** An alkaloidal purine in coffee, tea, and cola drinks. A cardiac and renal stimulant which produces varying pharmacologic responses.

**Calciferol.** Vitamin $D_2$. A fat soluble vitamin produced by ergosterol irradiation. Prevents rickets.

**Calcium.** A major mineral, essential in bone formation, blood clotting, muscle tone, and nerve function. Deficiency may result in rickets or possibly osteomalacia.

**Caffeine.** An alkaloidal purine in coffee, tea, and cola drinks. A cardiac and renal stimulant which produces varying pharmacologic responses.

**Calciferol.** Vitamin D2. A fat soluble vitamin produced by ergosterol irradiation. Prevents rickets.

**Calcium.** A major mineral, essential in bone formation, blood clotting, muscle tone, and nerve function. Deficiency may result in rickets or possibly osteomalacia.

**Calorie.** The amount of heat energy required to raise the temperature of one kilogram of water one degree Centigrade. This is the large Calorie, or kilocalorie as used in nutrition. Calories come from carbohydrate, protein, fat, alcohol, and alcohol derivatives (like sorbitol).

**Calculus.** Commonly called stone.

**Carbohydrate.** One of three major energy sources in food. Contains carbon, hydrogen, and oxygen. *Available carbohydrates*, such as sugar and starch, provide glucose and glycogen to the body and supply four Calories per gram. *Indigestible carbohydrate* is primarily indigestible plant cellulose.

**Carob powder**. A powder that looks and tastes like chocolate but does not contain lactose. It may be used as a substitute for chocolate on lactose and galactose restricted diets.

**Carotene**. Yellow-red plant pigment converted in the body to vitamin A. Two international units of betacarotene are equivalent to one international unit of vitamin A. Abundant in green leafy, and yellow vegetables.

**Casein**. A milk protein which can contain large amounts of lactose. A phosphoprotein.

**Casein hydrolysate**. Chemical decomposition of the principal protein of milk.

**Catabolism**. Opposite of anabolism. Metabolic process in which complex substances are broken down into simpler substances, usually yielding energy. Destructive metabolism.

**Catecholamines**. Chemicals synthesized in the brain, sympathetic nerve endings, peripheral tissues, and adrenal medulla.

**Celiac disease**. Malabsorptive syndrome due to sensitivity to gluten and resulting in decreased jejunal mucosa absorption of fat, carbohydrates, protein, vitamins, and minerals. See Wheat Elimination, paragraph 11-3.

**Cellulose**. The structural fibers in plants. Indigestible polysaccharide which provides bulk to the diet.

**Cholecalciferol**. Vitamin $D_2$. Initiates production of a calcium-binding protein.

**Cholesterol**. Fat-like steroid alcohol found in all tissues. It may be synthesized in the body, but is usually absorbed from the digestive tract in the presence of fat. It is excreted in bile. Foods of animal origin are dietary sources of cholesterol. It is a key part of the fatty deposits in the arterial wall in atherosclerosis.

**Choline**. A component of lecithin. Necessary for fat transport, preventing accumulation of fat in the liver. Occurs in all plant and animal cells and may be synthesized from glycine (an amino acid) in the presence of a methyl group.

**Chylomicron**. A blood lipoprotein containing primarily triglycerides from dietary fat and smaller amounts of cholesterol, phospholipid, and protein.

**Chyluria**. The presence of a fat globule emulsion, formed in the small intestine after digestion, in the urine giving it a milky appearance.

**Clinical nutrition**. That branch of the health sciences having to do with the diagnosis, treatment, and prevention of human disease caused by deficiency, excess, or metabolic imbalance of dietary nutrients.

**Cobalamin**. Vitamin $B_{12}$. Antipernicious anemia factor; extrinsic factor.

**Coffee oils**. Possible cause of gastrointestinal irritation, diarrhea is a common symptom.

**Colloid**. A material whose particles are between 1 and 100 millimicrons in size and dispersed throughout a medium. The particles in dispersion are larger than ordinary crystalloid molecules but are not large enough to settle out under the influence of gravity. Examples are blood protein and gelatin.

**Connective tissue**. Collagen and elastin. Collagen is converted to gelatin by moist heat cookery. Elastin is not broken down or softened in cooking.

**Creatinine**. One of the end products of food protein breakdown. The amount excreted in the urine is an index of muscle mass and may be used as a measure of basal heat production. **Clear liquid dessert**. Desserts that provide little or no residue, including plain gelatin and Popsicles.

**Crystalloid**. Small molecules dissolved in a medium such as salt dissolved in water. Other examples are $Na^+$, $K^+$, other electrolytes, BUN, uric acid, and creatinine dissolved in the blood.

**Curds**. The clumped part of curdled milk which contains lactose.

**Cyanocobalamin**. Vitamin $B_{12}$.

**Cyclamates**. A noncaloric sweetener with 30 to 60 times the sweet taste of sucrose. A sodium or calcium salt of cyclohexylsulfamic acid. Cyclamate was changed from the GRAS (generally recognized as safe by the Food and Drug Administration) list to drug status, permitting use only under medical supervision. A suspected carcinogen.

**Dehydration**. Removal of water from food, tissue, or substrate.

**Dehydroascorbic acid**. Oxidized vitamin C; biologically active; reversibly oxidized and reduced. **Deciliter**. One-tenth of a liter.

**Denaturation**. To change the chemical,

physical, or biologic properties of protein by heating, freezing, irradiation, pressure, or organic solvent application.

**Dextrin.** The intermediate product of starch breakdown; a polysaccharide.

**Dialysis.** To separate substances in a solution by using a semipermeable membrane; small substances will pass through and larger molecules will not. As used in food preparation, see attachment 5.

**Diet.** Food and drink consumed. See specific types in text.

**Dietary consultation.** Individualized professional guidance provided to assist patients in adapting food consumption to meet health needs. The patient's background, socioeconomic needs, and personal preferences are considered when instructing patients on the physician-prescribed diet.

**Dietary history.** Record of an individual's food intake taken by 24-hour recall or repeated food records. Basis for individualized dietary consultation.

**Dietary status.** Bodily condition resulting from the utilization of the essential nutrients available to the body. Dietary history provides some indication of dietary status.

**Dietetics.** The science and art of planning, preparing, and serving meals to individuals and groups according to the principles of nutrition and management; economic, social, cultural, psychological, and health or disease conditions are considered.

**Dietitian.** A professional who practices dietetics after following a prescribed academic program for a baccalaureate degree in an accredited institution and completing an accredited internship, or equivalent.

**Dietitian, Registered (R.D.).** A qualified dietitian who has also successfully completed the examination for professional registration and maintains continuing education requirements by completing 75 clock hours of professional education every 5 years.

**Digestibility.** The amount of nutrient absorbed by the body and not excreted in the feces.

**Digestion.** Process of converting food into substances which can be absorbed by the body.

**Disaccharidase.** An enzyme which hydrolyzes disaccharides to yield two single sugars.

**Diuresis.** Increased secretion of urine.

**Dumping syndrome.** Postgastrectomy epigastric discomfort resulting when a large amount of hypertonic, concentrated food draws large quantities of fluid from the bloodstream into the intestine.

**Duodenum.** The first segment of small intestine between the pylorus and jejunum. Pancreatic juice and bile are secreted into the duodenum.

**Edible portion (EP).** The trimmed weight of food that is normally eaten.

**Effusion.** Fluid escaping into a part or tissue.

**Endogenous.** Originating within the cell or tissue.

**Endogenous protein.** Body or tissue protein.

**Energy.** Capacity to do work, such as muscular activity, maintaining body temperature, and operating metabolic processes. As obtained from food oxidation, energy is expressed in calories.

Enrichment. The addition of one or more nutrients to a food to attain a higher level of those nutrients than normally present in the food. Bread and flour are often enriched.

**Enteral.** Within or by way of the intestine. Often used to refer to supplemental oral, or tube feedings.

**Enzyme.** An organic compound (usually protein) which accelerates metabolic reactions (such as digestion).

**Epinephrine.** A hormone released primarily in response to hypoglycemia. It increases blood pressure, stimulates the heart muscle, accelerates the heart rate, and increases cardiac output.

**Ergosterol.** A plant steroid converted to vitamin $D_2$, calciferol, upon irradiation or exposure to ultraviolet light.

**Essential amino acid.** Those amino acids that cannot be synthesized by the body; they must be obtained from food to ensure normal growth, development, and tissue repair.

**Essential fatty acid.** Fatty acids that cannot be synthesized in adequate amounts by the body to ensure growth, reproduction, skin health, and proper fat utilization.

**Ethanol.** See alcohol.

**Ethylenediamine-tetraacetate.** A non-nutritive food additive used to separate a part from a whole, or to act as a metal scavenger.

**Exchange list.** Grouping of foods similar in nutrients together so they may be used interchangeably.

**Excipient.** Any addition to a medicine designed to permit proper shaping or consistency.

**Exogenous.** Originating outside, externally caused. Extrinsic factor. Vitamin $B_{12}$.

**Exudative enteropathics.** Any disease of the intestine with material escaped from the blood vessels deposited in the intestine.

**Fat.** One of three major sources of food energy, which provides nine Calories per gram. A mixture of glyceryl esters of fatty acids; an oily, yellow, or white substance of animal or vegetable sources.

**Fatty acid.** Organic acids which combine with glycerol to form fat.

**Favism.** An acute hemolytic anemia resulting from ingestion of fava beans (horse or broad beans).

**Ferment.** Chemical change caused by digestive enzymes of micro-organisms.

**Fiber.** An indigestible part of fruits, vegetables, cereals, and grains important in the diet as roughage, or bulk.

**Flatulence.** Excessive gas in the stomach or intestines.

**Focacin.** Folic acid. Pteroylglutamic acid. A water-soluble vitamin of the B complex group needed for normal growth and hemopoiesis. Widely distributed in plant and animal tissues. Deficiency may be induced by sulfonamides or folic acid antagonists.

**Food habit.** Usual pattern of an individual or group for choosing, preparing, and eating food resulting from family, cultural, economic, and religious influences.

**Fortification.** The addition of one or more nutrients to a food whether or not they are naturally present. An example is margarine fortified with vitamin A.

**Full liquid dessert.** Desserts that are fluid or that easily become fluid, including plain gelatin, ice cream, soft custard, and pudding.

**Galactose.** A six carbon monosaccharide.

**Galactosemia.** Galactose in the blood due to an inborn error of metabolism in which the enzyme galactose-l-phosphate uridyl transferase is absent; thus, galactose is not converted to glucose. Mental and growth retardation, liver and spleen enlargement, cataracts, jaundice, weight loss, vomiting, and diarrhea result unless dietary modification eliminates lactose-and galactose-containing foods from the diet.

**Gavage.** Feeding via insertion of a tube through the mouth into the stomach.

**Gelatin.** An incomplete protein obtained from partial hydrolysis of collagen.

**Geriatrics.** Study and treatment of diseases and problems occurring in old age.

**Glomerular filtration rate (GFR).** Milliliters of blood which pass through the kidney glomeruli in one minute; may be used to estimate kidney function.

**Glucose.** Dextrose. Grape sugar. Blood sugar. A monosaccharide which may be absorbed into the bloodstream and is the major source of energy for the brain and nervous tissues.

**Glutathione.** A tripeptide believed to assist sulfhydryl containing enzymes to stay in the reduced state essential for their activity.

**Gluten.** A cereal grain protein; gluten provides elasticity to bread dough.

**Glycogen.** A polysaccharide composed of glucose units. The main form of carbohydrate stored by man and animals in liver, muscles, and other tissues.

**Gram.** A unit of mass and weight in the metric system. An ounce is approximately 28 grams.

**Gravidity.** Pregnancy.

**Hemicellulose.** A largely indigestible plant polysaccharide that absorbs water. Pectin is a hemi-cellulose that may lower serum cholesterol.

**Hemodialysis.** Dialyzing blood to remove waste products.

**Hepatosplenomegaly.** Enlargement of both liver and spleen.

**High biological value (HBV) protein.** A protein readily digested, absorbed, and utilized by the body, such as the protein in eggs.

**Homeostasis.** Balance of the internal environment including fluid, pH, body temperature, blood sugar level, heart and pulse rates, and hormonal control.

**Hydrogenated oil.** Addition of molecular hydrogen to double bonds in unsaturated fatty acids creating saturated solid fat with reduced essential fatty acid biological value.

**Hypercholesterolemia.** Elevated blood cholesterol associated with cardiovascular diseases.

**Hyperchylomicronemia.** Elevation of chylomicron lipoproteins circulating in the blood.

**Hyperkalemia.** Increased potassium in the blood. Hyperlipidemia. An elevation of one or

more lipid constituents of the blood.
**Hyperlipoproteinemia.** Elevation of blood lipoproteins.
**Hypernatremia.** Excessive amount of sodium in the blood.
**Idiopathic.** Without known origin.
**Ileum.** The part of the small intestine between the jejunum and large intestine.
**Inborn error of metabolism.** A metabolic defect existing at birth due to missing genes.
**Incomplete protein.** A protein lacking one or more essential amino acids.
**Ingestion.** Eating or drinking; taking in.
**Inorganic.** Minerals that do not contain carbon.
Inositol. A water soluble alcohol found primarily in cereal grains which combines with phosphate to form phytic acid.
**Instant cereal.** Pregelatinized (precooked) cereal requiring addition of water before serving.
**Insulin.** A hormone secreted by the beta cells of the islets of Langerhans in the pancreas. It is essential to carbohydrate metabolism in the body. Exogenous insulin is injected by some diabetics to provide proper carbohydrate metabolism.
**Insulin shock (or) reaction.** Very low blood sugar level resulting from overdose of insulin. Symptoms include hunger, weakness, nervousness, double vision, shallow breathing, sweating, headache, dizziness, mental confusion, muscular twitching, convulsion, loss of consciousness, coma, and eventually death. Fruit juice or intravenous glucose are often used to counteract insulin reaction.
**International unit.** A measure of biologic activity of a nutrient.
**Interpolate.** To determine intermediate values in a series based on observed values or to introduce new material in a given subject.
**Intrinsic factor.** Chemical in gastric juice that facilitates vitamin $B_{12}$ (extrinsic factor) absorption. Lack of intrinsic factor results in pernicious anemia.
**Iodine.** A trace mineral essential in regulating basal metabolism. Deficiency results in goiter.
**Iodine number (or) value.** The number of grams of iodine absorbed by 100 grams of fat. Indicates the amount of fatty acids and degree of unsaturation of a fat. The iodine number of saturated coconut oil is 10, and that of polyunsaturated safflower oil is 100.

**Iodized salt.** Table salt with one part sodium or potassium iodide per 5,000 to 10,000 parts sodium chloride.
**Irradiation.** Exposure to ultraviolet rays used for destroying microorganisms in food and converting provitamin D to active vitamin D.
**Isocaloric.** Containing an equal number of Calories.
**Jejunum.** The part of the small intestine between the duodenum and ileum.
**Joule.** A metric measure of energy equaling 4.184 Calories.
**Junket.** The precipitated protein of milk casein and fat.
**Ketogenic-antiketogenic ratio.** The ratio of the amount of ketogenic factors, such as fatty acids and ketogenic amino acids, to the amount of anti-ketogenic factors, such as carbohydrates, glucogenic amino acids, and the glycerol of fat.
**Ketosis.** An accumulation of ketone bodies (beta-hydroxybutyric acid, acetoacetic acid, and acetone) from incomplete fatty acid oxidation. Uncontrolled ketosis may result in acidosis.
**Kosher foods.** Foods prepared and served by Orthodox Judaism dietary laws which include: (1) milk and meat are not consumed at the same meal, (2) meat must be slaughtered in a special ordained manner and cleaned (koshered) by soaking in water, salting, and washing, (3) meat from cud-chewing, cloven-hooved animals (cows, sheep, goats) may be eaten, (4) finfish may be eaten. No pork or shellfish are eaten.
**Kwashiorkor.** Severe protein malnutrition in children resulting in retarded growth, anemia, edema, fatty liver, lack of pigment in the hair and skin, gastrointestinal disorders, muscle atrophy, and psychomotor wasting.
**Labile.** Unstable.
**Lactase.** Enzyme that splits lactose to glucose and galactose.
**Lactate, lactic acid, lactalbumin.** Substances related to lactose but which cannot be changed into galactose by the body.
**Lacto-ovo-vegetarian.** Person subsisting on grains, legumes, vegetables, fruits, milk, and eggs. Meat, poultry and fish are avoided.
**Lactose.** "Milk sugar." Disaccharide occurring in milk products. Contains one glucose and one galactose group.
**Lactose intolerance.** Lactose malabsorption due to lactase deficiency. Results in

diarrhea.

**Lecithin**. Phosphatidyl choline. A phospholipid containing glycerol, fatty acids, phosphoric acid, and choline. Involved in fat transport, lecithin is found in many cells, especially nerves. Lecithin synthesis in the body depends upon dietary intake of methyl groups or choline.

**Leucine**. An essential amino acid with ketogenic properties.

**Licorice**. Black flavoring extract containing glycyrrhizic acid which, in large amounts, can cause hypertension and hypokalemia.

**Lignin**. A constituent of crude fiber. An indigestible cellulose. With cellulose, the principal Part of the woody plants. Unlike cellulose, lignin can combine with bile to form insoluble complexes which are not absorbed.

**Linoleic acid**. Polyunsaturated essential fatty acid with 18 carbon atoms and two double bonds.

**Linolenic acid**. A nonessential polyunsaturated fatty acid with 18 carbon atoms and three double bonds.

**Lipid**. Fat or fat-like substances. Includes fatty acids, triglycerides, phosphatides (such as lecithin), terpenes, and steroids (such as cholesterol).

**Lipoprotein**. A compound consisting of a simple protein and lipid and involved in lipid transport. Types of lipoprotein circulating in the blood include chylomicrons, alpha lipoproteins (high density lipoproteins, HDL), prebeta lipoproteins (very low density lipoproteins, VLDL), and beta lipoprotein (low density lipoprotein, LDL). All are composed of phospholipid, triglyceride, cholesterol, and protein.

**Long-chain fatty acid**. Fatty acids containing 12 or more carbon atoms, such as stearic (18 carbon) and palmatic (16 carbon) acids.

**Low sodium milk**. Milk processed by ion-exchange process to remove approximately 90 percent of the naturally occurring sodium. Thiamin, riboflavin, and calcium are also decreased with an increase in potassium.

**Lycine**. An essential amino acid and the limiting amino acid in many cereal products.

**Magnesium**. An essential mineral. A cofactor in metabolism.

**Malabsorption syndrome**. A condition caused by failure of the body to absorb nutrients such as fats, calcium and other minerals, and vitamins. Examples include celiac disease, chronic pancrea-titis, sprue, cystic fibrosis, and carbohydrate intolerance.

**Malnutrition**. Lack or excess of absorbed nutrients resulting in impaired health status.

**Manganese**. An essential trace mineral.

**Mannitol**. A partially absorbed sugar alcohol with a sweet taste equal to sugar but with half the calories.

**Maple syrup urine disease**. Inborn error of metabolism treated with dietary restriction of leucine. isoleucine, and valine.

**Marasmus**. Severe protein-calorie malnutrition of infants and young children.

**Medium chain fatty acid**. Fatty acids containing 8 to 10 carbon atoms, such as caprylic (8 carbon) and capric (10 carbon) acids.

**Medium chain triglyceride (MCT)**. A fat composed primarily of saturated fatty acids with 8 to 10 carbon atoms. A commercially prepared food product for persons not able to digest or absorb food fats and oils.

**Menadione**. A synthetic, vitamin $K_2$ is much more potent biologically than vitamin K.

**Metabolism**. Chemical changes in the body: anabolism and catabolism.

**Methionine**. An essential amino acid important in protein and fat, metabolism.

**Methylcellulose**. Indigestible polysaccharide which provides bulk and satiety without. calories.

**Micronutrient**. Nutrients present. in less than 0.005 percent of body weight, such as trace minerals. Also, nutrients present in very small amounts in food.

**Microgram**. A metric system unit of mass representing one one-millionth of a gram or one one-thousandth of a milligram.

**Milk-alkali syndrome**. Ingestion of large quantities of milk and alkalies resulting in hyper-calcemia, calcium in soft tissues, vomiting, gastrointestinal bleeding, and high blood pressure.

**Milliosmole**. One thousandth of an osmole.

**Mineral**. Inorganic elements that build and repair body tissue or control body functions. The ones known to be essential to man are calcium, chlorine, chromium, cobalt, copper, fluorine, iodine, iron, magnesium, manganese, molybdenum, phosphorus, potassium, selenium, sodium, sulfur. and zinc.

**Mineral oil**. Liquid petroleum substance which is not absorbed by the gastrointestinal tract but interferes with absorption of fat soluble vitamins.

**Monosaccharides.** Carbohydrates composed of single simple sugars that cannot be hydrolyzed (broken) into smaller units. Examples are fructose, galactose, glucose, and ribose.

**Monounsaturated fat.** Fat that neither raises nor lowers blood cholesterol. Examples are olive oil and peanut oil.

**Monounsaturated fatty acid.** Fatty acids with only one unsaturated double bond.

**Monosodium glutamate (MSG).** A sodium-containing flavoring used in Asian cookery.

**Nasogastric tube.** Used in tube feeding; a tube inserted via the nose and esophagus into the stomach.

**Nausea.** Stomach discomfort with a tendency to vomit.

**Negative nitrogen balance.** Daily nitrogen excretion greater than nitrogen intake which may be brought about by fever, surgery, or burns.

**Niacin.** Nicotenic acid. A water-soluble B complex vitamin. Antipellagra factor. Necessary to cell respiration, carbohydrate and protein metabolism, and lipid synthesis; thus, requirement varies with caloric intake.

**Niacin equivalent.** The sum of nicotinic acid and niacin is the niacin equivalent. Sixty milligrams tryptophan may be converted to one milligram nicotinic acid.

**Nicotinic acid.** Niacin.

**Nitrogen balance/equilibrium.** An individual is in nitrogen balance when the nitrogen intake from food protein each day is approximately equal to the nitrogen loss in feces and urine.

**Non-nutritive sweetener.** A noncaloric synthetic sugar substitute. Examples are saccharine and cyclamate.

**Norepinephrine.** A hormone released primarily in response to hypotension to raise blood pressure.

**Nutrient.** Any chemical substance useful in nutrition for providing heat and energy, building and repairing tissues, and regulating life processes.

**Nutrition.** The study of food in relation to health. Combination of processes by which the body receives and uses the materials necessary for body functions, energy, growth, and tissue renewal.

**Nutrition history.** Laboratory and clinical findings, and a dietary history.

**Nutritional status.** The condition of the body resulting from consumption and utilization of nutrients.

**Nutriture.** Tissue nutrient balance of supply and demand.

**Obesity.** Fat. Body weight approximately 20 percent or more above desirable weight due to adiposity.

**Oil.** A lipid that is liquid at room temperature.

**Oleic acid.** An 18 carbon monounsaturated fatty acid abundant in fats and oils.

**Oliguria.** Decreased urinary output in relation to fluid intake.

**Oral hypoglycemic agents.** Orally administered compounds that stimulate beta cells in the islands of Langerhans of the pancreas to secrete endogenous insulin that reduces blood glucose in diabetics. Contraindicated for some patients.

**Osmolality.** A property of a solution which depends on the concentration of the solute per unit of solvent.

**Osmolarity.** A property of a solution which depends on the concentration of the solute per unit of total volume of solution.

**Osmole.** The standard unit of osmotic pressure. Overweight. Fat. Body weight approximately 10 to 20 percent above desirable weight due to adiposity.

**Oxalate.** Salt of oxalic acid. When combined in insoluble calcium salts. oxalate renders calcium unavailable for absorption.

**Pancreatic juice.** A digestive juice produced by the pancreas and secreted into the duodenum; contains enzymes involved in digestion of protein, carbohydrate. and fat.

**Pantothenic acid.** A water-soluble B complex vitamin that is part of coenzyme A. It is essential for growth. normal skin. nervous system development, and adrenal cortex function.

**Papain.** A proteolytic enzyme of papaya often used as a meat tenderizer.

**Parenteral feeding.** Food provided without use of the mouth and digestive tract, such as intravenous feeding.

**Pasteurized.** Heat treated to kill most pathogenic microorganisms. For example. pasteurized eggnog prevents the potential of salmonella infection from eggnog made with raw eggs.

**Pellagra.** Multiple B vitamin deficiency, notably

of niacin. Symptoms include dermatitis, diarrhea, dementia, and death.

**Peristalsis.** Alternate contraction and relaxation pf the gastrointestinal tract which moves contents toward the anus.

**Pernicious anemia.** Chronic macrocytic anemia due to $B_{12}$ and intrinsic factor deficiency.

**pH.** A measure of acidity and alkalinity.

**Phenylalanine.** An essential amino that may be converted to tyrosine. It can be ketogenic, glycogenic, and participate in transamination.

**Phenylketonuria (PKU).** Inborn error in metabolism resulting in the lack of the enzyme phenylal-anine hydroxylase. Phenylalanine cannot be converted to tyrosine without this enzyme. The resultant high levels of phenylalanine result in permanent mental retardation and poor growth and development unless there is close dietary control of phenylalanine ingestion.

**Phosphorus.** An essential mineral.

**Polysaccharide.** A complex carbohydrate containing more than four monosaccharides. Examples are glycogen, starch, and cellulose.

**Polyunsaturated fatty acids (PUFA).** Fatty acids with more than one unsaturated bond in the molecule.

**Polyunsaturated: saturated fatty acid ratio (P/S ratio).** The relative amount of polyunsaturated linoleic acid to total saturated fatty acids.

**Positive nitrogen balance.** Nitrogen intake exceeds nitrogen output, such as during infancy and childhood (tissue anabolism).

**Potassium.** An essential mineral of the intracellular fluids.

**Pressor agent.** Any substance that raises blood pressure.

**Protein.** The primary structure of plant and animal bodies. It is composed of amino acids and is approximately 16 percent nitrogen. Protein provides four Calories per gram.

**Protein hydrolysate.** A mixture of "predigested protein" in the form of amino acids and polypep-tides. Used for oral or parenteral feeding in cases of impaired digestion, such as pancreatic diseases.

**Protein calorie malnutrition.** A condition of severe tissue wasting, subcutaneous fat loss, and dehydration caused by inadequate protein and calorie intake.

**Protein quality.** A complete protein contains all the essential amino acids for growth and life. A partial protein maintains life but not growth. An incomplete protein can support neither growth nor life. If two incomplete proteins each supply the limiting amino acid(s) of the other, together they may be capable of supporting growth and life.

**Protein-sparing.** Refers to calories supplied by carbohydrates and fat. These calories save protein from being "burned" as energy so it may be used for anabolism.

**Provitamin.** A substance related to a vitamin but with no vitamin activity until it is converted to the biologically active form.

**P/S ratio.** Ratio of polyunsaturated to saturated fatty acids.

**Pureed.** A food blenderized to a paste consistency. Most baby foods are pureed.

**Purine.** Nitrogenous compounds of dietary or endogenous origin catabolized to uric acid in the body.

**Pyridoxine.** An alcohol form of vitamin 136, a B complex vitamin.

**Quick-cooking cereal/rice.** Cereals and rice that have disodium phosphate added to reduce their preparation time.

**Raffinose.** Trisaccharide containing glucose, galactose, and fructose. It is found in beets, roots, underground stems, cottonseed meal, and molasses.

**Recommended (Daily) Dietary Allowances (RDA).** Suggested amounts of nutrients to provide when planning diets. Designed to maintain good nutrition in healthy persons of average build and activity in a temperature climate with a margin of safety 10 to 50 percent above normal dietary requirements.

**Reconstitute.** To restore to the normal state, usually by adding water.

**Refuse.** Inedible, discarded foodstuffs.

**Residue.** Amount of bulk remaining in the digestive tract after digestion and absorption.

**Retinol.** A vitamin A alcohol.

**Retinol equivalent (RE).** Unit expressing vitamin A activity. One RE = 1 u retinol, 6 u beta-carotene, and 12 u for other provitamin A carotenoids.

**Riboflavin.** Vitamin $B_2$. Heat stable, water soluble vitamin essential to the health of skin and eyes.

**Rickets.** Vitamin D deficiency or disturbance of calcium-phosphorus metabolism.

**Saccharin.** A noncaloric artificial sweetener 700 times sweeter than sugar.

**Salt.** Table salt; sodium chloride; NaCl.

**Satiety.** Sense of fullness or comfort; gratification of appetite.

**Saturated fat.** A fat with no double bonds; chemically satisfied. Often solid at room temperature and usually of animal origin. Examples are butter, lard, and steak fat.

**Scurvy.** Vitamin C deficiency disease resulting in swollen bleeding gums, hemorrhage of the skin and mucous membranes, and anemia.

**Secretagogue.** An agent that stimulates secretion.

**Short-chain fatty acid.** Those containing four to six carbon atoms, such as caproic (6 carbon) and butyric (4 carbon) acids. Yields only about 5 Calories per gram.

**Skinfold measurement.** Measurement of the thickness of skin at body sites where adipose is normally deposited. Measured with a caliper and compared against a standard chart, it provides an estimate of degree of fatness.

**Sodium.** An essential mineral important in extra-cellular body fluids and in regulating many body functions.

**Soft.** Any easily digested food that is soft in texture and provides no harsh fibers or connective tissue.

**Sorbitol.** A sugar alcohol apparently metabolized without insulin. It contains 4 calories per gram and can be converted to utilizable carbohydrate in the form of glucose. Excessive use may cause gastrointestinal discomfort and diarrhea.

**Specific dynamic action.** Increased metabolism from heat of digesting, absorbing, and metabolizing food. Approximately 30 percent for protein, 13 percent, for fat, and 4 to 5 percent for carbohydrate.

**Standard of identity of foods.** Standards established by a government agency, primarily the US Food and Drug Administration, to define quality and container fill for foods.

**Stachyose.** Tetrasaccharide containing glucose, fructose, and two molecules of galactose. It is found in tubers, peas, lima beans, and beets.

**Starch.** Plant storage form of carbohydrate (just as the animal storage form is glycogen). A complex polysaccharide. Food sources include breads, cereals, and starchy vegetables.

**Sucrose.** Table sugar. A disaccharide composed of glucose and fructose.

**Sugar.** Sucrose. A sweet, soluble carbohydrate that provides 4 Calories of energy per gram.

**Sulphur.** An essential mineral.

**Supplement.** A concentrated source of nutrients, such as vitamins or minerals.

**Supplementary feeding.** Food provided in addition to regular meals to increase nutrient intake.

**Sweetening agent (or) sweeteners.** Natural sweeteners, such as sugar, or synthetic sweeteners, such as saccharin.

**Synthesis.** Putting elements together to form a whole.

**Tea tannin.** Possible cause of constipation.

**Textured vegetable protein.** Vegetable protein that is flavored, colored, and textured to resemble meat and poultry products.

**Theobromine.** The alkaloidal stimulant in cocoa beans, tea leaves, and cola nuts that acts as a diuretic, arterial dilator, and myocardial stimulant.

**Thiamin.** Vitamin $B_2$, a B complex vitamin and part of a coenzyme important in carbohydrate metabolism. Prevents beriberi.

**Threonine.** An essential amino acid.

**Tocopherols.** An alcohol-like group of substances. Four forms have vitamin E activity.

**Tofu.** Soybean curd; usually available in oriental grocery stores.

**Trace minerals.** Minerals required by the body in minute amounts.

**Triglyceride.** A fat composed of a glycerol molecule with three fatty acids.

**Tryptophane.** An essential amino acid. May be converted to niacin, and a source of the vasoconstrictor serotonin.

**Tyramine.** A decarboxylation product of tyrosine found in fermented cheeses, wines, and other foods. Produces severe hypertensive reaction if consumed in conjunction with monoamine oxidase inhibitory drugs.

**Underweight.** Body weight 10 percent or more below the established standards.

**Unsaturated fatty acids.** Those with one or more double bonds. Abundant in vegetable oils.

**Urea.** Major nitrogen containing product of protein metabolism and chief nitrogenous constituent of the urine.

**Uremia**. A toxic condition caused by the retention in the blood of urinary constituents including urea, creatine, uric acid, and other end products of protein metabolism.

**Vasopressor**. Any agent that causes contraction of the muscular tissue lining the arteries and capillaries.

**Vegetarian (or) vegan**. Person subsisting entirely or in a large part on fruits, grains, legumes, and vegetables. If eggs, fish, meat, milk, and poultry are totally excluded, a vegetarian diet may be deficient in calcium, phosphorus, riboflavin, and vitamins $B_{12}$ and D. Pure vegetarian diets are usually inadequate in protein for children.

**Viosterol**. Vitamin $D_2$, a product of ergosterol irradiation.

**Vitamin**. Organic substance provided in minute amounts in food or endogenuously synthesized. Essential in metabolic functions.

**Vitamin A**. Fat-soluble vitamin necessary for normal skin and bone development, maintenance of vision, and synthesis of mucopolysaccharides.

**Vitamin B complex**. Water soluble vitamins often found together in nature. Vitamins $B_1$ (thiamin), $B_2$ (riboflavin), $B_6$ group (pyridoxine, pyridoxal, and pyridoxamine), $B_{12}$ group (cobalamins), nicotinic acid (niacin), pteroylglutamic acid (PGA, folacin, or folic acid), pantothenic acid, and biotin. All except $B_{12}$ are coenzymes.

**Vitamin C**. Water-soluble vitamin. Ascorbic acid.

**Vitamin D**. Fat-soluble vitamins including ergocalciferol ($D_2$) and cholecalciferol ($D_3$).

**Vitamin E**. Fat-soluble vitamin. Tocopherols.

**Vitamin K**. Fat-soluble vitamin consumed in food and produced endogenously by intestinal flora. Necessary for blood clotting.

**Water**. A major nutrient required by the body. Endogenous water is provided as a byproduct of metabolism. Exogenous water may be in the fluid form or contained in food.

**Water requirement**. Water functions by removing body heat and urinary excreta. One milliliter water per calorie is usually sufficient unless there is a pathological condition such as fever or burn.

**Whey**. A clear, watery liquid remaining when milk curdles. It contains lactose, but little or no fat.

**Zanthine**. Weakly basic alkaloid chemicals including caffeine, theophylline, and theobromine.

**Zinc**. An essential trace mineral involved in growth, digestion, and metabolism. Deficiency results in retarded growth, delayed sexual maturity, and delayed wound healing.